Philosophy and Psychiatry

This groundbreaking volume of original essays presents fresh avenues of inquiry at the intersection of philosophy and psychiatry. Contributors draw from a variety of fields, including evolutionary psychiatry, phenomenology, biopsychosocial models, psychoanalysis, neuroscience, neuroethics, behavioral economics, and virtue theory. *Philosophy and Psychiatry*'s unique structure consists of two parts: in the first, philosophers write five lead essays with replies from psychiatrists; in the second, this arrangement is reversed. The result is an interdisciplinary exchange that allows for direct discourse, and a volume at the forefront of defining an emerging discipline. *Philosophy and Psychiatry* will be of interest to professionals in philosophy and psychiatry, as well as mental health researchers and clinicians.

Daniel D. Moseley co-founded and coordinates the University of North Carolina, Chapel Hill Philosophical Issues in Psychiatry Research Group. He is a philosopher who is currently a postdoctoral fellow in a joint Duke University and University of North Carolina, Chapel Hill program in mental health research.

Gary Gala co-founded and coordinates the University of North Carolina, Chapel Hill Philosophical Issues in Psychiatry Research Group. He is Associate Chair for Education and Training in Psychiatry. He is also a visiting scholar in the Department of Philosophy at University of North Carolina, Chapel Hill.

Philosophy and Psychiatry

Problems, Intersections, and New Perspectives

Edited by
Daniel D. Moseley and Gary Gala

Routledge
Taylor & Francis Group
NEW YORK AND LONDON

First published 2016
by Routledge
711 Third Avenue, New York, NY 10017

and by Routledge
2 Park Square, Milton Park, Abingdon, Oxon, OX14 4RN

Routledge is an imprint of the Taylor & Francis Group, an informa business

Library of Congress Cataloging in Publication Data
Philosophy and psychiatry (Moseley)
Philosophy and psychiatry: problems, intersections, and new perspectives / edited by Daniel Moseley and Gary Gala.
p.; cm.
Includes bibliographical references and index.
I. Moseley, Daniel, editor. II. Gala, Gary, editor. III. Title.
[DNLM: 1. Psychiatry. 2. Philosophy. WM 100]
RC454.4
616.89–dc23
2015007721

ISBN: 978-0-415-70816-6 (hbk)
ISBN: 978-1-315-68872-5 (ebk)

Typeset in Bembo
by Taylor & Francis Books

For Bernie Gert

Contents

Preface

The philosophy of psychiatry is an exciting and rapidly expanding field of study. One of the central aims of this volume is to identify topics at the intersection of philosophy and psychiatry that have not been exhaustively discussed in the current literature. We have invited ten philosophers and ten psychiatrists, whose work has not been primarily in the philosophy of psychiatry, to venture out of their respective disciplines to discuss the implications or assumptions that their work has for the other field. We are grateful to all of the contributors for writing original essays for this volume and taking the risk of stepping outside of their ordinary comfort zones to boldly explore new territory. For each of those essays, we have also recruited commentators from the other discipline (philosophers commentating on psychiatrists' essays, and vice versa) in order to create a dialogue format for the volume. We would like to thank all of the commentators for their work on this project. We discuss the rationale for this format in our introductory essay, "Beyond the Philosophy of Psychiatry."

Our work with the University of North Carolina at Chapel Hill Philosophy and Psychiatry Research Group (PPRG) was the main inspiration for this volume. We formed the group in September 2010. Bernard Gert was a helpful mentor for us in the early days of the group before he passed away in 2011. The structure of this volume is largely influenced by the structure of our PPRG meetings. We are grateful to the faculty, clinicians, graduate and undergraduate students, medical students, psychiatric residents, and others, from both UNC-CH and Duke University, who have attended these meetings. We also thank Andrew Beck of Routledge for approaching us to put together this volume. His advice and support of this project have been invaluable. We would also like to thank the Departments of Philosophy and Psychiatry at UNC-CH and the Center for Bioethics at UNC-CH for their support of PPRG.

Moseley would like to acknowledge the financial support of grant number (2T32NR008856, PI: Barbara Mark), which was funded by the National Institute of Nursing Research and the National Institutes of Health.

We also have debts of personal support to acknowledge. Gala would like to extend a personal acknowledgement to Liz Dreesen. Moseley would like to thank Joy Meyer for her patience and support.

List of Contributors

Richard A. Chefetz is a psychiatrist in private practice in Washington, D.C. He is a Distinguished Visiting Lecturer at the William Alanson White Institute of Psychiatry, Psychoanalysis, and Psychology. He is also a faculty member at the Washington School of Psychiatry, the Institute of Contemporary Psychotherapy and Psychoanalysis, and the Washington Center for Psychoanalysis. Dr. Chefetz is a Certified Consultant at the American Society of Clinical Hypnosis, and is trained in Level I and II EMDR. He is the author of *Intensive Psychotherapy for Persistent Dissociative Processes: The Fear of Feeling Real* (2015).

Alex Cohen is Associate Professor in the Department of Psychology at Louisiana State University, and an Adjunct Professor at the University of Louisiana Health Sciences Center and Pennington Biomedical Research Center. His work has been funded by the National Institute of Mental Health, the Norway Research Council, and the Louisiana Board of Regents. He has over 80 peer-reviewed scientific publications on serious mental illness. Additionally, he is a licensed clinical psychologist in the state of Louisiana, and he oversees treatment teams at public and private treatment facilities in the southern Louisiana region.

Alison Denham is jointly appointed to the Departments of Philosophy and Political Economy at Tulane University, New Orleans. She is a Senior Research Fellow and former Tutorial Fellow in Philosophy at St Anne's College, Oxford, and a Visiting Professor in the Faculty of Philosophy, University of Oxford. She is also the editor of *Plato on Art and Beauty* (2011).

Gary Gala is co-founder and coordinator of the Philosophical Issues in Psychiatry Research Group at the University of North Carolina at Chapel Hill (UNC-CH). He is also Associate Chair for Education and Training in Psychiatry, and Visiting

Scholar in the Department of Philosophy at UNC-CH. His writing has been published in journals such as *The American Journal of Psychiatry* and *Iris. European Journal of Philosophy and Public Debate.*

Justin Garson is Assistant Professor of Philosophy at Hunter College of the City University of New York. He is the author of the recently published *The Biological Mind: A Philosophical Introduction* (Routledge 2015), and his articles have appeared in journals such as *Science in Context* (forthcoming) and the *British Journal for the Philosophy of Science.*

Valerie Hardcastle is Professor of Philosophy, Psychology, and Psychiatry & Behavioral Neuroscience; Scholar-in-Residence, Weaver Institute for Law and Psychiatry; Director, Program in Medicine, Health, and Society; Executive Director and Co-PI of the University of Cincinnati LEAF. She is the author of five books and over 130 essays.

Jennifer Hawkins joined the faculty at Duke University in January 2010 with a joint appointment in Philosophy and the Department of Medicine. She is co-editor with Ezekiel J. Emanuel of *Exploitation and Developing Countries: The Ethics of Clinical Research* (2008).

Mardy S. Ireland is a psychoanalyst and psychologist in clinical practice in Raleigh, N.C. She taught psychology and psychoanalysis for over 20 years in graduate and post-graduate institutions in Northern California before returning to her home state of North Carolina in 2009. She is the author of two books, several book chapters, and multiple articles on psychoanalysis.

Scott Y. H. Kim is a Senior Investigator in the Department of Bioethics, National Institutes of Health (NIH), USA. Prior to joining the NIH in 2013, he was Co-Director, Center for Bioethics and Behavioral Sciences in Medicine at the University of Michigan. Dr. Kim's work has been supported by the NIH, Michael J. Fox Foundation, American Association for Geriatric Psychiatry, and Greenwall Foundation. He is the author of *Evaluation of Capacity to Consent to Treatment* (2010).

Warren Kinghorn is Assistant Professor of Psychiatry and Pastoral and Moral Theology at Duke University Medical Center and Divinity School, and a staff psychiatrist at the Durham VA Medical Center. He is Co-director of the Initiative in Theology, Medicine, and Culture at Duke Divinity School, and a faculty associate of the Trent Center for Bioethics, Medical Humanities and the History of Medicine at the Duke Center for Spirituality, Theology, and Health. He is also a Faculty Scholar of the University of Chicago Program on Medicine and Religion.

Nicholas Kontos is Assistant Professor of Psychiatry at Harvard Medical School. He is also an attending physician on the Avery D. Weisman, MD Psychiatric

Consultation Service at the Massachusetts General Hospital, where he is currently the Director of the Fellowship in Psychosomatic Medicine.

Benjamin Kozuch is currently a Lecturer in the Department of Philosophy at The University of Arizona. His work has been published in journals such as *Mind and Language* and *Philosophical Studies.*

Marc Lange is Theda Perdue Distinguished Professor of Philosophy and Philosophy Department Chair at the University of North Carolina at Chapel Hill. His books include *Laws and Lawmakers: Science, Metaphysics, and the Laws of Nature* (2009) and *An Introduction to the Philosophy of Physics: Locality, Fields, Energy, and Mass* (2002). He is Associate Editor of *The British Journal for the Philosophy of Science*, and three of his papers have been recognized by *The Philosophers' Annual* as among the ten best philosophy papers published in their years.

Ken Levy is the Holt B. Harrison Associate Professor of Law at LSU Law Center in Baton Rouge, Louisiana. His most recent publications focus on the relationship between criminal responsibility and moral responsibility, the role of revenge in the criminal justice system, and the impossibility defense.

Michael McKenna is Professor of Philosophy and the Keith Lehrer Chair at University of Arizona in the Department of Philosophy and the Center for the Philosophy of Freedom. He is the author of *Conversation and Responsibility* (2012) and numerous articles on free will and moral responsibility.

Daniel D. Moseley is a fellow in the National Research Service Award (NRSA) Mental Health Postdoctoral Research Fellowship Program, which is a collaborative project between The Cecil G. Sheps Center for Health Services Research at the University of North Carolina at Chapel Hill (UNC-CH) and the Duke University Medical Center. Moseley co-founded the UNC-CH Philosophy and Psychiatry Research Group (PPRG) in September 2010.

Abraham M. Nussbaum is Assistant Professor in the Department of Psychiatry at the University of Colorado School of Medicine, and Director of Adult Inpatient Psychiatry at Denver Health. With his colleagues, Dr. Nussbaum conducts clinical research into psychiatric diagnosis and treatment that has appeared in journals including *Academic Medicine, The American Journal of Psychiatry, The Cochrane Library, JAMA, Literature and Medicine*, and *The Journal of General Internal Medicine.* He authored the best-selling *Pocket Guide to the DSM-5 Diagnostic Exam* (2013) and is co-writing a sequel, *The DSM-5 Pocket Guide to Pediatric Mental Health,* with Robert J. Hilt. His next book, *Seeing Wisely: A Physician's Search for A Renewed Vision of Medicine*, is forthcoming.

Christian Perring is Professor of Philosophy at Dowling College, New York. He is Co-editor (with Lloyd Wells) of *Diagnostic Dilemmas in Child and Adolescent Psychiatry: Philosophical Perspectives* (2014). He is also Editor of *Metapsychology Online*

Reviews, and a member of the Executive Council of the Association for the Advancement of Philosophy and Psychiatry.

Hanna Pickard is a Reader in Philosophy at the University of Birmingham, and a Fellow of All Souls College in Oxford. She has developed a *Responsibility without Blame* framework that articulates the concepts and practices informing the clinical stance of holding patients responsible and accountable for problematic behavior without blaming them, in order to facilitate learning and change. She has published in journals and volumes such as *Notre Dame Philosophical Reviews*, *The Oxford Handbook of Philosophy and Psychiatry*, and the *Journal of Applied Philosophy*.

C. D. C. Reeve is Delta Kappa Epsilon Distinguished Professor of Philosophy at the University of North Carolina at Chapel Hill. He has recently published books such as *Aristotle on Practical Wisdom* (2013), *Blindness and Reorientation: Problems in Plato's Republic* (2012), and *Action, Contemplation, and Happiness: An Essay on Aristotle* (2012). He has also translated Plato's *Euthyphro*, *Apology*, *Crito*, *Meno*, *Cratylus* and *Republic* (2005), as well as Aristotle's *Politics* and *Nicomachean Ethics*.

David R. Rubinow is the Assad Meymandi Professor and Chair of the Department of Psychiatry in the School of Medicine at the University of North Carolina at Chapel Hill. He has served as a mentor for an extensive number of trainees, and received numerous awards for his research, including the A. E. Bennett Neuropsychiatric Research Foundation Award, Research Award of the Academy of Psychosomatic Medicine, Gold Medal Award of the Society of Biological Psychiatry, Mood Disorders Research Award of the American College of Psychiatrists, Menninger Award of the American College of Physicians, NIH Distinguished Clinical Educator Award, NIMH Mentor of the Year 2002, and USPHS Outstanding Service Medal. He was inducted into the Institute of Medicine in 2012.

Walter Sinnott-Armstrong is Chauncey Stillman Professor of Practical Ethics in the Philosophy Department and the Kenan Institute for Ethics at Duke University. He is also core faculty in the Duke Institute for Brain Sciences and the Center for Cognitive Neuroscience. He has served as vice-chair of the Board of Officers of the American Philosophical Association, and co-director of the MacArthur Project on Law and Neuroscience.

Chandra Sripada holds a joint appointment at the University of Michigan. One appointment is in the Department of Psychiatry, where he studies brain mechanisms of attention and self-regulation. The other appointment is in the Department of Philosophy, where he tries to understand how emerging results from the sciences impact our picture of ourselves as free and rational agents. His writing has appeared in journals such as *Nous* and the *International Journal of Neuropsychopharmacology*.

Jesse S. Summers is a post-doctoral fellow at the Kenan Institute for Ethics, Adjunct Assistant Professor in the Philosophy Department, and Fellow in the

Thompson Writing Program at Duke University. He received his PhD in Philosophy from UCLA. His work is on compulsion, addiction, and various other forms of irrationality, particularly on their moral implications. He has published in journals such as *Philosophy, Psychiatry, & Psychology* (forthcoming), *Oxford Studies in Normative Ethics*, and *Notre Dame Philosophical Reviews*.

George Szmukler is Professor of Psychiatry and Society at the Institute of Psychiatry, King's College London, and previously an honorary consultant psychiatrist at the South London and Maudsley NHS Foundation Trust. He is an Associate Director of the NIHR – Mental Health Research Network, with special responsibility for patient and public involvement in research.

Franklin Worrell is a PhD candidate in Philosophy at Tulane University, where he is completing a dissertation on responsibility and brain deviance, particularly as concerns the paraphilic disorders. He has previously published (with Alison Denham) on the fracturing of identity in David Lynch's *Mulholland Drive*. He has been the recipient of fellowships from the Murphy Institute's Center for Ethics and Public Affairs and Freie Universität Berlin.

Introduction

Beyond the Philosophy of Psychiatry

Daniel D. Moseley and Gary Gala

This volume of originally written essays presents a dialogue that examines issues at the intersection of psychiatry and philosophy. Some of the central questions include: What is a mental disorder? Is a psychiatric diagnosis just a tool used by psychiatrists to enforce social norms on people that have "problems in living"? Is there any ethical justification for coercing a person who has been diagnosed with a mental disorder to compel that person to comply with medication or treatment? Can a person who has been diagnosed with a severe mental disorder be held morally responsible for her or his actions? These questions are not new, but the arguments and perspectives formulated in this volume are. The volume consists of ten lead essays and ten commentaries. Half of the lead essays are written by philosophers, and the other half are written by psychiatrists (or other clinicians and researchers that work in psychiatry). Philosophers have provided commentaries on the psychiatrists, and psychiatrists have provided commentaries on the philosophers.

The essays have not been written in the spirit of providing the final word on the topics that are discussed. The chapters are also not intended to function as encyclopedia, handbook, or guidebook entries that provide an overview of a specific topic. The authors of the lead essays in this volume bring their own particular background and expertise from their respective disciplines. They have generously accepted the opportunity to discuss themes from their own research that intersect with philosophy and psychiatry. The commentators on the lead essays also draw from their own disciplinary background and research interests to evaluate the strengths and weaknesses of the lead essays.

Our aim in putting together this volume is to produce a conversation that will inspire students, professors, clinicians, and researchers to reflect on the philosophical assumptions and implications of psychiatric care, research, and services. Readers who approach this volume with a background (or primary interest) in medicine, psychology, or social science may want to begin by reading the lead essays by the psychiatrists: Kontos, Kinghorn, Szmukler, Kim, and Rubinow. These psychiatrists were invited to reflect on philosophical dimensions of their work. Their essays are not intended to be works in philosophy. The philosophical commentaries help to further initiate those who are intrigued by the questions that are examined into the philosophical complexities of those essays. These commentaries are intended to engage with psychiatry and to explore constructive directions for future research. Readers of this volume with a background (or primary interest) in philosophy may want to begin by reading the lead essays by the philosophers: Lange; Kozuch and McKenna; Summers and Sinnott-Armstrong; Worrell and Denham; and Reeve. The psychiatric commentaries on their essays reveal how clinical experience and training can elucidate philosophical theorizing. Most of the commentaries in this volume can also be read as stand-alone works. We intend for the volume to present a conversation that shows the give and take between the disciplines.

Rather than summarize the contents of this volume, we shall present a framework for examining different points of intersection between philosophy and psychiatry.[1] We discuss three types of conversations:

1. philosophy *of* psychiatry;
2. philosophy *in* psychiatry;
3. philosophy *out of* psychiatry.

These forms of discussion are not mutually exclusive. The second and third types of discussion also reveal a range of problems and perspectives that fall outside the purview of the philosophy of psychiatry. Our characterization of these three different types of conversations focuses on differences between their methods and subject matter. The methods of psychiatry include the statistical and scientific tools of psychology, medicine, epidemiology, neuroscience, and genetics. The methods of philosophy include the tools of conceptual, linguistic, and logical analysis and the theories and interpretative techniques that have been developed in the various traditions of philosophy. (Psychoanalysis deploys methods that are both philosophical and psychiatric.) The characteristic subject matter of psychiatry includes investigating the causes of psychopathologies and providing treatment for psychopathologies. The characteristic subject matter of philosophy includes certain paradigm questions of inquiry: What is justice? Does God exist? Do we have free will? Is immortality possible?

The Philosophy of Psychiatry

The first kind of conversation, the philosophy *of* psychiatry, uses the methods of philosophy to investigate the subject matter of psychiatry. There is a large group of sub-fields in philosophy that discuss "the philosophy of" in which the blank is filled by numerous possible areas of inquiry: philosophy of art; of film; of physics; of history; of literature; of economics; of mind, and so on. The philosophy of psychiatry is a familiar, and expanding, field of inquiry that often takes the tools of contemporary epistemology, ethics, or philosophy of mind, and applies those tools to the subject matter of psychiatry—psychopathology, mental health services and research, and mental health law and policy.[2] Philosophers who contribute to work at the intersection of philosophy and psychiatry often adopt this approach to the field. The following two types of discussions reveal ways in which future research may go beyond the philosophy of psychiatry.

Philosophy in Psychiatry

The second type of conversation, philosophy *in* psychiatry, examines philosophical assumptions that are widespread in the methods of psychiatric research and practice. For instance, the *Diagnostic and Statistical Manual of Mental Disorders* (DSM) adopts a symptom-based approach to psychiatric nosology. The symptom-based approach that it advances and the revision process of the various editions of the DSM have been the subject of widespread controversy.[3] Discussions of the scientific validity of the DSM nosology raise challenging questions about explanation and reduction in psychiatry. The use of the DSM by clinicians and the revision process of the various editions have moral and political implications for society: such as whether the "grief exemption" in the DSM-5 is turning ordinary grief into a pathological process that should be treated with antidepressants.[4] Discussions that fall under the rubric of "philosophy *in* psychiatry" reveal the philosophical assumptions and implications of the everyday practice of psychiatry.

Philosophy out of Psychiatry

The third type of conversation, philosophy *out of* psychiatry, aspires to develop philosophical theories that are informed by, and continuous with, the practice of psychiatry. These discussions focus on how insights, hypotheses, and conclusions from the history and contemporary practice of psychiatry can inform reflection on central philosophical issues, such as naturalism and human nature. The work of Ian Hacking and Jonathan Lear provide contemporary examples of this type of conversation. The essay by David Rubinow and the commentary by Valerie Hardcastle reveal how rigorous bench-work in psychiatry can lead to keen observations about the limitations and scope of neurological explanations of human behavior. The essay by C. D. C. Reeve and the commentary by Mardy S. Ireland show how philosophical film analysis and psychoanalytic theory can reveal insights into human nature and practical reasoning.

Philosophy and psychiatry are separated by the intellectual division of labor, but the practitioners of the disciplines do share a common interest in making sense of themselves. We hope that the dialogue that emerges from this volume will launch future research in the philosophy *of* psychiatry, philosophy *in* psychiatry, and philosophy *out of* psychiatry. Philosophers and psychiatrists should not try to go at it alone in the project of rendering ourselves and the world intelligible. Philosophy and psychiatry need each other.

Notes

1 The framework for the three conversations that is provided in this essay builds on a similar framework developed for examining the points of intersection between economics and ethics in Brennan and Moseley (2013).

2 For introductions to the philosophy of psychiatry, see Graham (2013), Fulford et al. (2013), and Radden (2004).
3 See Olbert, Gala, and Tupler (2014) for a crisp articulation of the worries about the heterogeneity of the symptom-based approach. See Kendler and Parnas (2012) for an overview of the current debates.
4 Kinghorn's contribution to this volume formulates a moral and political defense of the DSM. See Moseley (2015) for a discussion of the moral and political implications of the DSM-5.

References

Brennan, Geoffrey and Daniel Moseley. 2013. "Economics and Ethics." In *The International Encyclopedia of Ethics*, edited by Hugh LaFollette. Oxford: Wiley-Blackwell.

Fulford, K. W. M., Martin Davies, Richard Gipps, George Graham, John Sadler, Giovanni Stanghellini, and Tim Thornton, Eds. 2013. *The Oxford Handbook of Philosophy and Psychiatry*. Oxford: Oxford University Press.

Graham, George. 2013. *The Disordered Mind, 2nd Edition*. New York: Routledge.

Kendler, Kenneth and Josef Parnas, Eds. 2012. *Philosophical Issues in Psychiatry II: Nosology*. Oxford: Oxford University Press.

Moseley, Daniel, Ed. 2015. *The Moral and Political Implications of the DSM-5*. Special Issue of *Public Affairs Quarterly*. 29 (1).

Olbert, Charles, Gary Gala, and Larry Tupler. 2014. "Quantifying Hetereogeneity Attributable to Polythetic Diagnostic Criteria: Theoretical Framework and Empirical Application." *Journal of Abnormal Psychology*. 123 (2): 452–62.

Radden, Jennifer, Ed. 2004. *The Philosophy of Psychiatry: A Companion*. Oxford: Oxford University Press.

Part 1

Psychiatric Diagnosis and Agency

1a

Can What's in Your Head be "All in Your Head?"

Possibilities and Problems of Psychological Symptom Amplification

Nicholas Kontos

> One can never be sick enough. Even the stricken can milk it.
>
> Ben Marcus (Marcus 2013)

1. Introduction

The imperative to act in situations of uncertainty is a core characteristic of clinical medicine. In the presence of a suffering, scared, usually trusting, sometimes demanding, and always-expectant patient, a physician does not have the luxury of indefinite restraint (Montgomery 2006). Even if the required action is "just" the provision of explanation, a doctor often must perform it without the comfort of standing on solid factual ground (Pender 2006).

In psychiatry, this dilemma achieves a level of near absurdity that is, if not unheard of elsewhere in medicine, then distinguished by its pervasiveness. A psychiatrist's daily role involves making mostly unprovable diagnoses, and mobilizing therapies about which one can at best assert what they do rather than how they work. Still, unless the brain is assigned a status of immunity from pathology denied to every other bodily organ (including its own motor and sensory components), the role is a necessary one.

Lacking confirmatory biomarkers, most psychiatric diagnosing starts and stops at the level of symptoms and signs. Signs tend to be evident and useful in only the most severe mental illness states (e.g., the motor signs of catatonia, disorganized thought in psychotic disorders). When it comes to other prevalent psychopathological entities, particularly mood and anxiety disorders, psychiatric diagnoses are almost exclusively based on the volunteered and elicited complaints of patients – that is, symptoms.

It is often said that the vast majority of medical diagnoses can be found in the history alone; that is, in the facilitated reporting of symptoms and their circumstantial and longitudinal contexts. This received wisdom may be somewhat overblown, though. In a recent study of emergency-room visits, history alone was considered diagnostically sufficient in only about 20 percent of patients. While symptoms probably are the "most potent single tool" in patient assessment (Paley et al. 2011), that potency is relative. Further, in outpatient settings, at least one third of symptoms end up medically unexplained (Kroenke et al. 2002), suggesting that in and of themselves, patient reports can be the packaging for contents that do not come "as advertised."

Given our dependence on symptoms and magnified environment of uncertainty, psychiatrists ought to find these statistics troubling. Yet, one seldom encounters skepticism about the meaning or magnitude of patients' expressions of their psychological complaints. Instead, for better or for worse, patients are said to "meet criteria" for one or another condition in the *Diagnostic and Statistical Manual of Mental Disorders* (DSM) (American Psychiatric Association [APA] 2013). Those criteria largely involve the accumulation of symptom endorsements, often obtained via a questionnaire, inventory, or mnemonic originally derived from those same criteria. The psychiatric diagnostic process thus becomes a circular one in which unexplained symptoms are impossibilities.

This chapter attempts to examine the idea of whether the medically unexplained symptom (MUS) concept, traditionally reserved for somatic symptoms, can or should be extended to psychological complaints. In alternative terms, this means asking if there exists a psychological analogue of somatizing. This is a fortuitous but potentially confusing time to pose such a question since the recently released DSM-5 reconfigured the MUS/somatization concept in its "Somatic Symptom and Related Disorders" category. In the current environment of controversy and flux regarding these terms, the reader will hopefully forgive their use in this chapter. Discussion of the psychological variant of MUS/somatization will use these terms in analogy; otherwise, the term "psychological symptom amplification" (PSA) will be used. This term is intended to be purely descriptive and to lack implication of intentionality, PSA refers to excessive symptom reports and impact regardless of the presence or absence of corresponding psychopathology as determined via reasonable and responsible medical assessment.

The issue of whether psychological symptoms are subject to amplification raises difficult questions touching upon dualism, identity, the nature of the doctor–patient relationship, and the validity of psychiatric diagnosing. Considering the possibility of PSA will not make psychiatric practice or research any easier, but hopefully this chapter will demonstrate how ignoring it might be making things harder.

2. Current Concepts of Somatic Symptom Amplification

The idea that psychological symptoms such as "depression," "anxiety," and "racing thoughts" may be over-endorsed or impactful in certain patients has not been accounted for. On the other hand, patients have long been known to represent somatic experiences such as pain in ways that are not necessarily diagnostically helpful.

Examining a psychological analogue of this phenomenon requires taking a step back to look at some concepts of somatic symptom amplification.

"Medically" "Unexplained" "Symptoms"

Placing each of the component words of the term, MUS, in scare quotes is not intended to be cute or cynical. Instead, it highlights the contested status of each of these terms. How one thinks about "medically" depends upon what one considers to be the methods and objectives of medicine. Are they health-oriented, and directed toward the World Health Organization's view of "a state of complete physical, mental and social well-being and not merely the absence of disease or infirmity" (World Health Organization [WHO] 1946)? A slightly more limited perspective might be that of "whole person medicine," which attempts to identify and remove limitations of "functioning," defined as the "achievement of goals or the realization of purposes" (Cassell 2013). A more bounded view of medicine reverse engineers it from the existence of disease, thus confining its activities to pursuing "the absence (or alleviation) of disease and infirmity" (Cantor 2003).

Invoking disease in any definition of medicine begs the question of what disease is, and evokes complex arguments (Humber and Almeder 1997) that are beyond the scope of this chapter. The ambiguity is worth mentioning, though, since explanation-as-disease is pertinent to the "unexplained" element of MUS. For most physicians, an adequate explanation for a patient's symptom must be found in an anatomic lesion, a physiologic aberration, or a legitimized pattern of distress/impairment. The explanation ought to be sufficient in any patient with the same symptoms and clinical findings. Unfortunately, that explanation is often elusive or unsatisfactory to one or both parties in the doctor–patient relationship where "the physician and the great majority of his patients no longer share a similar view of the body and the mechanisms which determine health and disease" (Rosenberg 1979). This is especially true when the explanation is a negative one – that is, "I cannot find a (disease-based) cause for your problem."

So the question of what constitutes medical explanation, and, by extension, its absence, is incompletely settled. It is nonetheless fair to say that people bring uncomfortable experiences to physicians when they believe them to fall within the purview of medicine – that is, when they consider those experiences "symptoms." Eisenberg has gone so far as to say that a person's presentation of an experience to a physician is enough to make that experience a symptom and that person a patient; that "patienthood is a psychosocial state … it is the patient who decides" (Eisenberg 1980). This formulation contrasts with others in which a person's distress is interpreted by a physician who determines whether and which diagnosis applies. When affirmative and clear, that determination grants the experience symptom status, and the person patient or sick role status (Parsons 1951; Rosenberg 2003).

Somatization and DSM

For as long as medicine has been practiced, there have been patients who presented to their physicians with cryptogenic symptoms. The term "somatization" was first used in the 1920s by the psychoanalyst Welhelm Stekel to capture the idea that unacceptable emotional states could be transformed into the otherwise inexplicable somatic signs of conversion hysteria. Applications of the term expanded dramatically in the 1960s and 1970s, coming to refer not just to conversion phenomena, but to any individual or collective tendency to experience emotional states through somatic symptoms (Berrios and Mumford 1995).

The writers of DSMs I and II avoided the word "somatization." This decision was apparently made in the interest of precision in delineating the psychodynamic mechanisms that underlie "psychophysiologic disorders" ("a chronic and exaggerated state of the normal physiological expression of emotion, with the feeling, or subjective part, repressed"), and "psychoneurotic reactions," particularly conversion or "hysterical neurosis" (where loss of function was instrumental and carried symbolic meaning) (APA 1952; APA 1968).

The diagnostic debut of "somatization" occurred in DSM-III. Given its psychoanalytic heritage, "somatization" is a surprising term to see avoided in earlier DSMs, yet considered ready for prime time in DSM-III; the latter edition ostensibly being characterized by a commitment to an "atheoretical," purely descriptive stance in the service of diagnostic reliability (Wilson 1993). Yet little attempt was made to alter somatization's conceptual trajectory, with explicit mention made of the "positive evidence, or a strong presumption, that the (somatic) symptoms are linked to psychological factors or conflicts." This explanation for why "the specific pathophysiologic processes involved are not demonstrable or understandable by existing laboratory procedures" (APA 1980) was used to explain not only conversion signs, but also the multi-organ-system complaints of patients with all manner of MUS, as seen in somatization disorder and hypochondriasis.

DSM-IV did not alter this "official" stance on somatization, but it did make at least one important change. Previously diagnoses of exclusion, somatoform diagnoses in DSM-IV could be made in situations where the *presence* of a patient's complaint was medically explainable but its *impact* was not (APA 1994). Nearly 20 years later, this allowance has become the diagnostic standard. Responding in part to research indicating that it is the secondary impact, rather than the etiology, of symptoms that correlates with functional impairment and distress (Tomenson et al. 2013), and in accordance with voices raised against the "dualism" that informs distinctions between somatic and psychological etiologies of MUS, DSM-5 does away with terms derived from "somatization" (APA 2013).

Moving Forward

Ultimately, these changes in how the DSMs characterize MUS are more about American psychiatry's own struggles with the psychoanalytically inherited somatization construct than they are about effacing all potential psychological explanations of MUS expression. Without declaring the extinction of the psychoanalytically informed version of somatization, a more integrative model has been in ascendance for a while now. In this model of somatization (Barsky and Borus 1999), patients presenting with MUS are thought to have low sensation thresholds as understood through biological mechanisms such as central sensitization (Cagnie et al. 2014) and/or more psychological ones such as low distress tolerance (Leyro et al. 2010). The "second hit" in this model involves a propensity to attach medical significance, concern, and responses to the experiences in question. This propensity has been observed in multiple studies of patients with hypochondriasis (Barsky et al. 1993; Weck et al. 2012; Gropalis et al. 2013).

Hypochondriasis is only one manifestation of MUS and the somatizing tendency, and fear is only one influence upon individuals' responses to distressing sensations. Integrating the ideas of MUS, somatization, and current diagnostic and mechanistic frameworks for them, one can envision not so much a somatizing as a medicalizing tendency.

3. Medicalization and Psychological Symptom Amplification

For MUS to have any staying power in an individual, or for somatization or medicalization to be stable social options, there must be a perpetuating force available. What a person stands to gain from what otherwise appears to be bafflingly persistent suffering must be examined in any consideration of symptom amplification. One must also consider the ways and ease of accessing those gains.

Status of the Symptomatic

Socially, medicalization connotes the processes and products deployed by a culture to grant or impose medical status onto previously non-medical forms of suffering and deviance. That status includes "defining a problem in medical terms, usually as an illness or disorder, or using a medical intervention to treat it" (Conrad 2005). At the individual level, medicalization reveals itself in the propensity and intensity with which one seeks or claims sick role status for uncomfortable experiences. For physicians, medicalization means the socially or self-imposed expansion of one's job description (whether as opportunity or burden).

Appropriately utilized, medicalization can reduce suffering and preserve the humanity of the sick. The benefits of medicalization include explanation/diagnosis and relief/treatment, not only as applied to distressing experiences themselves, but also to the fear and worry they engender. Medicalization's benefits extend into other material and immaterial domains. Often invoked in medicine, but seldom linked to its sociological heritage, the sick role was described in detail by Talcott Parsons in his 1951 book, "The Social System" (Parsons 1951), and in his and others' subsequent work (Parsons 1975; Williams 2005). For the purposes of this chapter, the patient-seated privileges of sick role status are most pertinent. These include blamelessness for the presence of symptoms, relief from obligations incompatible with sickness, and both expectation and entitlement to receive care. While Parsons confined "care" to medical care, there is some face validity to its extension into sympathy and succor from family and peers.

These desirable accompaniments of sickness, when not outweighed by the joys of healthier living, could account for the momentum that medicalization has culturally and, for many, individually. Who among us could not at one time or another use a little absolution, release, and nurturing? When viewed from the perspective of those already feeling "unworthy, beleaguered, and unloved," the nature of primary gain in the context of somatization becomes much less mysterious (Gerstenblith and Kontos, 2015), as does the notorious chronicity of somatizing patients.

Stigma and Destigmatization

Sick role status does not come easily. Not merely a transaction in which suffering and effort are exchanged for relief and benefits, the sick role is granted only to categories of suffering that society (and medicine as a powerful subgroup of society) deems worthy. Selectivity in the sick role is necessary in order to avoid diluting its power. However, one person's selectivity is another's exclusivity. For many people with medically ambiguous states of suffering such as chronic fatigue syndrome (recently redubbed "systemic exertion intolerance disease" [Institute of Medicine 2015]), the need and longing for sick role status exists in tension with resentment over the experience of it being withheld. As Rosenberg points out, "the social legitimacy – and often social resources – associated with the sickness role constitutes a prize worth contesting" (Rosenberg 2006).

Contesting the "prize" of sick role legitimacy has long been a project for the mentally ill and their professional and personal advocates. Stigma is a heterogeneous phenomenon, significant aspects of which include prejudice and ostracism. Also, with mental illness itself being heterogeneous, stigma is expressed differently towards different forms of psychopathology (e.g., addiction versus schizophrenia). Nevertheless, a great deal of stigma could be construed as the non-legitimization of psychiatric sick role status. Blaming the psychiatrically sick for their symptoms, attributing sub-adequate role fulfillment to sloth, and impeding access to medical care and sympathy are all targets of destigmatization-related education efforts.

While the mentally ill, and particularly those with chronic psychotic disorders and other severe and persistent mental illnesses, continue to suffer the disadvantages of stigma, there are signs of change. Public education initiatives, greater information accessibility/availability, and commercial influences may be both contributors to and products of an alteration in social attitudes toward mental illness and its treatment. Significant recent increases have occurred in public endorsement of the biological basis of depressive illness (Blumner and Marcus 2009), as well as in favorable attitudes toward seeking mental health care (Mojtabai 2007; Mojtabai 2009). Linkages have been noted between increased knowledge/belief in disease models of mental illnesses and likelihood of help-seeking (Rüsch et al. 2011; Blumner and Marcus 2009). The medical mainstreaming of mood and anxiety disorders is also evident in their portrayal in the media as things to "discuss with your doctor," and in their being objects of health care screening akin to hypertension and hyperlipidemia (Kroenke et al. 2010; Hahn et al. 2006).

An ideal outcome of these trends and efforts is that those afflicted with mental illnesses are granted the sick role status that they deserve. A great deal of the effort exerted in the service of this goal is in accord with the dominant disease model of specific, biological disease entities (Temkin 1977; Rosenberg 2003). Of course, propagation of biological models of mental illness, such as the "chemical imbalance," is a two-edged sword. On the one hand, it might bring unnecessarily suffering stoics into the treatment they need by reducing self-stigmatization. On the other hand, it expands the medicalization options of those prone to amplified, pathologized experiences into the psychiatric domain. Lurie identifies this latter potential as a "defense of externalization" akin to somatization (Lurie 1991). His impression is supported by the association between "medical behavior, including antidepressant use," and a decrease in self-stigma that unfortunately is not linked to any increased sense of empowerment (Evans-Lacko et al. 2012).

In short, destigmatization through medicalization makes PSA fair game.

4. The Invisibility of Psychological Symptom Amplification

Psychiatry's efforts at medical legitimization might contribute not only to making a psychological analogue of somatization possible, but also to the field's unawareness of that possibility. Like the rest of medicine (Snelders et al. 2006; Ackerknecht 1962), psychiatry goes through cycles of discovery, excess, and readjustment in its employment of various diagnostic and therapeutic methods (Pressman 1998; Luhrmann 2001). A distinguishing characteristic of psychiatry's participation in these processes is the ever-present need to establish or reinforce its medical *bona fides* through them. Two ways of doing this are by accentuating the impact of mental illness, and by linking psychopathology to other contemporary medical trends. Neither of these is absolutely "wrong" in a moral or ontological sense, but they do contribute in important ways to how psychiatry views and constructs people/patients.

Understanding Need

With regard to establishing need, worldwide estimates of the burden of major depressive disorder (MDD) have been sufficiently publicized so as to not require reiteration here. Further, a large literature cites a massive prevalence of "depression and anxiety" in primary care settings, a failure of primary care providers to identify it, and a failure to effectively treat it even when identified. Responses to these findings have been robust in terms of screening practices and psychotropic prescription rates. However, a separate literature demonstrating up to 40 percent rates of "false" positive diagnoses of MDD by non-psychiatrists (Klinkman et al. 1998; Boland et al. 1995) gets little attention. Also, while antidepressant prescriptions have skyrocketed, the prevalence of active MDD remains unchanged (Mojtabai 2011). Many factors might underlie this population-level inefficacy in MDD treatment, but it is interesting to note that a sizeable percentage of these medications are being prescribed in the absence of documented psychiatric diagnoses (Mojtabai and Olfson 2011; Pagura et al. 2011).

A link between these findings and the invisibility of PSA might be found in the high rates at which patients endorse statements indicating that psychotropic medications are effective at reducing "stress," smoothing relationships, and coping with life stressors – all alongside and on a par with their belief in the drugs' efficacy in treating disorders such as MDD and panic disorder (Mojtabai 2009). Primary care physicians certainly have the impression that patients are initiating more and more requests for psychotropic medications (Paterniti et al. 2010; Kravitz et al. 2005), but their focus has been more on prescription than diagnosis trends. Synthesizing these findings suggests that a sizeable number of patients may be presenting to their doctors with depressive complaints misattributed to depressive disorders.

A Pathologizing Bias?

How doctors interpret symptom reports depends on a complex blend of medical knowledge, clinical experience, and, unavoidably, values and biases (Fulford 2004; Klerman 1972; Fogel et al. 1992). A relevant question is whether or not people who bring their complaints to doctors are met by a profession that thinks critically about their self-reports. Is a "depressed" mood as volunteered or checked off on an inventory to be taken at first as a "depressive symptom" or as sadness? Likewise, how does a physician interpret a patient's complaints of "anxiety?" The overlap between lay and jargon terms in psychiatry does not help matters. Physicians can certainly impose pathological meaning onto patients' experiences (Ring et al. 2005). However, as the literature on "somatizing" has long pointed out, physicians must also be attentive to the possibility of patients prematurely imposing pathological interpretations on their own experiences. A bias against this type of caution may enlarge psychiatry's blind spot to the possibility of PSA.

Being more concerned with symptom interpretation than with broader debates about disease "construction," this chapter will not address the influences of professional and economic interests. Even absent these formidable pathologizing forces, it can be argued that medical school primes the pump of pathologizing bias. The teaching of patient examination typically begins with an orientation to what is being examined. For example, auscultation of the heart is demonstrated first via the discrimination of normal heart sounds and how they are best appreciated; only after these normal findings and techniques are established does one learn the characteristics of murmurs, rubs, gallops, and so on. In contrast to this sequence of training in normal function, exam technique, and pathological findings, the psychiatric interview and exam is generally taught, right from the start, with reference to abnormality.

Instruction in affect, behavior, and cognitive phenomena and methods of probing them tends to use their anomalous expressions (e.g., lability, agitation, and inattention) as the didactic baseline. In worse cases, mental status is reverse engineered from DSM criteria as when affect is taught as part of an inquiry (often mnemonic based) into depressive and (hypo)manic episodes. The illness-based "checklist" approach to psychological exam training (Freudenreich et al. 2004) can produce physicians whose pathological bias may be a product of never having appreciated basic concepts such as mood and affect (Serby 2003) as existing outside of a disordered context. One need only look at the American Psychiatric Press's definition of insight to drive this point home – "capacity to understand one's illness." Assessment of judgment is proposed in the same text as best achieved through assessment of compliance with treatment (Andrews 2008).

Phenomenologically attuned psychiatrists make attempts to balance out this trend in psychiatric training (Sims 2003; Taylor and Vaidya 2009; Broome et al. 2012), but they face an uphill battle. For example, the sixth edition of an influential introductory book on psychiatric diagnosis places its chapter on "The Psychiatric Evaluation" last after each preceding one lays out a major domain of psychopathology. According to the authors, "to elicit enough information about the disorder(s) to make a diagnosis, one must know the signs, symptoms, course, and complications. This is the primary reason this chapter concludes the book" (North and Yutzy 2010). Most medical evaluations start with history and exam, then conclude with an assessment. Here the order is not only reversed, but the presence of "the disorder(s)" is assumed.

Concern about a pathologizing bias in psychiatry is a longstanding one that has often centered on the field's gravitation to interventionist and dogmatic fads (Ghaemi 2010). Even before the publication of DSM-I, concern existed about "Education Versus Indoctrination in Psychiatric Teaching," and its linkage to the desire for medical legitimation of the field (Ebaugh 1951). Decades ago, Kendall noted powerful biases in depression diagnoses, concluding "that, because the effect of the bias is always to cause the observer to find what he is expecting, he becomes progressively more convinced he is right" (Kendall 1968).

Kendall hoped that "these sources of error could all be eliminated if structured interviewing schedules were used." However, Maj recently noted the imperatives and problems of using clinical judgment in an era of criterion-based diagnosing in both clinical and scientific domains, especially given the latter's frequent use of "lay interviewers, who by definition are unable to exercise clinical judgment" (Maj 2013). With pure criterion-based interviewing, reliability is achieved, but bias is skewed toward the assumed presence of pathology.

Other suggestions of a pathologizing bias in psychiatry exist. The general acceptance of the term "self-medication" in addictive disorders implicitly uses diagnosis–treatment terminology (Bolton et al. 2009), when "self-regulation" is a less presumptive alternative. Increased rates of prescribing (Mojtabai 2008), and particularly non-evidence-based poly-prescribing (Mojtabai and Olfson 2010; Freudenreich et al. 2012), may be proxies for physicians' willingness to accept face-value psychological symptom endorsements as representations of pathology.

Selective Anti-Dualism

If PSA is made possible by successes in medicalizing psychiatry, then shouldn't that high tide have raised all boats and brought a psychological analogue of somatization to the same level of recognition as somatization itself? Psychiatry's exceptionalist approach to dualism might provide some answer as to why not. A meaningful discussion of the philosophical and clinical implications of "dualistic" versus "non-dualistic" considerations in disease/illness is too complex for this chapter. Suffice to say that there are very few card-carrying dualists on the record in psychiatry. Mind–body dualism is categorically written off as a bad thing, especially regarding MUS-related terminology (Sharpe 2013; Creed et al. 2010; Mayou et al. 2003).

Looking down one's nose at the MUS concept, however, is presumptuous; it assumes that the "medically" part is settled as "reductionist" and accepted as such across the board by the great unwashed of medicine (Kontos 2011). Crombez and colleagues (2009) note that MUS and somatization are multi-faceted entities that can be subdivided into components oriented toward etiology, symptom expression, and help-seeking.

Those who support a non-dualistic view of MUS/somatizing seem unperturbed by the purely etiologic focus of their anti-dualism sentiments. As noted earlier, DSM-5 deemphasizes concerns about the psychogenesis versus somatogenesis of symptoms. The disordered element of somatic symptom disorders is not a mechanism of symptom production, but rather maladaptive or abnormal (Pilowsky 1990) illness behaviors (Mechanic 1995). This formulation is expressed in a way that casually and paradoxically makes a distinction between somatic and psychological symptoms. Only somatic symptoms are taken to be potential objects of maladaptive illness behavior patterns. Hence we have "*somatic* symptom and related disorders." If psychiatry is serious about its non-dualistic rhetoric, then those principles ought to be applied to symptoms as much as to etiologic concerns. When these principles are combined with those underlying psychiatric medicalization, the possibility of PSA becomes harder to ignore.

5. Manifestations and Detection

If physicians entertained idea of PSA, what would they see? To be sure, just as MUS/somatization is multi-faceted, so too should be its psychiatric analogue.

Attribution of Experience

The hypochondriacal "restrictive concept of good health" (Weck et al. 2012) seems intuitively and experientially to be an important part of PSA. Just as a somatically preoccupied patient believes healthy living to be incompatible with aches, pains, dyspepsia, and the like (Salkovskis et al. 2002), the psychological symptom amplifier might (also) expect or require freedom from sadness, worry, distractedness, and volatile temperament. That these experiences are easily, sometimes eagerly, referred to by patients and doctors alike as "depression," "anxiety," "attention-deficit," and "bipolar" fertilizes ideas that these complaints can and ought to be labeled and treated; and that to not do so is to consign oneself or one's patient to an unfairly compromised existence. (The somewhat related issue of enhancement "therapies" will not be addressed here.)

Individuals and cultures vary in their somatic versus psychological symptom experiences (Kirmayer and Sartorius 2007). Parker and Parker found the tendency to attribute somatic experiences to psychological sources to be associated with the self-labeling of dysphoric mood as "depression" (Parker and Parker 2003). Perhaps tellingly, their report accentuates the challenge of finding depressive illness in under-reporters, and not the equally valid one of misdiagnosing it in over-reporters. Subsequent studies reveal patient populations that are prone to high endorsement of both somatic and psychological symptoms (Smith et al. 2005; Haug et al. 2004), though some interpret these findings as evidence of comorbidity between somatoform, mood, and anxiety disorders (Löwe et al. 2008).

Handling of Experience

The abnormal or maladaptive illness behavior aspect of MUS/somatization/somatic symptom disorders takes us beyond attributional aspects of these conditions and into consideration of patients' experiences themselves. Zanarini and colleagues describe "emotional hyperchondriasis" in borderline (Zanarini and Frankenburg 1994) and other personality-disordered patients (Zanarini et al. 2013). Here, "hyperbolic" expressions of psychological distress serve complex functions of metabolizing other unbearable feeling states and managing relationships. The former element might involve distortion and representation of psychological distress as mood and anxiety "disorders" that are then aggressively but futilely treated by providers. The latter element involves securing attachments via sick role privilege while simultaneously casting others in helpless and/or uncaring roles. High rates of personality disorder or maladaptive personality traits among patients with somatoform disorders (Rost et al. 1992; Russo et al. 1994) suggest that phenomena akin to emotional hypochondriasis are worth consideration in the interpretation of these patients' psychological self-reports.

Mentioned earlier, distress tolerance and related concepts such as anxiety sensitivity and discomfort intolerance are other psychological variables that influence the tendency to report, and ability to function with, somatic and psychological discomfort. Those with unfavorable levels of these variables are more likely to manifest emotion amplification and avoidance coping (Bernstein et al. 2009), misuse alcohol when experiencing "depressive symptoms" (Gorka et al. 2012), and report experiences meeting psychopathology criteria (Leyro et al. 2010). These findings highlight the possibility of a given psychological experience, disordered or not, being handled very differently by different individuals, both in terms of presentation to health care professionals and overall sense of impairment.

In keeping with the current conception of somatic symptom disorders, phenomena such as emotional hypochondriasis and distress (in)tolerance can facilitate PSA regardless of whether or not psychopathology is "truly" present. Thus, one might encounter a patient whose persistent, myriad, and exaggerated complaints lead to a false positive diagnosis of major depressive disorder, or one whose mild depressive illness leads to inordinate impairment. Both would be manifesting PSA.

Assessment of Experience

These last few possibilities lead to some frustrating yet fascinating clinical and philosophical conundrums. In the Western model of diseases as "specific entities" (Rosenberg 2002), a patient either does or does not "have" a given mental disorder. Even within a "spectrum" model of somatic (e.g., hypothyroid), or psychiatric (e.g., attention deficit) disorder, severity cutoffs impose an entity model. Even if one does not adhere to this model of diagnosis, the evidence base that guides care is. How does one sift through the amplifying patient's report or, even more complex, observable behavior, to get to an accurate and meaningful diagnosis? How does one prescribe treatments for symptom amplifiers while possessing and conveying accurate, responsible expectations about their efficacy? Further, given the pathological status of somatic symptom disorders, many patients with PSA would technically "have" a mental illness – a "symptom disorder" – simply by virtue of their PSA itself. With the somatic symptom and related disorders said to have high comorbidity rates with mood and anxiety disorders, the dilemmas just cited become circular ones.

Nonetheless, a maxim in the care of somatizing patients is to curb strong forces favoring aggressive workups and symptom-targeted interventions. One must take care not to be lulled into complacency by the over-endorsing patient's relentless stream of symptoms, but physicians learn early on that the endorsements uncovered in a "pan-positive" review of systems are not necessarily what they seem. Instruction in medical history-taking has long included attention to the frequent need to tease out "patients' feelings and subjective sensations from (their) erroneous ideas and opinions" (Gillis 2006). This advice contrasts sharply with contemporary psychiatric diagnosing. Much has been made of polypharmacy trends in psychiatric treatment, but one must bear in mind that polypharmacy at best begins with poly-diagnosis, and at worst with the accumulation of symptomatic treatments for uncontextualized complaints. Both practices imply assumptions about the face-value medical meanings of individual patients' multi-domain symptom endorsements.

Heavier handed interpretive history-taking also bucks against trends in medical education and practice that encourage egalitarian or "patient-centered" care and discourage the kind of conscious exercise of physician authority that is necessary for reframing patients' experiences (Chew-Graham et al. 2004). "If the patient experiences it, it's 'real'" is a frequent invocation in discussions of symptoms. This perspective caters to conflation between the presence of a symptom and its meaning. A physician can respect the former while questioning or even correcting a patient's beliefs about the latter. Indeed, this authority is arguably fundamental to diagnosis and to medical practice generally (Måseide 1991). Physicians reluctant to apply it to objectively unverifiable psychological symptoms should note that they already do so on a regular basis in the assessment of pain. Mismanagement of that responsibility in the direction of overly credulous and/or aggressive medical attention to pain can have lethal consequences (Bohnert et al. 2011).

6. Consequences of Ignoring Psychological Symptom Amplification

Still, since most mood and anxiety disorders are more readily treatable than most symptom amplification presentations (Kroenke 2007; Sumathipala 2007), there can be a strong moral imperative for physicians to give patients hope and "the benefit of the doubt" by diagnosing and treating the former class of illnesses based on the idea that "it can't hurt but it might help" (Kontos et al. 2003). The oft-reported prevalence of undiagnosed mental illness (WHO 2004; Kessler et al. 2003) provides added impetus to stress detection over discrimination. Neither of these is an invalid perspective, but assuming them without also considering PSA might come at many different currencies of cost.

Illness and Identity in the Clinic

Overlapping as they do with important parts of identity such as temperament, motivation, and mood, psychiatric disorders can influence sense of self in profound ways. A patient diagnosed, accurately or not, with bipolar disorder may come to see himself as mercurial and irresponsible in a variety of ways that do not necessarily flow forth from the "actual" pathology. Excessive symptom impact can be present before the given doctor–patient interaction even begins. Physicians face considerable challenges and duties in handling these circumstances.

A physician's premature closure or fixation on a particular diagnostic-therapeutic stance in the absence of expected signs, longitudinal patterns, or benefit from aggressive treatments reinforces similar closure and fixation by certain patients. Inattention to or unintended encouragement of patient beliefs about their symptoms can cement both parties in restricted role identities. Especially for the patient, these roles do not end at the clinic's walls and are analogous to those seen in the "total institutions" of old (Kontos et al. 2014).

Balint's "apostolic function" of the physician (Balint 1972) involves conveying to patients (hopefully adaptive) attitudes and behaviors about managing their sick role status. The functional somatic syndromes (FSS) provide some clues as to what happens when this role is mismanaged in PSA. Considered by many to be closely related to somatic symptom disorders, FSS include entities such as irritable bowel syndrome, chronic fatigue syndrome, and fibromyalgia. Regardless of their individual or collective validity, these controversial illnesses seem marked less by their symptoms or cryptogenesis (which, after all, are not unique to them) than by the illness behaviors of the afflicted. Of particular interest here are frequent findings of *worse* functioning and quality of life in these states after medical "labeling" (Huibers and Wessely 2006; Riedl et al. 2009). Negative expectations and illness behaviors in chronic fatigue syndrome are reflected in dampened placebo (Cho et al. 2005) and symptomatic treatment responses (Blockmans et al. 2006), and in the adverse effects of support group participation on functioning (Friedberg et al. 2005).

Striving for correct diagnoses is a necessary but insufficient execution of one's apostolic function. Agreement can be hard to come by with many patients with ambiguous symptom etiology (Greer and Halgin 2006). Explanations of symptoms that do not reinforce pre-existing, medicalized beliefs (Stone et al. 2002) and which are not "exculpating" are prone to offend; and those that satisfy patients can be seen by physicians as "colluding" (Salmon et al. 1999). Physicians' apostolic function includes gauging patients' illness beliefs and behaviors in order to promote accuracy and proportionality. This can be an uphill task. Containment strategies form much of the evidence base for handling MUS/somatization (Smith et al. 2003). The difficulty, or occasional futility, of the task does not remove physicians' obligations to avoid harm and provide expert advice. The rhetorical popularity of patient-as-person practice in the clinic might well be complemented by advice against person-as-patient existence in the broader world.

"Caseness" and Scientific Accuracy

The potential effects of undetected PSA in scientific psychiatry can be insidious and far-reaching for two main reasons. First, the study of psychopathology depends upon correct initial classification of subjects as having the disorder in question (i.e., "caseness"). Second, the results of clinical and epidemiologic studies guide downstream patient care and resource allocation decisions.

Possible effects of undetected PSA in psychiatric research are illustrated by the proposed subpopulation of subjects with "anxious depression" in the Sequenced Treatment Alternatives to Relieve Depression (STAR*D) project. These subjects are believed to have a subtype of major depressive disorder identified via threshold number/severity of symptom endorsements on the "anxiety/somatization factor" of the Hamilton Depression Rating Scale (HDRS-17) (Hamilton 1960; Fava et al. 2004). This factor addresses a panoply of somatic symptoms, including gastroenterologic, cardiovascular, respiratory, neurologic, urinary, and constitutional. A standardized structured interview for the HDRS-17 surveys these via the question, "Tell me if you've had any of the following physical symptoms in the past week (READ LIST)," followed by, "How much has (the symptom) been bothering you in the past week" (Williams 1988).

Subjects meeting this criterion represented approximately 45 percent of the depressed sample in STAR*D. This subgroup was characterized by greater endorsement of nearly every HDRS symptom and was more likely to endorse symptoms consistent with generalized anxiety disorder, panic disorder, obsessive-compulsive disorder, post-traumatic stress disorder, agoraphobia, hypochondriasis, and "somatoform disorder" (Fava et al. 2004). Further analysis revealed the anxious depression subgroup to demonstrate greater chronicity, poorer treatment response rates, and seemingly poorer treatment tolerance and/or adherence as reflected in time spent in treatment and on final medication dosages (Fava et al. 2008). Many of these findings are replicated in subsequent samples (Fava et al. 2006; Papakostas et al. 2008; Wiethoff et al. 2010) that also reveal greater side-effect vulnerability (Chan et al. 2012), though not unerringly (Wiethoff et al. 2010). The malleability, or treatment responsiveness, of the somatic complaints correlates with ultimate antidepressant responsiveness (Farabaugh et al. 2005; Farabaugh et al. 2010).

It seems possible that "anxious depression" is a heterogeneous category containing a significant proportion of patients characterized by amplification and over-endorsement of somatic and psychological symptoms. From a "caseness" point of view, this possibility makes sense if one compares case identification methods in anxious depression and somatization. Like the HDRS-17 anxiety/somatization subscale, the Patient Health Questionaire 15 (PHQ-15) surveys the presence and severity of respondents' gastrointestinal, cardiac, pulmonary, genitourinary, musculoskeletal, and constitutional symptoms. Here, however, threshold endorsements correlate with the presence of somatoform disorders (Kroenke et al. 2002; Kroenke et al. 2010). It may be risky to assume that a symptom is a depressive symptom merely by virtue of its having been elicited by a depression inventory.

Especially given recent controversy over the superiority of antidepressants over placebos in major depressive disorder (Kirsch et al. 2008), the possibility of large numbers of symptom-amplifying subjects negatively skewing active drug response rates is an important one. The problem for these subjects might be that their lesser response rates result from initial misdiagnosis. A non-mutually-exclusive factor may be that the side-effect vulnerability, negative expectations, and abnormal illness behaviors that characterize symptom amplifiers (Barsky et al. 2002) dampen their responses to even appropriately directed interventions.

Another important research domain, psychiatric epidemiology, is too far afield of the clinical thrust of this chapter to delve into in any detail. That investigator interpretations of symptom endorsements on even a "gold standard" inventory like the HDRS-17 (Cusin et al. 2010) can be questioned based on a symptom amplification hypothesis suggests some challenges and opportunities in this area. Is PSA a partial explanation for staggering findings whereby nearly a quarter of the mentally ill population meets criteria for three or more diagnoses (Kessler et al. 2005), or over half of those with major depressive disorder "have" multiple psychiatric morbidities (Melartin et al. 2002)? Perhaps there are ways of addressing allegations of diagnostic and therapeutic excesses in psychiatry that do not invite overhaul so much as revised application of current concepts.

7. Conclusion

Hopefully, this chapter has supplied some basis for considering the possibility that psychological symptoms are subject to the same distortions as somatic ones. In a sense, this idea is nothing new. Though a cognitive-behavioral model of somatization/MUS has been leaned on here, older psychoanalytic concepts of ego defenses provide precedent for the idea that one's experiences and behaviors are not necessarily always (or even usually) representative of underlying psychological "truth."

Ultimately, if PSA has conceptual legs, clinicians are left with the conundrum of proving negatives – the absence of *prima facie* psychopathology – in situations where they are without means of even proving positives. There is appropriate discomfort with a diagnostic mode in which one is an umpire whose ball and strike calls dictate practical reality (Murray pers. comm.). However, a "benefit of the doubt" mode, in which every pitch/complaint is a strike/symptom-of-disorder, is disempowering for physicians, a disservice to patients, and a distorting force exerted on the pursuit of knowledge.

Acknowledgments

The author would like to thank John Querques and Oliver Freudenreich for their help and encouragement in developing the ideas behind this essay.

References

Ackerknecht, Erwin H. 1962. "Aspects of the History of Therapeutics." *Bulletin of the History of Medicine* 36: 389–419.

American Psychiatric Association. 1952. *Diagnostic and Statistical Manual of Mental Disorders*. Washington, DC: American Psychiatric Association.

——1968. *Diagnostic and Statistical Manual of Mental Disorders, 2nd Edition*. Washington, DC: American Psychiatric Association.

——1980. *Diagnostic and Statistical Manual of Mental Disorders, 3rd Edition*. Washington, DC: American Psychiatric Association.

——1994. *Diagnostic and Statistical Manual of Mental Disorders, 4th Edition*. Washington, DC: American Psychiatric Association.

——2013. *Diagnostic and Statistical Manual of Mental Disorders, 5th Edition*. Arlington, VA: American Psychiatric Publishing.

Andrews, Linda B. 2008. "The Psychiatric Interview and Mental Status Examination." In *The American Psychiatric Publishing Textbook of Psychiatry, 5th Edition*, edited by Robert E. Hales, Stuart C. Yudofsky, and Glen O. Gabbard. Arlington, VA: American Psychiatric Publishing.

Balint, Michael. 1972. *The Doctor, His Patient, and the Illness, 2nd Edition*. New York: International Universities Press, Inc.

Barsky, Arthur J., and Jonathan F. Borus. 1999. "Functional Somatic Syndromes." *Annals of Internal Medicine* 130: 910–21.

Barsky, Arthur J., Remy R. Coeytaux, Marilyn K. Sarnie, and Paul D. Cleary. 1993. "Hypochondriacal Patients' Beliefs About Good Health." *American Journal of Psychiatry* 150: 1085–89.

Barsky, Arthur J., Ralph Saintort, Malcolm P. Rogers, and Jonathan F. Borus. 2002. "Nonspecific Medication Side Effects and the Nocebo Phenomenon." *Journal of the American Medical Association* 287: 622–27.

Bernstein, Amit, Michael J. Zvolensky, Anka A. Vujanovic, and Rudolf Moos. 2009. "Integrating Anxiety Sensitivity, Distress Tolerance, and Discomfort Intolerance: A Hierarchical Model of Affect Sensitivity and Tolerance." *Behavior Therapy* 40: 291–301.

Berrios, German E., and David Mumford. 1995. "Somatoform Disorders, Clinical Section." In *A History of Clinical Psychiatry*, edited by German Berrios and Roy Porter. New Brunswick, NJ: Athlone Press.

Blockmans, Daniel, Philippe Persoons, Boudewijn Van Houdenhove, and Herman Bobbaers. 2006. "Does Methylphenidate Reduce the Symptoms of Chronic Fatigue Syndrome." *American Journal of Medicine* 119: e23–30.

Blumner, Kate H., and Steven C. Marcus. 2009. "Changing Perceptions of Depression: Ten-Year Trends From the General Social Survey." *Psychiatric Services* 60: 306–12.

Bohnert, Amy S.B., Marcia Valenstein, Matthew J. Bair, Dara Ganoczy, John F. McCarthy, Mark A. Ilgen, and Frederic C. Blow. 2011. "Association Between Opioid Prescribing Patterns and Opioid Overdose-Related Deaths." *Journal of the American Medical Association* 305: 1315–21.

Boland, Robert J., Susan Diaz, Ruth M. Lamdan, Dilip Ramchandani, and James R. McCartney. 1995. "Overdiagnosis of Depression in the General Hospital." *General Hospital Psychiatry* 18: 28–35.

Bolton, James M., Jennifer Robinson, and Jitender Sareen. 2009. "Self-Medication of Mood Disorders With Alcohol and Drugs in the National Epidemiologic Survey on Alcohol and Related Conditions." *Journal of Affective Disorders* 115: 367–75.

Broome, Matthew R., Robert Harland, Gareth S. Owen, and Argyris Stringaris. 2012. *The Maudsley Reader in Phenomenological Psychiatry*. New York: Cambridge University Press.

Cagnie, Barbara, I. Coppieters, S. Denecker, J. Six, L. Danneels, and M. Meeus. 2014. "Central Sensitization in Fibromyalgia? A Systematic Review on Structural and Functional Brain MRI." *Seminars in Arthritis and Rheumatism* epub ahead of print. Accessed March 20, 2014. Doi: 10.1016/j.semarthrit.2014.01.001.

Cantor, David. 2003. "The Diseased Body." In *Companion to Medicine in the Twentieth Century*, edited by Roger Cooter and John Pickstone, 347–66, New York: Routledge.

Cassell, Eric J. 2013. *The Nature of Healing*. New York: Oxford University Press.

Chan, Herng Nieng, A. John Rush, Andrew A. Nierenberg, Madhukar Trivedi, Stephen R. Wisniewski, G.K. Balasubramani, Edward S. Friedman, Bradley N. Gaynes, Lori Davis, David

Morris, and Maurizio Fava. 2012. "Correlates and Outcomes of Depressed Out-Patients with Greater and Fewer Anxious Symptoms: A CO-MED Report. *International Journal of Neuropsychopharmacology* 15: 1387–99.

Chew-Graham, Carolyn A., Carl R. May, Martin O. Roland. 2004. "The Harmful Consequences of Elevating the Doctor-Patient Relationship to Be a Primary Goal of the General Practice Consultation. *Family Practice* 21: 229–31.

Cho, Hyong Jin, Matthew Hotopf, and Simon Wessely. 2005. "The Placebo Response in the Treatment of Chronic Fatigue Syndrome: A Systematic Review and Meta-Analysis." *Psychosomatic Medicine* 67: 301–13.

Conrad, Peter. 2005. "The Shifting Engines of Medicalization." *Journal of Health and Social Behavior* 46: 3–14.

Creed, Francis, Elspeth Guthrie, Per Fink, Peter Henningsen, Winfried Rief, Michael Sharpe, and Peter White. 2010. "Is There a Better Term Than 'Medically Unexplained Symptoms?'" *Journal of Psychosomatic Research* 68: 5–8.

Crombez, Geert, Koen Beirens, Stefaan Van Damme, Christopher Eccleston, and Johnny Fontaine. 2009. "The Unbearable Lightness of Somatisation: A Systematic Review of the Concept of Somatisation in Empirical Studies of Pain." *Pain* 145: 31–35.

Cusin, Cristina, Huaiyu Yang, Albert Yeung, and Maurizio Fava. 2010. "Rating Scales for Depression." In *Handbook of Clinical Rating Scales and Assessment in Psychiatry and Mental Health*, edited by Lee Baer and Mark A. Blais, 7–35, New York: Humana Press.

Ebaugh, F.G. 1951. "Education Versus Indoctrination in Psychiatric Training." *American Journal of Psychiatry* 107: 633–34.

Eisenberg, Leon. 1980. "What Makes Persons 'Patients' and Patients 'Well?'" *American Journal of Medicine* 69: 277–86.

Evans-Lacko, S., E. Brohan, R. Mojtabai, and G. Thornicroft. 2012. "Association Between Public Views of Mental Illness and Self-Stigma Among Individuals With Mental Illness in 14 European Countries." *Psychological Medicine* 42: 1741–52.

Farabaugh, Amy H., Stella Bitran, Janet Witte, Jonathan Alpert, Sarah Chuzi, Alisabet J. Clain, Lee Baer, Maurizio Fava, Patrick J. McGrath, Christina Dording, David Mischoulon, and George I. Papakostas. 2010. "Anxious Depression and Early Changes in the HAMD-17 Anxiety-Somatization Factor Items and Antidepressant Treatment Outcome." *International Clinical Psychopharmacology* 25: 214–17.

Farabaugh, Amy, David Mischoulon, Maurizio Fava, Shirley L. Wu, Alessandra Mascarini, Eliana Tossani, and Jonathan E. Alpert. 2005. "The Relationship Between Early Changes in the HAMD-17 Anxiety/Somatization Factor Items and Treatment Outcome Among Depressed Outpatients." *International Clinical Psychopharmacology* 20: 87–91.

Fava, Maurizio, John A. Rush, Jonathan E. Alpert, Cheryl N. Carmin, G.K. Balasubramani, Stephen R. Wisniewski, Madhukar H. Trivedi, Melanie M. Biggs, and Kathy Shores-Wilson. 2006. "What Clinical and Symptom Features and Comorbid Disorders Characterize Outpatients With Anxious Major Depressive Disorder: A Replication and Extension." *Canadian Journal of Psychiatry* 51: 823–35.

Fava, Maurizio, Jonathan E. Alpert, Cheryl N. Carmin, Stephen R. Wisnewski, Madhukar H. Trivedi, Melanie M. Biggs, Kathy Shores-Wilson, Don Morgan, Terry Schwartz, G.K. Balasubramani, and John A. Rush. 2004. "Clinical Correlates and Symptom Patterns of Anxious Depression Among Patients With Major Depressive Disorder in STAR*D." *Psychological Medicine* 34: 1299–308.

Fava, Maurizio, A. John Rush, Jonathan E. Alpert, G.K. Balasubramani, Stephen R. Wisniewski, Cheryl N. Carmin, Melanie M. Biggs, Sidney Zisook, Andrew Leuchter, Robert Howland, Diane Warden, and Madhukar H. Trivedi. 2008. "Difference in Treatment Outcome in Outpatients With Anxious Versus Nonanxious Depression: A STAR*D Report." *American Journal of Psychiatry* 165: 342–51.

Fogel, Barry S., James Duffy, Eileen M. McNamara, and Steven Salloway. 1992. "Skeptics and Enthusiasts in Neuropsychiatry." *Journal of Neuropsychiatry* 4: 458–62.

Freudenreich, Oliver, Nicholas Kontos, and John Querques. 2012. "Psychiatric Polypharmacy: A Clinical Approach Based on Etiology and Differential Diagnosis." *Harvard Review of Psychiatry* 20: 79–85.

Freudenreich, Oliver, John Querques, and Nicholas Kontos. 2004. "Checklist Psychiatry's Effect on Psychiatric Education." *American Journal of Psychiatry* 161: 930.

Friedberg, Fred, Debbie W. Leung, and Joyce Quick. 2005. "Do Support Groups Help People With Chronic Fatigue Syndrome and Fibromyalgia? A Comparison of Active and Inactive Members" *Journal of Rheumatology* 32: 2416–420.

Fulford, K.W.M. (Bill). 2004. "Facts/Values: Ten Principles of Values-Based Medicine." In *The Philosophy of Psychiatry: A Companion*, edited by Jennifer Radden, 205–34, New York: Oxford University Press.

Gerstenblith, Theodore A., and Nicholas Kontos. 2015. "Somatic Symptom and Related Disorders." In *Massachusetts General Hospital Comprehensive Clinical Psychiatry*, edited by Theodore A. Stern, Maurizio Fava, Timothy E. Wilens, and Jerrold F. Rosenbaum. Philadelphia, PA: Mosby Elsevier.

Ghaemi, S. Nassir. 2010. *The Rise and Fall of the Biopsychosocial Model: Reconciling Art & Science in Psychiatry*. Baltimore, MD: The Johns Hopkins University Press.

Gillis, Jonathan. 2006. "The History of the Patient History." *Bulletin of the History of Medicine* 80: 490–512.

Gorka, S.M., B. Ali, and S.B. Daughters. 2012. "The Role of Distress Tolerance in the Relationship Between Depressive Symptoms and Problematic Alcohol Use." *Psychology and Addictive Behavior* 26: 621–26.

Greer, Joseph, and Richard Halgin. 2006. "Predictors of Physician-Patient Agreement on Symptom Etiology in Primary Care." *Psychosomatic Medicine* 68: 277–82.

Gropalis, Maria, Gaby Bleichhardt, Wolfgang Hiller, and Michael Witthöft. 2013. "Specificity and Modifiability of Cognitive Biases in Hypochondriasis." *Journal of Counseling and Clinical Psychology* 81: 558–65.

Hahn, Daniela, Katrin Reuter, and Martin Harter. 2006. "Screening for Affective and Anxiety Disorders in Medical Patients: Comparison of HADS, GHQ-12 and Brief-PHQ." *Psychosocial Medicine* 11: 1–9.

Hamilton, Max. 1960. "A Rating Scale for Depression." *Journal of Neurology, Neurosurgery and Psychiatry* 23: 56–62.

Haug, Tone Tangen, Arnstein Mykletun, and Alv A. Dahl. 2004. "The Association Between Anxiety, Depression, and Somatic Symptoms in a Large Population: The HUNT-II Study." *Psychosomatic Medicine* 66: 845–51.

Huibers, Marcus J.H., and Simon Wessely. 2006. "The Act of Diagnosis: Pros and Cons of Labelling Chronic Fatigue Syndrome." *Psychological Medicine* 36: 895–900.

Humber, James M., and Robert F. Almeder, editors. 1997. *What Is Disease?* Totowa, NJ: Humana Press.

Institute of Medicine of the National Academies. 2015. *Beyond Myalgic Encephalomyelitis/ Chronic Fatigue Syndrome: Redefining an Illness*. Washington, DC: National Academy of Sciences.

Kendall, R.E. 1968. "An Important Source of Bias Affecting Ratings Made by Psychiatrists." *Journal of Psychiatric Research* 6: 135–41.

Kessler, Ronald C., Patricia Berglund, Olga Demler, Robert Jin, Doreen Koretz, Kathleen R. Merikangas, A. John Rush, Ellen E. Walters, and Philip S. Wang. 2003. "The Epidemiology of Major Depressive Disorder: Results From the National Comorbidity Survey Replication." *Journal of the American Medical Association* 289: 3095–105.

Kessler, Ronald C., Wai Tat Chiu, Olga Demler, and Ellen E. Walters. 2005. "Prevalence, Severity, and Comorbidity of 12-Month DSM-IV Disorders in the National Comorbidity Survey Replication." *Journal of the American Medical Association* 62: 617–27.

Kirmayer, Laurence J., and N. Sartorius. 2007. "Cultural Models and Somatic Syndromes." *Psychosomatic Medicine* 69: 832–40.

Kirsch, Irving, Brett J. Deacon, Tania B. Huedo-Medina, Alan Scoboria, Thomas J. Moore, and Blair T. Johnaon. 2008. "Initial Severity and Antidepressant Benefits: A Meta-Analysis Submitted to the Food and Drug Administration." *PLoS Medicine* 5: e45.

Klerman, Gerald L. 1972. "Psychotropic Hedonism vs. Pharmacological Calvinism." *Hastings Center Report* 2: 1–3.

Klinkman, Michael S., James C. Coyne, Susan Gallo, and Thomas L. Schwenk. 1998. "False Positives, False Negatives, and the Validity of the Diagnosis of Major Depression in Primary Care." *Archives of Family Medicine* 7: 451–61.

Kontos, Nicholas. 2011. "Perspective: Biomedicine – Menace or Straw Man? Reexamining the Biopsychosocial Argument." *Academic Medicine* 86: 505–15.

Kontos, Nicholas, Oliver Freudenreich, and John Querques. 2014. "Outpatient Institutionalization – 100 Words." *British Journal of Psychiatry* 205: 339.

Kontos, Nicholas, Oliver Freudenreich, John Querques, and Edward Norris. 2003. "The Consultation Psychiatrist as Effective Physician." *General Hospital Psychiatry* 25: 20–23.

Kravitz, Richard L., Ronald M. Epstein, Mitchell D. Feldman, Carol E. Franz, Rahman Azari, Michael S. Wilkes, Ladson Hinton, and Peter Franks. 2005. "Influence of Patients' Requests for Direct-to-Consumer Advertised Antidepressants." *Journal of the American Medical Association* 293: 1995–2002.

Kroenke, Kurt. 2007. "Efficacy of Treatment for Somatoform Disorders: A Review of Randomized Controlled Trials." *Psychosomatic Medicine* 69: 881–88.

Kroenke, Kurt, Robert L. Spitzer, and Janet B.W. Williams. 2002. "The PHQ-15: Validity of a New Measure for Evaluating the Severity of Somatic Symptoms." *Psychosomatic Medicine* 64: 258–66.

Kroenke, Kurt, Robert L. Spitzer, Janet B.W. Williams, and Bernd Löwe. 2010. "The Patient Health Questionnaire Somatic, Anxiety, and Depressive Symptom Scales: A Systematic Review. *General Hospital Psychiatry* 32: 345–59.

Leyro, Teresa M., Michael J. Zvolensky, and Amit Bernstein. 2010. "Distress Tolerance and Psychopathological Symptoms and Disorders: A Review of the Empirical Literature Among Adults." *Psychological Bulletin* 136: 576–600.

Löwe, Bernd, Robert L. Spitzer, Janet B.W. Williams, Monika Mussell, Dieter Schellberg, and Kurt Kroenke. 2008. "Depression, Anxiety and Somatization in Primary Care: Syndrome Overlap and Functional Impairment." *General Hospital Psychiatry* 30: 191–99.

Luhrmann, T.M. 2001. *Of Two Minds: An Anthropologist Looks at American Psychiatry*. New York: Vintage Books.

Lurie, Scott N. 1991. "Psychological Issues in Treatment of the 'Chemical Imbalance.'" *American Journal of Psychotherapy* 3: 348–58.

Maj, Mario. 2013. "'Clinical Judgment' and the DSM-5 Diagnosis of Major Depression." *World Psychiatry* 12: 89–91.

Marcus, Ben. 2013. *The Flame Alphabet*. New York: Vintage Books.

Måseide, Per. 1991. "Possibly Abusive, Often Benign, and Always Necessary. On Power and Domination in Medical Practice." *Social Health and Illness* 13: 545–61.

Mayou, Richard, Laurence J. Kirmayer, Greg Simon, Kurt Kroenke, and Michael Sharpe. 2003. "Somatoform Disorders: Time for a New Approach in DSM-V." *American Journal of Psychiatry* 162: 847–55.

Mechanic, David. 1995. "Sociological Dimensions of Illness Behavior." *Social Science and Medicine*. 41: 1207–16.

Melartin, Tarja K., Heikki J. Rytsälä, Ulla S. Leskelä, Paula S. Lestelä-Mielonen, T. Petteri Sokero, and Erkki Isometsä. 2002. "Current Comorbidity of Psychiatric Disorders Among DSM-IV Major Depressive Disorder Patients in the Vantaa Depression Study." *Journal of Clinical Psychiatry* 63: 126–34.

Mojtabai, Ramin. 2007. "Americans' Attitudes Toward Mental Health Treatment Seeking: 1990–2003." *Psychiatric Services* 58: 642–51.

——2008. "Increase in Antidepressant Medication in the US Adult Population Between 1990 and 2003." *Psychotherapy and Psychosomatics* 77: 83–92.

——2009. "Americans' Attitudes Toward Psychiatric Medications: 1998–2006." *Psychiatric Services* 60: 1015–23.

——2011. "The Public Health Impact of Antidepressants: An Instrumental Variable Analysis." *Journal of Affective Disorders* 134: 188–97.

Mojtabai, Ramin, and Mark Olfson. 2010. "National Trends in Psychotropic Medication Polypharmacy in Office-Based Psychiatry." *Archives of General Psychiatry* 67: 26–36.

——2011. "Proportion of Antidepressants Prescribed Without a Psychiatric Diagnosis Is Growing." *Substance Abuse & Mental Health* 30: 1434–42.

Montgomery, Kathryn. 2006. *How Doctors Think: Clinical Judgment and the Practice of Medicine.* New York: Oxford University Press.

North, Carol S., and Sean H. Yutzy. 2010. *Goodwin & Guze's Psychiatric Diagnosis, 6th Edition.* New York: Oxford University Press.

Pagura, Jina, Laurence Y. Katz, Ramin Mojtabai, Benjamin G. Druss, Brian Cox, and Jitender Sareen. 2011. "Antidepressant Use in the Absence of Common Mental Disorders in the General Population." *Journal of Clinical Psychiatry* 72: 494–502.

Paley, Liza, Taiba Zornitzki, Joel Cohen, Joshua Friedman, Natalia Kozak, and Ami Schattner. 2011. "Utility of Clinical Examination in the Diagnosis of Emergency Department Patients Admitted to the Department of Medicine of an Academic Hospital." *Archives of Internal Medicine* 171: 1393–400.

Papakostas, George I., Patrick McGrath, Jonathan Stewart, Dana Charles, Ying Chen, David Mischoulon, Christina Dording, and Maurizio Fava. 2008. "Psychic and Somatic Anxiety Symptoms as Predictors of Response to Fluoxetine in Major Depressive Disorder." *Psychiatry Research* 161: 116–20.

Parker, Gordon, and Kay Parker. 2003. "Influence of Symptom Attribution on Reporting Depression and Recourse to Treatment." *Australian and New Zealand Journal of Psychiatry* 37: 469–74.

Parsons, Talcott. 1951. *The Social System.* USA: Free Press.

——1975. "The Sick Role and the Role of the Physician Reconsidered." *Milbank Memorial Fund Quarterly of Health and Society* 53: 257–78.

Paterniti, Debora A., Tonya L. Fancher, Camille S. Cipri, Stefan Timmermans, John Heritage, and Richard L. Kravitz. 2010. "Getting to 'No:" Strategies Primary Care Physicians Use to Deny Patient Requests." *Archieves of Internal Medicine* 170: 381–88.

Pender, Stephen. 2006. "Examples and Experience: On the Uncertainty of Medicine." *British Journal for the History of Science* 39: 1–28.

Pilowsky, Issy. 1990. "The Concept of Abnormal Illness Behavior." *Psychosomatics.* 31: 207–13.

Pressman, Jack D. 1998. *Last Resort: Psychosurgery and the Limits of Medicine.* New York: Cambridge University Press.

Riedl, Andrea, Julia Maass, Herbert Fliege, Andreas Stengel, Marco Schmidtmann, Burghard F. Klapp, and Hubert Mönnikes. 2009. "Subjective Theories of Illness and Clinical and Psychological Outcomes in Patients with Irritable Bowel Syndrome." 67: 449–55.

Ring, Adele, Christopher Dowrick, Gerry M. Humphris, John Davies, and Peter Salmon. 2005. "The Somatizing Effect of Clinical Consultation: What Patients and Doctors Say and Do Not Say When Patients Present Medically Unexplained Symptoms." *Social Science and Medicine* 61: 1505–15.

Rosenberg, Charles E. 1979. "The Therapeutic Revolution: Medicine, Meaning, and Social Change in Nineteenth-Century America." In *The Therapeutic Revolution: Essays in the Social History of American Medicine*, edited by Charles E. Rosenberg and Morris J. Vogel, 3–26, USA: University of Pennsylvania Press.

——2002. "The Tyranny of Diagnosis: Specific Entities and Individual Experience." *Milbank Quarterly* 80: 237–60.

——2003. "What is Disease? In Memory of Owsei Temkin." *Bulletin of the History of Medicine* 77: 491–505.

——2006. "Contested Boundaries: Psychiatry, Disease, and Diagnosis." *Perspectives in Biology and Medicine* 49: 404–24.

Rost, Kathyn M., Richard N. Akins, Frank W. Brown, and Richard G. Smith. 1992. "The Comorbidity of DSM-III-R Personality Disorders in Somatization Disorder." *General Hosptial Psychiatry* 14: 322–26.

Rüsch, Nicolas, Sara E. Evans-Lacko, Claire Henderson, Clare Flach, and Graham Thornicroft. 2011. "Knowledge and Attitudes as Predictors of Intentions to Seek Help for and Disclose a Mental Illness. *Psychiatric Services* 62: 675–78.

Russo, Joan, Wayne Katon, Mark Sullivan, Michael Clark, and Dedra Buchwald. 1994. "Severity of Somatization and its Relationship to Psychiatric Disorders and Personality." *Psychosomatics* 35: 546–56.

Salkovskis, P.M., K.A. Rimes, H.M.C. Warwick, and D.M. Clark. 2002. "The Health Anxiety Inventory: Development and Validation of Scales for the Measurement of Health Anxiety and Hypochondriasis." *Psychological Medicine* 32: 843–53.

Salmon, Peter, Sarah Peters, and Ian Stanley. 1999. "Patients' Perceptions of Medical Explanations for Somatisation Disorders: Qualitative Analysis." *British Medical Journal* 318: 372–76.

Serby, Michael. 2003. "Psychiatric Resident Conceptualizations of Mood and Affect Within the Mental Status Examination." *American Journal of Psychiatry* 160: 1527–29.

Sharpe, Michael. 2013. "Somatic Symptoms: Beyond 'Medically Unexplained.'" *British Journal of Psychiatry* 203: 320–21.

Sims, Andrew C.P. 2003. *Symptoms in the Mind: An Introduction to Descriptive Psychiatry*. London, UK: Saunders.

Smith, Robert C., Joseph C. Gardiner, Judith S. Lyles, Corina Sirbu, Francesca C. Dwamena, Annemarie Hodges, Claire Collins, Catherine Lein, William Given, Barbara Given, and John Goddeeris. 2005. "Exploration of DSM-IV Criteria in Primary Care Patients With Medically Unexplained Symptoms." *Psychosomatic Medicine* 67: 123–29.

Smith, Robert C., Catherine Lein, Clare Collins, Judith S. Lyles, Barbara Given, Francesca C. Dwamena, John Coffey, AnneMarie Hodges, Joseph C. Gardiner, John Goddeeris, and William Given. 2003. "Treating Patients With Medically Unexplained Symptoms in Primary Care." *Journal of General Internal Medicine* 18: 478–89.

Snelders, Stephen, Charles Kaplan, and Toine Pieters. 2006. "On Cannabis, Chloral Hydrate, and Career Cycles of Psychotropics Drugs in Medicine." *Bulletin of the History of Medicine* 80: 95–114.

Stone, Jon, Wojtek Wojcik, Daniel Durrance, Alan Carson, Steff Lewis, Lesley MacKenzie, Charles P. Warlow, and Michael Sharpe. 2002. "What Should We Say to Patients With Symptoms Unexplained by Disease? The 'Number Needed to Offend'." *British Medical Journal* 325: 21–28.

Sumathipala, Athula. 2007. "What is the Evidence for the Efficacy of Treatments for Somatoform Disorders? A Critical Review of Previous Intervention Studies." *Psychosomatic Medicine* 69. 889–900.

Taylor, Michael Alan, and Nutan Atre Vaidya. 2009. *Descriptive Psychopathology: The Signs and Symptoms of Mental Disorders*. New York: Cambridge University Press.

Temkin, Owsei. 1977. *The Double Face of Janus and Other Essays in the History of Medicine*. Baltimore, MD: The Johns Hopkins University Press.

Tomenson, Barbara, Cecilia Essau, Frank Jacobi, Karl Heinz Ladwig, Kari Ann Leiknes, Roselind Lieb, Gunther Meinischmidt, John McBeth, Judith Rosmalen, Winfried Rief, Athula Sumathipala, and Francis Creed. 2013. "Total Somatic Symptom Score as a Predictor of Health Outcome in Somatic Symptom Disorders." *British Journal of Psychiatry* 203: 373–80.

Weck, Florian, Julia M.B. Neng, Samantha Richtberg, and Ulrich Stangier. 2012. "The Restrictive Concept of Good Health in Patients With Hypochondriasis." *Journal of Anxiety Disorders* 26: 792–98.

WHO World Mental Health Survey Consortium. 2004. "Prevalence, Severity, and Unmet Need for Treatment of Mental Disorders in the World Health Organization World Mental Health Surveys." *Journal of the American Medical Association* 291: 2581–90.

Wiethoff, Katja, Michael Bauer, Thomas C. Baghai, Hans-Jürgen Moller, Robert Fisher, Dorothea Hollinde, Julia Kiermeir, Iris Hauth, Gerd Laux, Joachim Cordes, Peter Briefer, Klaus-Thomas Kronmüller, Joachim Zeiler, and Mazda Adli. 2010. "Prevalence and Treatment Outcome in Anxious Versus Nonanxious Depression: Results From the German Algorithm Project." *Journal of Clinical Psychiatry* 71: 1047–54.

Williams, Janet B. 1988. "A Structured Interview Guide for the Hamilton Depression Rating Scale." *Archives of General Psychiatry* 45: 742–47.

Williams, Simon J. 2005. "Parsons Revisited: From the Sick Role to … ?" *Health (London)* 9: 123–44.

Wilson, Mitchell. 1993. "DSM-III and the Transformation of American Psychiatry: A History." *American Journal of Psychiatry* 150: 399–410.

World Health Organization. *Preamble to the Constitution of the World Health Organization as Adopted by the International Health Conference*, New York, 19–22 June, 1946; signed on 22 July 1946 by the representatives of 61 States (Official Records of the World Health Organization, no. 2, p. 100) and entered into force on 7 April 1948.

Zanarini, Mary C., and Frances R. Frankenburg. 1994. "Emotional Hypochondriasis, Hyperbole, and the Borderline Patient." *Journal of Psychotherapy Practice and Research* 3: 25–36.

Zanarini, Mary C., Frances R. Frankenburg, and Garrett Fitzmaurice. 2013. "Defense Mechanisms Reported by Patients with Borderline Personality Disorder and Axis II Comparison Subjects Over 16 Years of Prospective Follow-Up: Description and Prediction of Recovery." *American Journal of Psychiatry* 170: 111–20.

1b

Commentary on Kontos: The Hiddenness of Psychological Symptom Amplification

Some Historical Observations

Justin Garson

Nicholas Kontos' contribution to this volume is provocative, for a number of reasons that I will develop below. As I understand him, he has three main goals. The first goal is to articulate the theoretical possibility and clinical reality of what he calls "psychological symptom amplification" (PSA). The second goal is to ask why PSA is so hidden from clinicians and psychiatric researchers. The third goal is to indicate the negative consequences, for patients and clinicians, of failing to recognize PSA.

What is PSA? As he puts it, psychological symptom amplification takes place when patients present symptoms to clinicians that they do not actually have, or, perhaps more commonly, they exaggerate symptoms they do have. Crudely put, PSA refers to the situation in which a patient thinks "there's something wrong," but, in fact, there's "nothing wrong" (or, alternately, the case in which there *is* something wrong, but it's different from, or not as bad as, what the patient thinks is wrong). There is no implication of intentionality here. A man who likes to keep a tidy kitchen says that he has a touch of OCD. A woman who is down about a recent job loss says she's depressed. People who get nervous before making presentations believe themselves to be afflicted with anxiety disorders. Someone with occasional mood fluctuations wonders if he's bipolar. Too often, clinicians are only happy to validate patients' erroneous interpretations of their problems. PSA is, as he puts it, the "psychological analogue of somatization."

In the following, I'm going to focus on the second problem that Kontos tackles: Why is PSA so unrecognizable? Why is it so hidden? Kontos provides a number of reasons why PSA has evaded the kind of clinical and research scrutiny that it deserves. In my view, the "hiddenness" of PSA has deep historical and institutional roots. My argument, in a nutshell, is this: A major transition that took place in American psychiatry in the 1970s was the transition from seeing the symptoms of mental disorders as (typically unconscious) *strategies* deployed by patients for coping with unpleasant situations, to seeing those symptoms as the outcome of inner *dysfunctions*, nothing more. But in order for the clinician to recognize PSA, he or she must, as Kontos notes, look at the patient's reports as the outcome of a kind of unconscious "strategy" for obtaining the benefits of the "sick role." To recognize PSA, then, the clinician must adopt a way of seeing that has been effectively abolished in American psychiatry. So to begin to recognize PSA where it occurs, we have to unearth the complex play of historical and institutional factors that tend to obscure it. I'll begin with Kontos' observations and then develop my historical points.

Kontos notes that there are a number of obstacles that prevent a clinician from recognizing that the patient's presented symptoms are exaggerated or nonexistent. There are additional obstacles that prevent the clinician from telling the patient the same. First, medical students in psychiatry are trained to assume that, if a patient presents with some complaint or another, then the patient must have a mental disorder. The clinician's job is merely to figure out what it is. As Kontos puts it, "medical school primes the pump of pathologizing bias." Students are not trained, first and foremost, to pose the following question: *Is* there, in fact, anything wrong? And is it possible that the symptoms are exaggerated or that the patient is misinterpreting them? Second, clinicians naturally want to help alleviate distress and suffering. If the clinician realizes that prescribing an antidepressant or anti-anxiety medication might alleviate the patient's distress, then that provides a strong incentive to do so, irrespective of whether the symptoms do, in fact, satisfy the criteria for a specific mental disorder.

Third, and most generally, one reason that PSA is hard to see is because of the very general process of "medicalization." Very roughly, "medicalization" takes place when a certain kind of problem goes from being what Thomas Szasz famously called a "problem in living" to a "medical problem." The process of medicalization has been, in some ways, very positive for society as a whole. Patients who struggle with depression, anxiety disorders, or other major mental disorders feel less stigmatized about consulting a clinician and getting the help that they need because they recognize that they have a bona fide medical issue. They don't have character defects or moral failings. "Medicalization" isn't a pejorative term. Yet for all the benefits that medicalization has brought, it also has its downside. It fosters PSA. People who don't actually have psychiatric problems turn up to clinicians in droves and believe themselves to be entitled to the same sorts of benefits that they see others enjoying. Being sick is not entirely without benefits! Kontos writes, "for [PSA] to have any staying power in an individual … there must be a perpetuating force available. What a person stands to gain from what otherwise appears to be bafflingly persistent suffering must be examined in any consideration of symptom amplification."

This claim – that PSA is hard to see because of the process of "medicalization" – is roughly correct, though it suffers form a certain degree of vagueness. This is perhaps due to the overuse of the term. Since the 1970s, clinical psychologists have lamented the degree to which professional psychiatrists in the United States have "medicalized" everyday problems. Historians routinely describe the complex transitions that took place in American psychiatry in the 1970s in terms of the imposition of the "medical model." We all recognize that the third edition of the DSM, the DSM-III of 1980, signaled a fundamental change in the way that psychiatry is practiced in the United States, and that the change had something to do with "medicalization." So what is this "medicalization," and what exactly took place in psychiatry in the 1970s that the term "medical model" is supposed to denote?

I'm going to suggest the following account of the transition that American psychiatry passed through in the 1970s. This is a transition that culminated with the publication of the DSM-III in 1980, and that makes PSA so hard to "see." I believe that what was most distinctive about this transition was that American psychiatrists went from seeing mental disorders as (generally unconscious) *strategies* to seeing disorders as *dysfunctions*. In other words, prior to the 1970s, many psychiatrists considered mental disorders to represent, at base, *various strategies that people deploy, unconsciously, to cope with unpleasant situations*. Mental disorders possessed a teleological dimension. They were "for" something. The characteristic symptoms of mental disorders represented the working out of various strategies to resolve, or deflect, or live with unpleasant situations. There was no implication that these "strategies" were consciously selected. Nor was there an implication that these "strategies" were successful. In fact, they were typically unconscious, harmful, and counterproductive. As the American psychoanalyst Harry Stack Sullivan (1962: 8) put it, the clinician's job reduced to the following: "We must understand what the patient is trying to do."

A few examples will suffice to demonstrate the point. Freud's own psychoanalytic theories need no introduction. For Freud, dreams, slips of the tongue, and neurotic symptoms all represented distorted fulfillments of repressed desires. Consider Freud's account, in 1917, of a young woman's protracted and compulsive bedtime routine, which involved arranging her pillows in a diamond-like shape (Freud 1966: 327–33). In Freud's view, her ritual was nothing more than a symbolic fulfillment of her wish to usurp her mother's place. The distortion, moreover, served the goal of preventing herself from becoming aware of the true nature of this desire. So, compulsions played various functions in her psychological economy. They represented the working out of a certain strategy. They were goal-driven and goal-directed.

The point here is not that Freud was right, or that we should bring back his form of psychoanalysis. The point is that Freud's work exemplified a type of reasoning that had a remarkable staying power throughout the first half of the twentieth century, namely, that symptoms of psychiatric problems represented a kind of strategy that the patient was adopting for dealing with something. A few more examples will suffice to illustrate that this concept of disorder-as-strategy was not merely a Freudian preoccupation.

The psychoanalysts who came after Freud also adopted this perspective, even those that differed significantly from Freud. Harry Stack Sullivan (whom I noted above) was largely responsible, in the 1920s and 1930s, for the attempt to carry Freudian insights from the clinic to the asylum, and to use psychoanalysis to illuminate, and treat, schizophrenia. Sullivan was well known for emphasizing the social dynamics of schizophrenia, that is, the extent to which schizophrenia was an interpersonal disease.

What is important for my purposes is that he viewed schizophrenia within a teleological framework. In his view, catatonic-type schizophrenia represented a regression to an earlier stage of psychological development. The function of this regression was to enable the patient to better incorporate distressing life experiences into his or her personal narrative (Sullivan 1962: 20). Again, the point here is not that Sullivan was right or that we should follow in his footsteps. The point is that he saw schizophrenia as a strategy, albeit a dangerous one, that people used to deal with specific problems. The patient was actively, though unintentionally, "conspiring" with his or her illness to "get a job done."

In the 1930s and afterwards, figures such as Wilhelm Reich (1972) and Anna Freud (1946) developed psychoanalytic theory substantially (before Reich's expulsion from the International Psychoanalytic Society) through the study of human character traits. A crucial idea here was that personality types, mannerisms, or even bodily postures could represent mechanisms for defending the ego against id impulses as well as for "interfacing" with other people. Reich referred to these mechanisms as "character armor" and summarized his view concisely: "[T]he neurotic character traits as a whole prove to be a compact *defense mechanism* against our therapeutic efforts, and when we trace the origin of this character 'armor' analytically, we see that it also has a definite economic function" (1972: 48). For Reich as well as Anna Freud, the elements of human character, even pathological ones, represented strategies for negotiating between the demands of the id, on the one hand, and the demands of the outside world, on the other. They were goal-directed and teleological.

In the 1950s, one of the most well-known theories of schizophrenia was the "double-bind" theory (Bateson et al. 1956). In this view, symptoms of schizophrenia such as delusions and disorganized thought represented mechanisms that people used for the purpose of resolving what the psychologist Gregory Bateson and his colleagues called a "double-bind" situation. In their view, as a child the patient was repeatedly confronted with a kind of "lose-lose" situation (typically imposed by the mother) in which any coherent response would be penalized, and which forced the patient to adopt more radical solutions, such as delusions and incoherent speech. Again, nobody wishes to return to the stigmatizing idea of the "schizophrenogenic" mother whose terrible nurturing practices drive her kids crazy. The point I am making is that, throughout the first half of the century, many psychiatrists took it for granted that symptoms of various mental disorders represented strategic moves in a complex puzzle that the patient was trying to solve.

Finally, the American Psychiatric Association (APA), in the first edition of the DSM, canonized this view that mental disorders of different stripes could be understood as coping mechanisms. They were seen as goal-driven and goal-directed. In that manual, the APA recognized three major types of non-organic mental disorders: psychotic, psychoneurotic, and personality disorders. Crucially, it depicted *each type* as representing a different sort of strategy for resolving inner psychological conflicts. The psychotic reactions are those in which "the personality, in its struggle for adjustment to internal and external stresses, utilizes severe affective disturbance, profound autism, and withdrawal from reality" (APA 1952: 12). Psychoneurotic reactions are defined in terms of the various mechanisms that the patient uses to combat anxiety, such as depression, phobias, and compulsions (1952: 12). The personality disorders take place when the patient "utilizes primarily a pattern of action or behavior in its adjustment struggle" (1952: 13).

Not everyone viewed mental disorders as strategies. For example, Emil Kraepelin, that pillar of the "medical model," believed that many mental disorders could be understood as diseases of the brain or nervous system or as hereditary conditions. The idea that they represented strategies for coping with psychological conflicts was almost absent from his viewpoint. Almost, but not entirely! Kraepelin himself recognized that certain symptoms might represent the working out of a strategy deployed by the patient. For example, in his discussion of acquired neurasthenia, he tells us that chronic invalidity can, in some cases, represent a strategy for perpetuating the sick role and acquiring its associated benefits. In the most extreme cases, he tells us, "the patients tend to become chronic invalids of a most distressing type ... They betake themselves to the seclusion of a charitable institution with its freedom from annoyances ... The increasing demand for sympathy leads to prevarications and to various assumed contortions, in order to assure the physicians or friends that they are in critical condition" (1912: 152–53).

All this changed in the 1970s, with the process that led to the publication of the DSM-III. The story has been told elsewhere; I will summarize it very briefly here (see Garson 2015, Chapter 8, and references therein). The APA was in the midst of several conflicts. Within the ranks of the APA itself, biologically and behaviourally oriented psychiatrists were in conflict with psychodynamically oriented psychiatrists (as well as with clinical psychologists associated with the American *Psychological* Association). The APA was also engaged in an ideological battle with the so-called "antipsychiatry" movement, which saw mental disorders as mere "problems in living," or as social deviance. As a strategy for responding to their critics, powerful individuals within the APA, notably Robert Spitzer and Donald Klein, worked tirelessly to promote a certain framework for thinking about mental disorders, namely, the perspective of disorder-as-dysfunction. This perspective was canonized in the DSM-III as part of a working definition of "mental disorder" itself (APA 1980: 6).

One of the consequences of the ready adoption of this viewpoint was that what I'm referring to as this teleological framework for thinking about psychiatric problems was effectively abolished. Psychiatric symptoms were simply the result of various sorts of "behavioral, psychological, or biological dysfunction[s]" (APA 1980: 6). Just as there's no sense in which cancer or diabetes represent the "working out of a strategy" on the part of the patient for accomplishing some unconscious goal, neither do mental disorders (which are, after all, merely physical disorders that manifest in a special way in the mind). This framework, for better or worse, persists to the present day. For example, recently, some psychiatric researchers have been advocating for a transition from the DSM system of classification to a new system of classification, the Research Domain Criteria (RDoC), promulgated by the National Institutes of Mental Health (NIMH). Advocates of RDoC, however, still insist, as loudly as ever, that mental disorders boil down to inner dysfunctions (Insel et al. 2010: 748).

What does this transition – from disorder-as-strategy to disorder-as-dysfunction – have to do with PSA? As Kontos points out, the ability to recognize the existence of psychological symptom amplification requires the ability to detect when the patient is enacting a certain strategy. Namely, it requires seeing the symptoms, or reported symptoms, as movements within a certain strategy for accomplishing a specific end. In a line that's reminiscent of Sullivan, Kontos tells us that "what a person stands to gain from what otherwise appears to be bafflingly persistent suffering must be examined in any consideration of symptom amplification." This is the point that Harry Stack Sullivan made: We must understand what the patient is trying to do. But this is precisely a way of seeing that has become a piece of heresy in professional American psychiatry, as represented by the APA and the NIMH. It requires seeing the patient as an active, goal-directed, goal-seeking agent, and potentially as an unwitting conspirator to the illness. And that's something that we rarely do anymore, for two reasons. The first reason is that we've learned to see symptoms as the expressions of inner dysfunctions, and nothing more. The second is that we're concerned, rightfully so, with the threat of stigma.

We've made extraordinary progress in destigmatizing mental disorder. Part of the process of destigmatizing mental disorder has involved changing the public perception of what it means to have a disorder. Specifically, as Kontos emphasizes, people who struggle with psychiatric problems are not malingerers. They're not making some kind of illegitimate bid for the benefits of the "sick role." They're not social parasites. This change in perception has led to huge benefits for society and for people with mental disorders, unquestionably. To suggest that a person reporting symptoms is engaging in a certain strategy for obtaining certain benefits raises the specter of stigma. It's a delicate matter. But there are other ways of avoiding or minimizing the threat of stigma than to simply ignore the possibility of PSA.

In light of the threat of stigma, I should emphasize here that nothing in the view of psychiatry that I've laid out, where mental disorders are seen as having a strategic or teleological dimension, should be an excuse for stigma. First, not all mental disorders have this feature. Some mental disorders probably should be described simply and solely as the result of some sort of inner dysfunction. Second, when we talk about strategies, there is no implication of conscious intentionality. The idea is not that these are consciously pursued. Third, people who exhibit PSA very often do have genuine psychiatric problems – just not the ones they believe themselves to have. Finally, people who exhibit PSA are often themselves victims of misinformation. Seeing PSA where it occurs requires promoting public education about the nature of psychiatric problems. It's not that people are trying to dupe the system by pretending to have something they don't have.

In short, I think Kontos should be applauded for facing up to a phenomenon that, owing to deep-rooted institutional and historical facts, often goes unnoticed. My goal here has merely been to complement his analysis by drawing out some very general historical observations about recent transitions in American psychiatry that contribute to making PSA so hard to see.

References

American Psychiatric Association. 1952. *Diagnostic and Statistical Manual of Mental Disorders.* Washington, DC: American Psychiatric Association.

——1980. *Diagnostic and Statistical Manual of Mental Disorders: DSM-III*. Washington, DC: American Psychiatric Association.

Bateson, G., Jackson, D. D., Haley, J., Weakland, J. 1956. "Toward a Theory of Schizophrenia." *Behavioral Science* 1: 251–64.

Freud, A. 1946. *The Ego and the Mechanisms of Defense*. New York: International Universities Press.

Freud, S. 1966. *Introductory Lectures on Psycho-Analysis*. New York: W. W. Norton.

Garson, J. 2015. *The Biological Mind: A Philosophical Introduction*. London: Routledge.

Insel, T. R., Cuthbert, B., Garvey, M., Heinssen, R., Pine, D. S., Quinn, K., Sanislow, C., Wang, P. 2010. "Research Domain Criteria (RDoC): Toward a New Classification Framework for Research on Mental Disorders." *American Journal of Psychiatry* 167: 748–51.

Kraepelin, E. 1912. *Clinical Psychiatry: A Textbook for Students and Physicians*. London: Macmillan and Co.

Reich, W. 1972. *Character Analysis*. New York: Farrar, Straus, and Giroux.

Sullivan, H. S. 1962. *Schizophrenia as a Human Process*. New York: W. W. Norton.

2a
How are Mental Illnesses Different?

Marc Lange

1. Introduction

How are mental illnesses (i.e., diseases of the mind) different? It depends … different from what? From

(i) … one another?
(ii) … mental health?
(iii) … unhealthful mental conditions that are not illnesses?
(iv) … somatic illnesses?

Let's consider each of these questions in turn.

Question (i) concerns the individuation of mental illnesses. Sometimes what had been considered a single disease is revealed to be in fact several diseases, as when Sydenham discovered that "the pox" includes smallpox and measles. On other occasions, what had been regarded as distinct diseases are discovered to be actually a single disease, as when Koch discovered that phthisis (involving the lungs), scrofula (involving the lymph glands of the neck), and Pott's disease (involving the spine) are all the same disease (tuberculosis). Like somatic medicine, psychiatry has been concerned with disease individuation. For example, *Schizophrenia Research* recently devoted its first "Current Controversies" issue to "whether schizophrenia is composed of multiple disorders with a common core clinical syndrome, or one disorder with variations in clinical presentation" (DeLisi and Nasrallah 1995: 133). Question (i) asks what makes one mental illness distinct from another. For instance, what facts are psychiatrists trying to ascertain when they are trying to find out whether all instances of schizophrenia involve the same disorder? The answer, presumably, is facts about etiology; different mental diseases are distinguished by having different etiologies. One of this paper's goals is to elaborate this answer.

If the individuation of mental illnesses is a fact that psychiatry aims to discover rather than a matter of convenience, then mental diseases are medical natural kinds:

> Psychiatric diagnosis enables a wealth of facts regarding a patient's history and current state to be communicated in just a word or two. But we ask more of diagnosis than efficient communication. We want it to be valid, by which we mean that we want it to correspond to what exists in nature – to describe a "real" disorder. … The trick is to find indirect indicators that a diagnostic definition maps closely on to the "real" underlying disorder.
>
> *(Robins and Barrett 1989: v)*

Diseases have long been treated as natural kinds in medical reasoning – for instance, in explanation and in confirmation. Just as two geological samples tend to share certain properties because they are samples of the same mineral, so two patients tend to share certain properties because they have the same disease. One patient's response to a given therapy is (ceteris paribus) evidence that another patient will have the same response because the two patients are believed to have the same disease.[1] Question (i), then, asks about what it is in virtue of which mental diseases constitute natural kinds.

Question (ii) concerns the distinction between health and illness. Is unwellness a departure from statistically normal functioning, or reduction of evolutionary fitness, or interference with human flourishing understood in irreducibly normative terms, or deviation from prevailing cultural ideals, or … ? I will not pursue this question, since question (i) leads us to focus on etiologies, and whether a mental condition is healthful or not makes no difference to how it is caused or to how biomedical scientists investigate its causes.[2]

Question (iii) recognizes that the diagnosis of a fractured rib might explain the patient's symptoms and be useful prognostically and therapeutically, for example, but is not a disease. Injuries, wounds, swelling, symptoms (e.g., fever), signs, syndromes, anatomical variants (flat feet), events (myocardial infarction), allergies, disabilities (blindness), impairments (myopia), congenital malformations (cleft palate), anatomical lesions (subdural haematoma), poisonings, burns, starvation, and drowning are not widely considered diseases. (See the survey conducted by Campbell *et al.* 1979.) Question (iii) asks how mental diseases differ from pathological mental conditions that are not diseases. From the fact that (e.g.) mauling by a lion is not a disease but *Streptococcus pneumoniae* infection is, Reznek (1987) and King (1981: 167) conclude that no natural distinction exists between diseases and other pathological categories. We shall be in a better position to judge after we have offered an answer to question (i).

Finally, question (iv) asks whether the answers to the preceding three questions regarding *mental* illness differ from the corresponding answers regarding *somatic* illness. I will examine whether mental and somatic illnesses differ in the grounds of their individuation, their status as medical natural kinds, and their distinction from pathological conditions that are not diseases. (Since I do not address question (ii), I will not examine whether mental and somatic diseases differ with regard to this question – e.g., whether values and culture play a greater role in determining the unhealthfulness of a mental than of a somatic condition. I will also not consider what, if anything, makes a disease mental rather than somatic or other respects in which mental diseases may differ from somatic ones, such as in constituting moral failings.)

To tip my hand: I will argue that diseases are distinct from some other pathological conditions (question (iii)) in being incapacities rather than states or processes. I will argue that a condition qualifies more fully as a distinct disease (question (i)) insofar as it is a natural kind of incapacity that figures in interesting function-analytic explanations of other, unhealthful incapacities. I will argue that these answers apply no differently to mental than to somatic diseases (question (iv)). In particular, I will argue that mental diseases do not differ from somatic diseases in being matters of degree, in being multifactorial, or in foreseeably becoming obsolete as medical natural kinds.

My concern throughout will be with the genuine mental illnesses (whatever they are), not with those categories that figure in current psychiatric classifications. Diagnostic categories in the *DSM* are adopted in the absence of complete information and reflect desiderata other than just the identification of natural kinds, such as facilitating medical communication, insurance, and agreement in diagnoses made by different clinicians. Furthermore, a disease's diagnostic criteria should not be confused with what the disease is or with a definition of the disease term. Kendell apparently intends to be putting the study of schizophrenia on a rigorous basis, rather than singling out schizophrenia as failing to constitute a natural kind, when he writes:

> We are just using words like schizophrenia as a convenient shorthand for what would otherwise be a statement running to two paragraphs about combinations of symptoms. There is no such thing as schizophrenia. It is just a shorthand symbol. *(Kendell 1989: 323)*

If Kendell were correct, then a patient's symptoms could not be explained by her schizophrenia (on pain of those symptoms explaining themselves) and the same (purported) disease could not have remained under discussion as the diagnostic criteria for schizophrenia were refined over successive editions of the *DSM*. This seems mistaken. Moreover, if the *DSM* gave definitions or essences rather than merely diagnostic criteria, then whether a patient has a given disease at a given moment would in some cases depend on whether her symptoms last longer than a certain period encompassing that moment. For example, if *DSM-IV-TR*'s requirement that a "manic episode" persist for at least one week were part of the definition of "manic episode" (rather than merely a diagnostic criterion), then a patient who died from a traffic accident before the requisite week had elapsed would not have had a manic episode despite being (until the accident) similar in all relevant respects to another patient who lived long enough to fall under the criterion.

2. What Individuates Diseases?

Plausibly, etiology unites various tokens of the same disease and differentiates them from tokens of other diseases. Infectious diseases are paradigmatic. Since different microbes cause measles and smallpox, they are different diseases. (Sydenham's evidence for this distinction was entirely clinical; what *makes* them distinct diseases is not the same as what counts as *evidence* of this distinction.) Phthisis and scrofula are both tuberculosis because the same microbe is responsible for both.

But how should we elaborate "same cause = same disease"? Different diseases can have the same cause. For example, exposure to cigarette smoke causes cancer and also causes emphysema; cases of cancer and emphysema that are both caused by exposure to cigarette smoke are not thereby united into a single disease. Cat bites can cause rabies, catch-scratch disease (infection by *Bartonella henselae*, a bacterium that is carried in cat saliva), and injuries that are not diseases. Distinguishing causes coarsely, we might even say that all genetic diseases have the same cause (namely, genes) and that a sedentary lifestyle is a cause of many diseases. Moreover, the same disease can have different causes. Some cases of rickets are caused by insufficient dietary vitamin D, others by an inborn error in renal synthesis of the hormone calcitriol, and still others by inherited disorders of renal phosphate transport. Some cases of emphysema are caused by exposure to cigarette smoke, whereas others are caused by alpha 1-antitrypsin deficiency (from a mutation on the long arm of chromosome 14); some are caused by both. Distinguishing causes finely, we might even say that some cases of emphysema are caused by cigarette smoking whereas others are caused by second-hand smoke.

In short, although there is presumably something correct in "same cause = same disease," it is not evident what should qualify as the "same cause." This difficulty is not always appreciated:

> The vexing problem [in psychiatric nosology] is that we do not, in general, know the etiology or pathophysiology necessary for the development of a psychiatric disorder. One could take a purely descriptive or syndromatological approach, eschew etiological speculations, and simply advance the belief that certain combinations of manifest symptoms, associated with particular demographic characteristics ... define a clinical picture worth attending to. The problem with this approach is that indefinitely many syndromes can be imaginatively stipulated. ... We need validity criteria to decide which syndromes are likely to reflect relatively uniform pathophysiologies and, hopefully, etiologies.
>
> *(Klein 1989: 203)*

Fair enough – but just as token combinations of symptoms can be grouped in various ways, not all of which correspond to real diseases, so likewise token etiologies can be grouped in various ways, not all of which correspond to real diseases. What counts as "uniform pathophysiologies"?

To understand how etiology individuates diseases, let's focus on a single somatic disease and ask: What is classical phenylketonuria (PKU)? In particular, let's consider what kind of thing we are trying to individuate. A disease – is it a process, a state, or an incapacity? If we understand the general ontological category to which diseases belong, then we may be better able to see what aspects of a disease's etiology are essential to it.

Consider first the view that "disease entities are complex processes not types of bodies" (Whitbeck 1977: 619; cf. Reznek 1987: 71–73; Wiggins and Schwartz 1994: 98). However, a disease can be present without any pathological process at all. Classical PKU is an autosomal recessive disease whose characteristic symptoms (notably impaired cognition, microcephaly, and motor dysfunction) and signs (phenylpyruvic acid in blood and urine, a distinctive "mousy" odor) result from elevated levels of L-phenylalanine and some of its metabolic derivatives in bodily fluids and tissues. Phenylketonurics who do not eat any phenylalanine (phe) lack elevated phe levels or any other PKU symptoms. Nowadays, infants are routinely screened at birth for PKU, and if they are found to have classical PKU, they are put on a phe-free diet for the remainder of their lives. As we will see, someone deficient in a certain enzyme necessary for phe metabolism has classical PKU – even if no pathological process has begun because she has not eaten any phe.

Accordingly, consider whether classical PKU is a particular natural kind of bodily state rather than process. Boorse (1977: 555; cf. 558, 562), for example, says that "a disease is a type of internal state which impairs health, i.e., reduces one or more functional abilities below typical efficiency." The disease is not the functional impairment that it explains, but rather the state responsible for the impairment. Different tokens belong to the same disease category by virtue of involving the same natural kind of state.

But some diseases are difficult to identify with particular bodily states. For example, an elevated level of phe (or its metabolic derivatives) in bodily fluids and tissues is not necessary for classical PKU, since, as we just saw, phenylketonurics who eat no phe avoid an elevated level. Moreover, an elevated phe level is not sufficient for classical PKU; there are other hyperphenylalanemias (HPAs) besides classical PKU. (They are termed "non-classical PKUs".) Classical PKU involves deficiency in the liver enzyme phenylalanine hydroxylase (pheOH), which catalyzes the first step in the catabolism of phe: its conversion to tyrosine. Another HPA involves deficiency in the other cofactor required by the same reaction: L-erythro-5,6,7,8-tetrahydrobiopterin (BH_4). Still other HPAs involve deficiencies in various enzymes that regenerate BH_4 from what it becomes as a result of helping to hydroxylate phe. Unlike classical PKU, symptoms of these other HPAs are not avoided by eliminating dietary phe, since BH_4 is also needed for tyrosine and tryptophan catabolism and to make various neurotransmitters.

Since having classical PKU is not having high phe levels, what other state might it be? Classical PKU cannot be the state of *synthesizing* too little pheOH, since some phenylketonurics produce plenty of pheOH, but the amino-acid sequence of their pheOH renders it unstable, so that at any moment, they have too little pheOH. Classical PKU cannot be the state of *having* too little pheOH, since some phenylketonurics have plenty of pheOH, but the amino-acid sequence of their pheOH renders it "inactive" (i.e., unable to catalyze the reaction at a sufficiently rapid rate).

Consider an amino-acid sequence for an active molecule of pheOH. Do you have classical PKU if and only if you lack pheOH with that particular amino-acid sequence? No: There are many amino-acid sequences that yield active pheOH. There is even greater diversity in the DNA base sequence coding for active pheOH.

The enzyme contains over 450 amino acids, and over 500 mutant alleles have been found so far, many of which are not pathological ("silent polymorphisms").[3]

Is classical PKU the state of having insufficient pheOH with this amino-acid sequence or that one or … (covering exactly the active forms of pheOH)? Although this state may be coextensive with classical PKU, it is not a natural kind of bodily state. It is motley. These forms of pheOH are distinguished from others merely by being all and only the active forms. A pheOH molecule's being active is not a state; it is a disposition.

We have thus arrived at the view that classical PKU is an incapacity. This incapacity may be present even when there is no opportunity to catalyze phe (and consequently there are no PKU symptoms) because of a phe-free diet. Classical PKU is not the incapacity to catabolize phe since all other HPAs also involve this incapacity. It is not the incapacity to hydroxylate phe since BH_4-deficiency also involves this incapacity. Rather, classical PKU is the incapacity to make enough active pheOH.[4]

How much is "enough"? There is no sharp distinction; there are milder and more severe cases of classical PKU.[5] What makes some amount of pheOH activity qualify as "enough"? (Why is a phenylketonuric on a phe-free diet still not making "enough" active pheOH?) A disease ascription takes place against a (generally tacit) understanding of the sorts of larger capacities that are part of good health. Just as there is a tacit understanding of what a "normal" diet is, roughly speaking, so there is a tacit understanding that the capacity to eat such a diet (without certain effects) is part of being in good health. This capacity is compromised by the incapacity to make enough active pheOH – and classical PKU's symptoms trace to this incapacity as a common cause.

Let's extend this proposal to other paradigmatic disease categories. The account of diseases as natural kinds of incapacities identifies an infectious disease with the host's incapacity to easily keep in check the given microbe's population within the host. ("Easily" admits of degrees and should not be understood to permit certain outside aids, such as medication – no matter how easily it can be taken.) For some kinds of microbes, the host ordinarily harbors a significant (though stable) population, but other factors (such as immunosuppression or a change in the population of other kinds of microbes within the host) can turn the population from colonizing to infectious. For other kinds of microbes, the host ordinarily loses the capacity to keep the population in check when even a small number of microbes of this kind enter the host; even a small population is out of control. In that case, the host already has one incapacity even before any such microbe has entered her body: the host is incapable of preventing the uncontrolled growth of the microbe's population *if a small number of these microbes enter her body*. But before any such microbes have entered, the host possesses this incapacity without possessing the disease. The host is afflicted with the disease only when she is incapable of controlling the microbe's current population in her body. Likewise, Typhoid Mary was "the bearer and distributer [sic] of the infecting agent of typhoid fever without developing the disease" (Reed *et al.* 1900: 202) because she was capable of easily keeping the typhoid microbe population in her body small enough. Someone else who is likewise asymptomatic and has a small typhoid microbe population in her body just as Mary does, but (unlike Mary) is incapable of easily keeping that population small, has (an early stage of) typhoid fever. She has the incapacity distinguishing that disease.

We thus have the start of an answer to question (i) regarding disease individuation: since a disease is an incapacity, diseases are distinguished by involving different incapacities, and a disease (the incapacity to X) is a natural kind insofar as X is not an arbitrary, gerrymandered category. For example, the incapacity to make enough active pheOH on Wednesdays is not a disease, and neither is the incapacity to make either enough active pheOH *or* enough active BH_4. There is no obvious reason why this answer cannot apply to mental illnesses as well as somatic ones (though I will consider some possible reasons in the next section). This proposal explains what was right about "same cause = same disease": the relevant "cause" is not an efficient cause, but rather the incapacity to X. That the same incapacity can have quite different efficient causes in different cases is no obstacle to its qualifying as a specific disease.

We also have the start of an answer to question (iii): since injuries, anatomical variant, burns, deformities, swelling, and anatomical lesions are states rather than incapacities, they are not diseases. However, as we saw earlier, not all incapacities are diseases: blindness, color blindness (Campbell *et al.* 1979), hemiplegia (paralysis of the arm and leg on the same side), and various other disabilities and impairments are definitely not diseases (though poliomyelitis, which can produce paralysis, definitely is). How can this be accounted for on the view that diseases are incapacities?

Cummins (1975) identifies an important variety of scientific explanation: explaining how a system has the capacity to X by decomposing that capacity into various subcapacities possessed by the system or its components. Calling this a "function-analytic explanation," Cummins says:

> The explanatory interest of [a function-analytic] account is roughly proportional to (i) the extent to which the analyzing capacities are less sophisticated than the analyzed capacities, (ii) the extent to which the analyzing capacities are different in type from the analyzed capacities, and (iii) the relative sophistication of the program appealed to, i.e., the relative complexity of the organization of component parts/processes which is attributed to the system.
>
> *(1975: 764)*

For example, an explanation of the heart's capacity to go "lub dub" in terms of its capacity to go "lub" and its capacity to go "dub" would lack any "interest" (i.e., not be a function-analytic explanation at all), whereas an explanation in terms of the atrial-ventricular node's capacity to conduct signals (and other similar capacities) would be more interesting (i.e., would possess greater explanatory power). (Though Cummins distinguishes them, I am not sure that (i), (ii), and (iii) are quite separate: Insofar as the components are simpler than the resultant, they must be different from the resultant and their organization must be sophisticated enough to produce a more complex resultant.)

I take a similar view of what makes an explanation supplied by an incapacity interesting. A disease is an incapacity that is explanatory. Insofar as the capacity to X can figure as a component in an interesting function-analytic explanation of the capacity to Y, the incapacity to X can figure in an interesting explanation of the incapacity to Y, and so tends to better qualify as a disease. Therefore, although Jones's incapacity to walk might be explained by Jones's incapacity to move his right leg, this explanation is far from interesting (and so paralysis of the right leg is not a disease) because the capacity to walk is not interestingly decomposed into the capacity to move the right leg and the capacity to move the left leg. (The incapacity produced by a broken leg is likewise not a disease.) In contrast, the incapacity to eat ordinary bread without various PKU symptoms is interestingly explained by the incapacity to synthesize enough active pheOH because the capacity to eat ordinary bread without various PKU symptoms is interestingly decomposed into the capacity to synthesize enough active pheOH and other such capacities.

In contrast (recalling an example I mentioned earlier that purportedly effaces the distinction between diseases and other pathological conditions), injury from an attacking lion is not a disease (since it is a state, not an incapacity), and the incapacity to repel easily an attacking lion is not a disease since the corresponding capacity does not figure in an interesting function-analytic explanation. Admittedly, Jones's capacity to repel easily an attacking lion might help to explain Jones's having been able to avoid serious injury during her recent safari. But this is not an interesting function-analytic explanation since the capacity to repel an attacking lion is not obviously much simpler than and different in kind from the capacity to avoid serious injury during a safari.

Blindness is an incapacity, and "Because Jones is blind" would in many contexts adequately answer why-questions such as "Why can't Jones drive?" Yet blindness is not a disease because the capacity to see is not a component in an interesting decomposition of (say) the capacity to drive. Recall point (iii) in Cummins's remark. Seeing does not occupy some subtle niche in a complex organizational scheme for driving; being able to see stands in no interesting relations to other capacities that together with it comprise an intricate network of interrelated capacities that amount to being able to drive. Rather, being able to see is simply a prerequisite for many of the capacities into which the capacity to drive might interestingly be decomposed. It is like being able to fit into a car. (I take a similar view of colorblindness,[6] shortsightedness, and suffocation.)

3. Does this Account Apply to Mental Illness?

I cannot consider all of the reasons why the foregoing account might appear not to apply to mental illnesses despite applying to somatic ones. But let's review and reject some of them.

One respect in which the individuation of mental disorders is sometimes believed to differ from the individuation of somatic ones is that a given mental disorder is more heterogeneous. The patients who meet the criteria for a given mental disorder in the *DSM* must have, for example, three symptoms from a list of fifteen, and so they tend to be less alike than patients with the same somatic illness (McNally 2011: 188–89). However, as I mentioned in section 1, the symptoms in the *DSM* are not supposed to be the essential, distinguishing feature of the given disease; they are merely diagnostic criteria. So patients may share a natural kind of incapacity despite differing symptomatically. Furthermore, as I also mentioned, a *DSM* category may well turn out not to be a genuinely distinct illness. Moreover, the heterogeneity within a given natural kind of somatic disease should not be underestimated. Classical PKU is one of many kinds of HPA, and there are also many amino-acid sequences that reduce the activity of pheOH and so cause classical PKU. The common cold involves infection with any of the rhinoviruses, and malaria can be caused by any of several species of *Plasmodium*. None of this heterogeneity prevents these categories from qualifying as natural kinds.[7]

It is often maintained that, unlike a somatic illness, a mental illness is not sharply distinguished from an extreme in normal variation, and so "the imposition of a diagnostic threshold … creat[es] a category where none exists in nature" (McNally 2011: 189). But of course, many somatic diseases are also matters of degree, with vague boundaries. Classical PKU is the incapacity to make enough active pheOH, where "enough" is not sharply defined. Medical communication may be facilitated by physicians' privileging some sharp threshold as diagnostic, but that convention does not purport to limn the natural kind. The DSM categories are not our best guesses of where the sharp thresholds between diseases lie, since our best guess may be that there is no sharp threshold. A vague boundary does not impugn a category's natural-kind status; as Sober (1980: 166) remarks, there is no specific moment at which a nitrogen atom and an approaching proton become an oxygen nucleus, yet chemical elements are paradigmatic natural kinds.

Some mental incapacities (such as being unable to quench anger) do not qualify as diseases because they do not supply interesting enough function-analytic explanations (just as the incapacity to move the right leg fails to supply an interesting function-analytic explanation of the inability to walk). But whether a function-analytic explanation is interesting is a matter of degree, and so the distinction between diseases and other medical conditions will not be sharp. Once again, there are intermediate cases among the somatic illnesses just as there are among the mental illnesses. Consider lead poisoning. On the one hand, having lead inside of your body is a state, and exposure to lead seems no more like a disease than does exposure to 600° temperatures. The capacity to withstand the heat of your current environment typically does not figure in any interesting function-analytic explanations, and the capacity to withstand the amount of lead in your current environment might well seem similar. However, the biochemical incapacities produced by lead poisoning are quite specific (since lead binds with enzymes that use zinc, iron, and calcium as cofactors, rendering them inactive) and the corresponding capacities figure in interesting function-analytic explanations. Nevertheless, part of what distinguishes lead poisoning, especially in the minds of those less familiar with these incapacities, is that it requires lead; if it was discovered that the same incapacities could also be produced by exposure to osmium, many of us would not say that a new cause of lead poisoning had been discovered. But we would if we had the biochemical incapacities primarily in mind. This result accords with the survey findings of Campbell *et al.* (1979): lead poisoning was regarded as a disease by almost 70 percent of general practitioners and nearly 90 percent of medical academics, but by only 30 percent each of non-medical academics and secondary-school students.

It may be suggested that a mental illness has a social and cultural context that a somatic illness does not have. Certain "transient mental illnesses" (Hacking 1998) seem to require a certain cultural context and so, it might be argued, are not natural kinds. However, I do not think that a cultural prerequisite is enough to keep a mental illness from qualifying as a natural kind. A disease, whether mental or somatic, may require certain causes, and those causes may be present only in certain circumstances, and human activity may be necessary to produce those circumstances. Silicosis, for instance, presumably did not afflict anyone before industrial techniques exposed workers to silica dust. Endstage renal disease did not exist until dialysis allowed patients without functioning kidneys to survive. That no one had endstage renal disease before dialysis was invented does not preclude its qualifying as a natural kind, just as a given chemical species (e.g., nylon) is a natural kind even though none existed before human beings discovered how to synthesize it.

Sometimes it is suggested that a mental illness, unlike a somatic one, cannot be individuated by its etiology because its symptoms have no single distinctive common cause:

> The main point ... is that current models of aetiology in psychopathology are essentially multifactorial, involving many kinds of causal pathway, with interactions between them. They include, in no particular order: genetic influences on traits, physical and interpersonal environmental impacts on early neural development, pre-, during and post-birth, subsequent adverse life events and chronic stressors, with effects through time evident in psychic life and the underlying neurochemistry, functional abnormalities of the brain, lesions to the brain, by disease processes or injury, styles of information processing evident in neuropsychological experimental paradigms, the operation of meanings drawn from the surrounding culture and subculture, and personal meanings deriving from individual learning histories and modes of interpretation.
>
> *(Bolton 2008: 73–74)*

> Our strongly held desires to find *the* explanation for individual psychiatric disorders are misplaced and counterproductive. Psychiatry has historically seen a few big explanations, most notably the discovery of the spirochete for general paresis. It is highly unlikely that spirochete-like big explanations remain to be discovered for major psychiatric disorders.
>
> *(Kendler 2005: 434)*

But being multifactorial and being brought about through feedback among several mechanisms are features of many somatic diseases, too – such as those where the infectious microbe is typically present and many different causes conspire to permit its population to get out of control. These causes can be of many kinds, including other illnesses, mental stressors, and environmental insults. Feedback occurs; a rise in the microbe's population causes the breakdown of other checks on its population growth, which enables its population to rise still further. Nonetheless, the disease can be understood as the incapacity to control the microbe's population.

Let's look at an example where a mental illness is thought to be impossible to individuate etiologically because it is multifactorial. Having asked "At what level of explanation should psychiatric disorders be etiologically defined?", Kendler reviews "the etiology of alcohol dependence (AD), a paradigmatically complex neuropsychiatric syndrome" (2012: 12). He identifies biological (e.g., genetic, metabolic), psychological (personality), social (childhood sexual abuse), cultural (beverage alcohol price), and other causes of AD. He concludes:

> Nature does not appear to have provided us one critical level of explanation for psychiatric illness that stands out from the background. … For [cystic fibrosis], explanatory power is highly concentrated in the level of DNA base-pair variation. For psychiatric disorders, explanatory power is dispersed and diffuse … [M]ost probably, the nature of psychiatric disorders themselves … does not yield up unambiguous choices for the best level at which to define psychiatric illness etiologically. … [Science] will not yield a single clear level of explanation on which to ground our nosology.
>
> *(Kendler 2012: 16–17)*

However, that a disease has many causes, at many levels, does not entail that the disease lacks a sharply defined essence. Causes of the disease must be distinguished from the incapacity that those causes cause; that the former are multifactorial and multi-level does not show that the latter is. Compare lead poisoning. An individual's lead poisoning might be explained socioculturally or in terms of her individual life-experiences or chemically. Nevertheless, lead exposure produces specific biochemical incapacities that are the common causes of the characteristic symptoms of lead poisoning. By the same token, a child's dental caries could be explained by the sociocultural influences leading to heavy sugar consumption among children, by the child's own particular behavior, or by the particular microorganisms (usually one or more varieties of *Streptococcus mutans*) responsible. In different contexts, different levels of explanation are appropriate (and so qualify as "*the* explanation"); nature fails to privilege one level. But that caries are properly considered in different contexts to be a public-health issue, an injury, or an infectious disease does not make the essential features of having dental caries "dispersed and diffuse."

What is AD, then? It is roughly the incapacity to maintain various homeostatic mechanisms in the absence of a certain level of alcohol consumption. All of the various risk factors for AD are risk factors for this incapacity. All of the various symptoms of AD are symptoms of this incapacity. Of course, the acquisition of this incapacity is grounded in a host of molecular changes, and different cases of AD may involve different changes (as I will mention again in the next section). One result of this incapacity is a tendency to consume enough alcohol to cause this incapacity to persist. But such molecular diversity and positive feedback do not entail that psychiatry should "shift from the quest for essences of psychiatric kinds among either biological and social facts about the disorders to a quest for the complex and multi-level causal mechanisms that produce, underlie and sustain psychiatric syndromes" (Kendler *et al.* 2011: 1146). We do not have to choose. Such causal mechanisms can be responsible for an incapacity that constitutes the essence of a psychiatric kind.

However, in the foreseeable future, new molecular tools will allow psychiatry to offer explanations and predictions without appealing to diseases as diagnoses at all. This *will* represent a "shift" in psychiatry – and in medicine generally – in which diseases are no longer called upon to serve as natural kinds. In facing obsolescence, mental illnesses are like diagnostic categories in other branches of medicine. This shift has already begun. Let's examine it more closely.

4. The End of Diseases

Diseases have long been central to medicine because the goals of medicine[8] have heretofore been best advanced by taking diseases to be natural kinds. For example, the best strategy for predicting what would happen if Jones were subjected to a given therapy has been to examine the past outcomes of so treating other patients similar to Jones, and an important respect of similarity has been their having the same disease as Jones. However, this role and others characteristic of medical natural kinds will in coming years be played less and less by diseases. Whereas medicine over the past few centuries has progressed partly by identifying and differentiating additional disease categories, genomic and proteomic medicine (and molecular medicine more generally) will instead lead to the end of diseases as useful medical categories. Let's see why this is so.

As we have seen, a disease is a natural kind of incapacity. But even when the incapacity is well defined at the molecular level, there will be heterogeneity in its molecular basis; it will be multiply realized. Medical explanations of a token illness's manifestations, predictions of its course, and choices among possible therapeutic strategies will increasingly be based not on the disease category to which the token belongs, but rather on the token's specific molecular subtype. A subtype will not be a natural kind of incapacity. Therefore, it will not be a distinct disease. Furthermore, many subtypes will contain only a single token illness. Predictions in medicine will be made not by drawing upon our past experience with other cases of the same subtype, but by inferences from chemical laws and the patient's biochemical state – that is, by modeling a given patient's (or organ's or cell's) "molecular signature," which includes its gene and protein activity patterns and the chemically specific environmental influences to which it is subject. Medical explanations will likewise appeal to chemical laws and initial conditions rather than to generalizations (even probabilistic or ceteris-paribus ones) covering all patients with a given disease. Clinical proteomics and pharmacogenomics combined with computationally sophisticated simulation techniques have initiated a revolution in patient care often called "individual medicine" (a.k.a. "personalized molecular medicine," "patient-tailored therapeutics," and "molecular diagnostics"): "In the next decade, patients are likely to have their individual genomes and transcriptomes stored as part of their medical records. Fine-tuning treatment on a case-by-case basis will become the norm" (Williams 2006: 53; cf. Liotta *et al.* 2001). Diseases will remain natural kinds, capable of grounding explanations and predictions, but medicine will no longer call upon them to serve as natural kinds.

Consider classical PKU. The Online Mendelian Inheritance in Man (OMIM) database currently lists over 65 alleles in the pheOH gene (on chromosome 12) that produce classical PKU. Each of these alleles (whether involving a missense or nonsense mutation, a single base-pair frame shift, or a larger deletion or insertion) creates the same incapacity: to make enough active pheOH. This incapacity can be created in different ways (e.g., by making pheOH that fails to bind phe, or making no pheOH at all, or making unstable pheOH), possibly leading to subtly different clinical manifestations. However, the different PKU allelic variants cannot all be distinguished as causing different incapacities – that is, separate diseases. The opportunity for biochemical and clinical heterogeneity among phenylketonurics is increased further by the fact that phenylketonurics are usually heterozygotes and may also differ in their capacities to exploit other metabolic pathways for catabolizing phe.

None of these facts undermines classical PKU's status as a natural kind of incapacity figuring in interesting function-analytic explanations of other incapacities. But these facts entail that as medicine increasingly tailors its explanations, predictions, and therapies to each patient's specific PKU allelic variant – or, rather, to each patient's entire genome – classical PKU can no longer serve as a medical natural kind. Some genomes will require phe-free diets, whereas others will tolerate somewhat greater dietary phe levels. Any therapy that aims to "fix" a PKU allele, to affect the regulation of its expression, to alter its product so as to augment that protein's activity, or to exploit other genes to compensate for pheOH deficiency will have to be targeted to a particular genome.

Analogous considerations apply to infectious diseases. Immunizations and therapies are now targeted not to particular diseases, but to particular microbial strains and serotypes. For instance, intensive research is currently directed at the strains of avian flu virus similar to the strain responsible for the 1918 pandemic. Although bacterial pneumonia, for example, could be subdivided into hundreds of different diseases, each involving a different strain of *Streptococcus pneumoniae*, medicine will not be using these as natural kinds. Rather, physicians will "soon" design individualized therapies from "first principles": by sequencing the genome of the strain infecting the patient, ascertaining the patent's immunological state (reflecting her genotype, current gene-expression profile, and personal history), and identifying the other genetic and environmental components of her unique individual susceptibility to infectious diseases and to adverse reactions from medication – "all this in 10 minutes using easy, inexpensive, office-based tests" (Hall 2003: 12).[9] Accordingly, there will be no need to try to predict a given possible therapy's effectiveness for a given patient by induction from that therapy's past results for similar serotypes or strains. It will not be medically relevant to ask (e.g.) whether the flu now common in Romania is a different disease from the flu now common in Southeast Asia, since scientists will not be predicting a given treatment's effectiveness for one by inferring from its effectiveness for the other – that is, by projecting across a natural kind. Pharmaceutical companies will attempt to develop novel vaccines or therapies only given precise genomic information regarding the intended infectious agent and infected host. Thus, rather than molecular medicine supplying merely "a new taxonomy of disease" by refining and narrowing disease categories (as predicted by Bell 2003: 215), I contend that molecular medicine is well on its way to rendering diseases obsolete as medical natural kinds.

Mental illnesses no less than somatic ones are likely to become obsolete as medical natural kinds. Computer-aided computation will allow simulation of a patient's brain at the level of neural networks or even at the molecular level so that features of a patient's brain in all of its individuality can be used to explain and to predict symptoms, course, and the effectiveness of and adverse reactions from various possible therapies. The bioinformatic computational algorithms in such *in silico* models will allow personalized therapies to be crafted (Kobeissy *et al.* 2013). For instance, individuals with AD differ in the neuroadaptive changes that have taken place in response to their chronic exposure to alcohol. These differences reflect differences in genetic and epigenetic factors and environmental experience; for instance, there are polymorphisms in the genes encoding for proteins involved in intoxication. Knowledge of these differences holds great promise in allowing individualized therapies to be developed (Lovinger and Crabbe 2005). Likewise, studies (Kirchheiner *et al.* 2001; Evers 2009) have recommended adjustments of the doses of antidepressants and antipsychotics based on the genotypes of certain cytochrome P450 enzymes involved in drug metabolism; these enzymes show considerable genetic polymorphism.

Although people will still be afflicted with diseases, and disease categories will remain natural kinds, diseases will be called upon less and less to serve as natural kinds in medical reasoning. In this respect, as in the others we have seen, mental illnesses are no different from somatic ones.

Notes

1 The ceteris paribus proviso is necessary because other information about differences between the patients can eliminate this confirmatory relevance – though therapeutic trials on individuals afflicted with a disease serve as evidence regarding how individuals even of another species having the same disease would respond.

2 Of course, the funding that such a study receives may depend on whether or not the condition is healthful.

3 The Phenylalanine Hydroxylase Locus Knowledgebase (www.pahdb.mcgill.ca) lists the known mutant alleles.

4 Of course, a disease can be discovered long before the precise incapacity individuating it is identified. By an "incapacity," I mean nothing more than the lack of a certain capacity, and a capacity is simply a disposition (i.e., a power). A fragile vase has the capacity to break and incapacity to speak, for example.

5 Indeed, there is also no sharp distinction between "active" and "inactive" pheOH, since there is a smooth continuum of rates at which various amino-acid sequences of pheOH catalyze hydroxylation. Classical PKU might better be described as the incapacity to make pheOH with enough activity. Both "incapacity" and "activity" refer to dispositions.

6 However, for some specific biochemical capacity that figures in a function-analytic explanation of the capacity to distinguish red from green, the corresponding incapacity would qualify as a disease. Accordingly, when red-green colorblindness is described as a hereditary, sex-linked trait, it is often characterized as a disease (e.g., by Bateson 1909).

7 A certain incapacity's homogeneity – and so its standing as a natural kind – can be a matter of degree. The rhinoviruses may be sufficiently alike to form a natural grouping – and so

the common cold may be a natural kind – even though there is (currently believed to be) no genus or other taxonomic category containing all and only the rhinoviruses and so the common cold is not as natural as could be. In holding that a disease may have an intermediate degree of "validity" (so that neither lumping it with another nor splitting it apart is entirely accurate), I am disagreeing with Jablensky (2012:89).

8 These goals include promoting a patient's health, relieving her suffering, predicting her future health, and preventing sickness.

9 There may also be important non-genomic influences on a therapy's effects, including nutritional status, other drugs being administered, and gut microbiota.

References

Bateson, William. 1909. *Mendel's Principles of Heredity*, 2nd ed. Cambridge: Cambridge University Press.

Bell, John I. 2003. "The Double Helix in Clinical Practice," *Nature* 421: 414–16.

Bolton, Derek. 2008. *What is a Mental Disorder?* Oxford: Oxford University Press.

Boorse, Christopher. 1977. "Health as a Theoretical Concept," *Philosophy of Science* 44: 542–73.

Campbell, E.J.M., J.G. Scadding, and R.S. Roberts. 1979. "The Concept of Disease," *British Medical Journal* 2: 757–62.

Cummins, Robert. 1975. "Functional Analysis," *Journal of Philosophy* 72: 741–65.

DeLisi, Lynn, and Henry Nasrallah. 1995. "Is Schizophrenia a Heterogeneous Disorder?" *Schizophrenia Research* 17: 133.

Evers, Kathinka. 2009. "Personalized Medicine in Psychiatry: Ethical Challenges and Opportunities," *Dialogues in Clinical Neuroscience* 11: 427–34.

Hacking, Ian. 1998. *Mad Travelers*. Cambridge: Harvard University Press.

Hall, Judith. 2003. "Individualized Medicine: What the Genetic Revolution Will Bring to Health Care in the 21st Century," *Canadian Family Physician* 49: 12–13.

Jablensky, Assen. 2012. "The Nosological Entity in Psychiatry: A Historical Illusion or a Moving Target?" in Kenneth Kendler and Josef Parnas (eds.), *Philosophical Issues in Psychiatry II: Nosology*, Oxford: Oxford University Press.

Kendell, R.E. 1989. "Clinical Validity," in Lee N. Robins and James E. Barrett (eds.), *The Validity of Psychiatric Diagnosis*, New York: Raven Press, pp. 305–21.

Kendler, Kenneth. 2005. "Toward a Philosophical Structure for Psychiatry," *American Journal of Psychiatry* 162: 433–40.

——2012. "Levels of Explanation in Psychiatric and Substance Abuse Disorders: Implications for the Development of an Etiologically Based Nosology," *Molecular Psychiatry* 17: 11–21.

Kendler, K.S., P. Zachar, and C. Craver. 2011. "What Kinds of Things are Psychiatric Disorders?" *Psychological Medicine* 41: 1143–50.

King, Lester. 1984. *Medical Thinking*, Princeton: Princeton University Press.

Kirchheiner, J., K. Brosen, M.L. Dahl, L.F. Gram, S. Kasper, I. Roots, F. Sjoqvist, E. Spina, and J. Brockmoller. 2001. "CYP2D6 and CYP2C19 Genotype-Based Dose Recommendations for Antidepressants: A First Step Towards Subpopulation-Specific Dosages," *Acta Psychiatrica Scandinavica* 104: 173–92.

Klein, Donald F. 1989. "The Pharmacological Validation of Psychiatric Diagnosis," in Lee N. Robins and James E. Barrett (eds.), *The Validity of Psychiatric Diagnosis*, New York: Raven Press, pp. 203–14.

Kobeissy, Firas, Ali Alawieh, Stafania Mondello, Rose-Mary Boustany, and Mark Gold. 2013. "Biomarkers in Psychiatry: How Close Are We?" *Frontiers in Molecular Psychiatry* 3: 114.

Liotta, Lance, Elise Kohn, and Emanuel Petricoin 2001. "Clinical Proteomics: Personalized Molecular Medicine," *Journal of the American Medical Association* 286: 2211–14.

Lovinger, David, and John Crabbe. 2005. "Laboratory Models of Alcoholism: Treatment Target Identification and Insight into Mechanisms," *Nature Neuroscience* 8: 1471–80.

McNally, Richard. 2011. *What is Mental Illness?* Cambridge: Harvard University Press.

Reed, Walter, Victor Vaughan, and Edward Shakespeare 1900, *Abstract of Report on the Origin and Spread of Typhoid Fever in U.S. Military Camps During the Spanish War of 1898*, Washington, DC: Government Printing Office.

Reznek, Lawrie. 1987. *The Nature of Disease*. London: Routledge.

Robins, Lee N., and James E. Barrett. 1989. "Preface," in Robins and Barrett (eds.), *The Validity of Psychiatric Diagnosis*, New York: Raven Press, pp. v–vi.

Sober, Elliott. 1980. "Evolution, Population Thinking, and Essentialism," *Philosophy of Science* 47: 350–83, reprinted in Sober (ed.), *Conceptual Issues in Evolutionary Biology*, 2nd ed., Cambridge, MA: Bradford, 1994, pp. 161–89.

Whitbeck, Caroline. 1977. "Causation in Medicine: The Disease Entity Model," *Philosophy of Science* 44: 619–37.

Wiggins, Osborn P., and Michael A. Schwartz. 1994. "The Limits of Psychiatric Knowledge and the Problem of Classification," in John Z. Sadler, Osborne P. Wiggins, and Michael A. Schwartz (eds.), *Philosophical Perspectives on Psychiatric Diagnostic Classification*, Baltimore: Johns Hopkins University Press, pp. 89–103.

Williams, Robert. 2006. "Animal Models in Biomedical Research," in Marschall Runge and Cam Patterson (eds.), *Principles of Molecular Medicine*, 2nd ed., Totowa, NJ: Humana, pp. 53–56.

2b

Commentary on Lange: How are Mental Incapacities Different?

Abraham M. Nussbaum

If we grant that diseases are natural kinds of incapacities, a question remains: Are mental diseases different kinds of incapacities than the incapacities characteristic of other kinds of disease?

I approach this question as a physician whose last philosophy class, a course in the philosophy of science during the spring of my freshman year, included a reading from Professor Lange on the syllabus. So being asked to respond to his essay brings up the old anxieties of the college freshman. *Will I misunderstand more than I understand? What can I possibly offer in reply? Will I fall asleep in the library again and miss dinner at the cafeteria?* I fear the historical answers—likely, little, and yes—will recur.

Yet as a practicing physician, I engage the questions of that philosophy course daily: *What does it mean to see, to measure, to test?* These questions return to me when I am sitting with a person with a mental disease such as, to use Lange's example, an alcohol use disorder. When I do, I find it impossible to neglect the ways in which it feels both like and unlike sitting with a person with a medical disease such as, to use Lange's other example, phenylketonuria (PKU). In both instances, I am aware of how the disease incapacitates the patient, but I experience the patient with alcohol use disorder differently from the way I experience the patient with PKU.

In this essay, I draw upon what I have learned in clinical practice to reflect upon Lange's argument. In exploring his account of PKU and alcohol use disorder, I propose that if mental diseases are natural kinds of incapacities, then they are different than other diseases because they affect a person's agency—her capacity to act in the world.

A great gift of following Professor Lange is that he has already shown many of the ways in which mental diseases are like other diseases. As a psychiatrist, I usually have to make this argument myself, as many people believe mental diseases are less "real" than somatic diseases. Yet, as Lange shows, mental diseases share many characteristics with "real" diseases. Mental diseases, like somatic diseases, are influenced by social and cultural factors. Our understanding of mental diseases, like somatic diseases, changes over time: Multiple diseases turn out to be manifestations of one disease, and one disease turns out to be caused by several distinct diseases. Psychiatrists, like other physicians, distinguish pathological conditions that are not themselves diseases from pathological conditions that occur as part of a disease; a person may be intoxicated on alcohol without experiencing alcohol use disorder. Psychiatrists, like other physicians, seek to distinguish disease from health. Psychiatrists, like other physicians, seek the etiology of the diseases they diagnose and treat.

Further, just as a psychiatrist's diagnostic manual may be superseded, so may the diagnostic manuals of other physicians. Lange considers diseases as natural kinds—their etiology distinguishing them as a set that truly belongs together—rather than as represented by their contemporary diagnostic criterion, which he characterizes as a pragmatic collection of signs, symptoms, and assumptions.[1] So one can agree or disagree with various aspects of contemporary diagnostic systems and still conclude, as Lange does, that mental diseases are like somatic diseases. Lange is interested in the natural incapacities that constitute a mental disorder rather than in the diagnostic criteria that may (or may not) correspond well to these natural incapacities. With this clarification, we can attend to the two diseases Lange examines in detail: PKU and alcohol use disorder.

First, phenylketonuria. PKU is an autosomal recessive condition in which a patient inherits an inability to produce necessary amounts of the liver enzyme phenylamine hydroxylase. Phenylamine hydroxylase is required to metabolize the amino acid phenylalanine—which is contained in high-protein foods such as dairy, eggs, legumes, meat, and nuts—into tyrosine. Without sufficient amounts of phenylamine hydroxylase, a patient with PKU experiences an accumulation of phenylalanine and a deficiency of tyrosine, which results in clinical signs and symptoms including growth restriction, elevated serum levels of phenylalanine, intellectual disability, osteopenia, visual abnormalities, and behavior problems. Lange argues that PKU cannot be defined as a pathological *process* because if a person with PKU scrupulously avoids phenylalanine-containing foods, she will not experience an accumulation of phenylalanine and a deficiency of tyrosine, so she will not develop the clinical signs and symptoms associated with PKU. Even without these clinical stigmata, though, a person still has PKU. Similarly, he observes that PKU cannot be defined as a *state* of having elevated levels of phenylalanine in bodily fluids and tissues because a person could have elevated levels of phenylalanine because of an alternate error in phenylamine synthesis. Finally, PKU cannot be defined as the *functional* impairments associated with it because, again, if a person does not eat phenylalanine-containing foods, she never develops the functional impairments. Accordingly, Lange concludes PKU is the *incapacity* to produce necessary amounts of the liver enzyme phenylamine hydroxylase. He observes that a person could have greater or smaller amounts of effective phenylamine hydroxylase, so she could be more or less incapacitated, and she could have a more or less severe case of PKU.

Lange then argues that not all incapacities are diseases. For incapacity to constitute a disease, Lange says, it must be explanatory on a functionally interesting level. To be this kind of explanation, Lange says, it must be capable of being decomposed into functionally interesting capacities that are interrelated such that all such capacities are necessary to complete an activity. So a person with PKU lacks the capacity to eat ordinary bread because ordinary bread contains phenylalanine, and when a person with PKU eats ordinary bread she will be unable to synthesize the phenylalanine she eats into tyrosine. In contrast, while blindness is surely an incapacity, Lange says it is not a disease. To be blind does not explain, on a functionally interesting level, why a blind person cannot, say, drive an automobile. Being able to see is not a functionally interesting component of driving, but a prerequisite for the interrelated capacities that together constitute driving. While Lange's account of why a disease like PKU is best considered an incapacity rather than a state, pathological process, or functional impairment is illuminating, I am less compelled by his argument about the limits of incapacities. It seems to me that this portion of his argument—not all incapacities are diseases—requires further elucidation, especially about what does and does not constitute a functionally interesting explanation.

Regardless, the first portion of his argument—diseases are incapacities—allows him to show many similarities between mental and somatic diseases. Just as mental diseases can be more or less severe, a somatic disease like PKU is an incapacity of degrees because people with PKU have differing amounts of effective phenylamine hydroxylase. Like many mental diseases, PKU may have vague boundaries and still be a disease. Lange observes that somatic diseases, like some mental diseases, can be more or less prevalent based upon changes in human activities; silicosis did not exist until people were exposed to silica dust, and end-stage renal disease did not exist until dialysis was available.[2] Lange also writes that somatic diseases, like mental diseases, may have multiple causes and yet also be a natural kind of incapacity.

This argument brings Lange to alcohol use disorder. Lange observes that an alcohol use disorder is considered a paradigmatic example of how mental diseases have too many causes—biologic, psychological, social, cultural, et cetera—to be defined on the basis of etiology. Yet Lange insists that a disease may have multiple causes and still be a disease if its multiple causes lead to an essential incapacity. Lange identifies the disease of alcohol use disorder as "the incapacity to maintain various homeostatic mechanisms in the absence of a certain level of alcohol consumption." In his account, the risk factors for an alcohol use disorder are risk factors for this incapacity, and the symptoms of an alcohol use disorder are symptoms of this incapacity. Lange also obliquely observes that alcohol use disorder, unlike PKU, is an acquired incapacity.

In Lange's reference to the acquisition of the incapacity of alcohol use disorder, I find a hint of the difference between alcohol use disorder and PKU. I am not claiming that only inborn diseases constitute medically natural kinds, but that his comment suggests a difference in the incapacities of mental diseases. In brief, I can readily imagine a person with PKU whose agency is not impaired by her disease, but I cannot imagine a person with alcohol use disorder whose agency is not impaired by her disease.

Locating the incapacities characteristic of a mental disease in a person's agency is dangerous because the stigmatization of persons with mental illness is pernicious and pervasive. An advantage of Lange's argument is that it implicitly reduces stigmatization, because if mental diseases are, like somatic diseases, natural kinds of incapacities, then a person with a mental disease is like a person with a somatic disease. In contrast, speaking of incapacities in a person's agency may suggest a person with a mental disease is the subject of her disease rather than an agent in her own life. I receive the criticisms of people like Thomas Szasz, who believes the diagnosis of a mental disease necessarily stigmatizes a person, as a vital warning (Bortolotti 2013).

In many medical settings, patients are relieved to receive a diagnosis, to know *why* they are ill. In my experience, this is less common in psychiatry. Many patients prefer to believe they have a medical disease or to deny the presence of any disease at all. A patient often avoids the dissonance between whom she perceives herself to be and whom she perceives herself as becoming if the psychiatrist has rightly diagnosed her problems. This avoidance points both to culturally constructed ways in which we respond differently to persons with mental disease and to something different about mental diseases themselves.

To speak of agency is to engage the debate about whether or not a person with mental illness is necessarily irrational—a characterization advanced by many critics of contemporary psychiatry. In her philosophical consideration of this question, Lisa Bortolotti observes that in much of the literature critical of psychiatry, the essential incapacity of a mental disease is a deviation from a norm of rationality. In this literature, the people whom psychiatry labels as mentally ill are people who are differently rational than other people, not people experiencing a disease. I agree with Bortolotti's counterarguments: Not all instances of irrationality indicate a mental disease, a person may have a mental disease without consistently behaving irrationally, and conceiving of mental disease as statistical deviations from norms of rationality does not account for what contemporary neuroscience teaches us about the interrelationship of the mind and the body. Indeed, contemporary neuroscience correlates mental diseases with specific deficits in neural circuits, structures, and functions, so Bortolotti concludes irrationality is neither a necessary nor sufficient definition of the essence of a mental disease (Bortolotti 2013).

A more qualified version of this account identifies impairments in decisional capacity as characteristic of mental diseases. So the philosopher Lubomira Radoilska observes a person with major depressive disorder has an impaired ability to engage in intentional actions, even actions she typically enjoys. Radoilska says the "distinctive paradox" of depression "is that the desirable is not desired and the choiceworthy does not get chosen" (Radoilska 2013: 1158). She observes that a person who is depressed "takes inappropriate responsibility for her misfortune" (1165). Radoilska concludes that a person experiencing depression is, to the extent she chooses against the activities and relationships that constitute her identity, being coerced by her disease.

I am not arguing that persons with mental illnesses are necessarily irrational, necessarily lack autonomy, or necessarily lack responsibility for their actions. I am arguing that persons with mental diseases have an impaired ability to actuate their desires. My aim is not to stigmatize, but to acknowledge, first, that a person with a mental disease possesses agency and, second, that her mental disease affects her agency. For the sake of brevity, I assume a person with a mental disease, as a person, possesses agency and responsibility like other persons, except to the extent her agency and responsibility are incapacitated.

If a host of factors—biological, psychological, cultural, et cetera—predispose a person towards a mental disease like alcohol dependence, it is also the case that several of these factors compromise her agency. For example, in their treatment of psychiatric ethics, Jennifer Radden and John Sadler write that persons with mental illness are especially vulnerable because they often experience impairments in

> their judgment in matters concerning their immediate and long-term self-interest, their reasoning ability, their insight into their own condition, their self-control, their personal and psychic integration, their capacity to communicate their concerns and needs to others, and their conception of other people's responses.
>
> *(Radden and Sadler 2010: 34–35)*[3]

While Radden and Sadler acknowledge that all persons at times suffer such impairments in judgment, they describe the characteristic impairments of mental diseases as those that compromise "the capabilities often associated with agency, self, and self-identity, and so that disorder seems to jeopardize traits we value, and to threaten moral categories forming our understanding of our humanity and personhood" (36). Mental diseases particularly incapacitate a person by threatening traits she identifies with her self.

Considering if and to what extent mental diseases impair judgment and agency is reflected in the debate about whether alcohol use disorder is a natural incapacity (e.g., Leshner 1997) or a biologically reinforced and influenced illness which involves an impairment of the will of the person with alcohol use disorder (e.g., Heyman 2009). While authors taking the former position emphasize addictions are diseases in part to reduce stigma, these well-intentioned arguments neglect the implications of initial voluntary behaviors and subsequent struggles to free oneself from addiction.

Lange's argument similarly neglects the fact that the incapacities of some mental diseases, like alcohol use disorder, involve voluntary behavior—a person choosing an incapacitating behavior. Even more, it neglects the ways all mental diseases impair the capacity to make choices, to be an agent acting in the world.

I experience this difference when seeing a patient with alcohol use disorder. I recognize a number of factors contributed to the development and maintenance of her alcohol use disorder. I work with a person to develop a treatment plan addressing each of these factors. I recognize that many of these factors, like incentive-sensitization and compulsive processes, impair her ability to choose her own well-being. So I work with her, using techniques such as motivational interviewing, to help her regain her agency and her capacity to make choices advancing her well-being.

Could not I do the same with a person with PKU? I could, for example, use motivational interviewing to help a person with PKU understand why she should not eat phenylalanine-containing foods. However, using motivational interviewing with a person with PKU addresses health behaviors that have developed in response to the disease of PKU, not the essential incapacity associated with PKU.

Since I believe alcohol use disorder involves an incapacity in agency, I find it helpful to receive a person with an approach I first encountered in the work of Paul

McHugh. When McHugh addresses alcohol use disorder, he characterizes it as a behavior that was initially chosen but has become biologically reinforced, even to the point of altering brain structure and function, while simultaneously remaining a chosen behavior, albeit a behavior that involves weaker choice as dependence increases. At some point, incapacity of agency is so profound that a choice becomes a compulsion. McHugh's account acknowledges the ways alcohol use disorder characteristically impairs the capacity of a person to seek her own well-being. The incapacity to choose well is not a symptom of the disease's later stages, as it would be, for example, in the neurocognitive disturbances associated with PKU, but incapacity essential to alcohol use disorder.

Now, if it is the case that diseases are incapacities, and that mental diseases are distinct from somatic diseases to the extent they are incapacities associated with a person's ability to be an agent in her own life, then at least three caveats must be observed. First, the contemporary division of diseases as mental and somatic often has more to do with historical accidents than with divisions between natural kinds. Second, the incapacitation of moral agency can occur outside of the context of mental disease; all people make choices against their own well-being at times. Third, different mental diseases incapacitate agency to greater and lesser degrees, and the degree of incapacity changes over time.

It is, of course, precisely because the degree of incapacity can change over time that we can offer medical hope to a person with mental disease. To me, acknowledging how agency is and is not impaired by a mental disease draws my attention to a patient's abilities and reminds me of her humanity. Rather than stigmatizing a person with a mental disease, I find that recognizing the ways mental disease affects agency reminds me of my responsibility to help a person reclaim her agency.

To conclude, I should acknowledge some particularities of my context and how I come to these questions. My clinical work is on the adult psychiatry unit of an academic safety-net hospital. Our unit is locked, and fewer than half of the patients are on the unit of their own choosing. The medical-legal term for this minority is "voluntary," and the term for the majority of the patients is "involuntary." We use these words, like so many other words in medicine, with little conscious consideration of what they reveal about our patients and ourselves. Writing this, I wonder to what extent my sense of mental diseases as especially involving incapacities in agency is related to my own context. I suspect it is substantial. At times, I experience a person with a mental disease as having such limited agency that she is profoundly vulnerable to threats from others, including the institutions in which we meet. In those moments, I find it almost overwhelming how much responsibility I have for a vulnerable ill person. It is not uncommon for me to meet a patient who is so impaired by her mental disease that she cannot communicate with other people, and I have the fearsome task of interpreting her speech and desires. This kind of patient lacks the capacity for intentional action; a deficiency caused by her mental disease.[4]

Almost as often, I work with a person who exhibits obvious effects of a mental disease yet has the capacity to decline treatment. In those instances, we recognize a person's freedom to choose against what we perceive to be her well-being, even if we believe her disease involves an incapacity in her ability to choose well. In those instances, I wonder what responsibility an agent has when their will is impaired but not fully incapacitated—if I recall that freshman philosophy course where I first read

Lange, I believe that was called the problem of the weak-willed agent. This is a problem I see daily, when I meet people with mental diseases—depression, mania, psychosis, and more—whose agency is impaired but not entirely incapacitated.

While I claim no certainty about precisely how mental diseases are different from somatic diseases,[5] my clinical experience teaches me that what marks mental diseases out from other kinds of diseases is also what binds them together: The incapacities of mental illness affect a person's agency.

Acknowledgments

I thank Gary Gala and Joel Yager for teaching me the psychiatric interview and how it opens up philosophical questions, Bridget Rector for editing this essay, and Professor Lange for the opportunity.

Notes

1 In this essay, I follow Lange's use of "mental diseases" to describe the condition that a psychiatrist diagnoses and treats, but as a practicing psychiatrist, I found myself tripping over his use of the word "diseases." Since DSM-III's introduction of the atheoretical model, psychiatrists have used "disorder" to describe the conditions a psychiatrist diagnoses (Wilson 1993). For now, this model endures as a way to unite the disparate etiological accounts endorsed by mental health practitioners. So the authors of DSM-5 describe it as a pragmatic text for clinical practice, writing that "DSM is intended to serve as a practical, functional, and flexible guide for organizing information that can aid in the accurate diagnosis and treatment of mental disorders" (American Psychiatric Association 2013: xli). Along with my friend and fellow psychiatrist Warren Kinghorn, I receive DSM as a text that must be read and utilized within the particular community for which it was designed. Kinghorn writes that DSM is the text that structures the communal life of American psychiatry; the DSM is "a pragmatic manual of clinical practice, bound to a particular time and cultural context, and exists as the expression of a particular community's way of 'going on' in research and patient care" (Kinghorn 2011: 14). By observing that DSM exists as the organizing text of a particular community, Kinghorn is able to enumerate why DSM must be used with humility (Nussbaum 2013) and to anticipate that DSM will be most problematic when exported outside of its particular context and community (Watters 2010). I typically use "disorder" to signify my acceptance of DSM-5 as our community's shared text, but since this essay is a response to Prof. Lange, I use "disease."

2 Silicosis, like the other occupational lung diseases, seems analogous to a broken limb, which Lange defines as a state rather than a disease. To me, silicosis seems more like an injured state than, say, the incapacity to maintain homeostasis after exposure to silica dust.

3 It is precisely because mental diseases can alter a person's ability to make autonomous decisions that persons with mental illness are considered a vulnerable population with regards to research (Kennett 2007).

4 Which is not to say that all the incapacities associated with mental diseases are intrinsic. Kennett writes, "Repeated experiences of illness, of hospital, of (perhaps coercive) treatment, of failed plans, of other ill people, and of the reactions of others to one's illness, must all over time profoundly affect the way the agent sees themselves and influence the ways in which they can project themselves into the future" (Kennett 2007: 97). Clearly, the cumulative blows of social stigma and mental health treatment itself can incapacitate a person's agency.

5 It seems arguable to me that the mental diseases (as well as the somatic diseases) will ever be elucidated in the manner Lange describes at the end of his paper. As a practicing psychiatrist, I am struck that while the technological hopes of grand round speakers are eternal, the

vessels of their hopes change yearly. Accordingly, I focused my efforts in this paper on his argument about mental diseases as incapacities.

References

American Psychiatric Association. 2013. *Diagnostic and Statistical Manual of Mental Disorders*. 5th ed. Arlington, VA: American Psychiatric Association.

Bortolotti, Lisa. 2013. "Rationality and Sanity: The Role of Rationality Judgments in Understanding Psychiatric Disorders." In *The Oxford Handbook of Philosophy and Psychiatry*, edited by K.W.M. Fulford, Martin Davies, Richard G.T. Gipps, George Graham, John Z. Sadler, Giovanni Stanghellini, and Tim Thornton, 480–96. New York: Oxford University Press.

Heyman, Gene M. 2009. *Addiction: A Disorder of Choice*. Cambridge, MA: Harvard University Press.

Kennett, Jeannette. 2007. "Mental Disorder, Moral Agency, and the Self." In *The Oxford Handbook of Bioethics*, edited by Bonnie Steinbock, 90–113. New York: Oxford University Press.

Kinghorn, Warren A. 2011. "Whose Disorder?: A Constructive MacIntyrean Critique of Psychiatric Nosology." *Journal of Medicine and Philosophy* 36 (2): 187–205. doi: 10.1093/jmp/jhr006.

Leshner, A.I. 1997. "Addiction Is a Brain Disease, and It Matters." *Science* 278 (5335): 45–47. doi: 10.1126/science.278.5335.45.

Nussbaum, Abraham M. 2013. "Interpreters or Teachers." *JAMA* 310 (3): 165–66.

Radden, Jennifer, and John Z. Sadler. 2010. *The Virtuous Psychiatrist: Character Ethics in Psychiatric Practice, International Perspectives in Philosophy and Psychiatry*. Oxford: Oxford University Press.

Radoilska, Lubomira. 2013. "Depression, Decisional Capacity, and Personal Autonomy." In *The Oxford Handbook of Philosophy and Psychiatry*, edited by K.W.M. Fulford, Martin Davies, Richard G.T. Gipps, George Graham, John Z. Sadler, Giovanni Stanghellini, and Tim Thornton, 1155–70. New York: Oxford University Press.

Watters, Ethan. 2010. *Crazy Like Us: The Globalization of the American Psyche*. 1st Free Press hardcover ed. New York: Free Press.

Wilson, Mitchell. 1993. "DSM-III and the Transformation of American Psychiatry: A History." *American Journal of Psychiatry* 150 (3): 399–410.

3a

The Political Science of Psychiatric Diagnosis

A Moral Defense of the DSM

Warren Kinghorn

1. Introduction

The fifth edition of the *Diagnostic and Statistical Manual of Mental Disorders* (*DSM-5*) is perhaps the most contested document in modern medicine and healthcare (American Psychiatric Association 2013). In the course of a planning and revision process spanning nearly 15 years, *DSM-5* was—and is still—the subject of intense scientific, political, and personal debate. Around the time of its publication in May 2013, the chair of the DSM-5 Task Force, David Kupfer, argued that *DSM-5* would "help clinicians more precisely identify mental disorders and improve diagnosis while maintaining the continuity of care", while prominent detractors charged that the *DSM-5* revision process had been a "debacle" (Frances 2013a, 2013b) and that the DSM, in all its editions, is a "flawed and fragile document" (Williams 2013). Prominent news outlets such as *The New York Times* and *The Wall Street Journal* greeted *DSM-5* with headlines like "Shortcomings of a Psychiatric Bible" (Editorial Board 2013) and "How Psychiatry Went Crazy" (Tavris 2013).

Criticism of the DSM—both *DSM-5* and its previous editions—has become a favored pastime of psychiatrists and psychiatric trainees; a sandlot sport that occasionally breaks into the big leagues.[1] Legions of clinicians, most of whom have not published their thoughts, note that the DSM is too categorical in its diagnoses (as opposed to dimensional or narrative), too formal and cookbookish, too quick to pathologize, too fixed on static and stigmatizing labels, too focused on experience and behavior rather than quantifiable biomarkers where these exist, and too broad-brush in its categories—to name only a few complaints. As a clinician I understand the allure of DSM-bashing, and have frequently participated in it to some degree. But criticizing the DSM, in most psychiatric contexts, is all too easy, because such criticism often goes uncontested. Much more uncommon are principled *defenders* of the DSM.

In this chapter I seek to provide a moral defense of the DSM from the perspective of a clinician who is well aware of the DSM's limitations. I will argue, in the end, that the DSM is an important clinical and moral document that usefully organizes a large body of empirical research and, more importantly, displays the collective judgment of American psychiatry about the boundaries and priorities of clinical practice. True to the founding premise of its third edition (*DSM-III*), it provides a common language for nosology and diagnosis that enables the very forms of argument that characterize its successive revisions—and, in this sense, serves as a unifying document for the field. But this defense of the DSM can emerge only after considering what the DSM is not but is sometimes mistaken to be. It is *not* apolitical or timeless. It is not value-free or culturally neutral. It is not a document that "cuts nature at its joints" in an objective, apolitical way, and therefore stands as a pinnacle of psychiatric progress. It is none of these things—which is to say that many, if not most, of the most common critiques of the DSM are valid.

In order to make sense of why the DSM is often misinterpreted as an apolitical and timeless scientific document, of how and why particular critiques of the DSM have emerged, and of how we might accurately understand the moral and clinical value of the DSM, I turn to a typology presented by moral philosopher Alasdair MacIntyre in his 1988 Edinburgh Gifford Lectures, published in 1990 as *Three Rival Versions of Moral Enquiry: Encyclopaedia, Genealogy, and Tradition* (MacIntyre 1990). MacIntyre's threefold typology of encyclopedia, genealogy, and tradition, which I will engage in more detail over the course of the essay, can be briefly stated as follows: MacIntyre charges that late nineteenth-century moral theorists went dangerously wrong by conceiving of moral enquiry as a progressive, rule-governed, scientific discovery process that would culminate in a timeless and universal ethical system ("encyclopedia"). This nineteenth-century project, MacIntyre charges, largely died in the nineteenth and twentieth centuries through the relentless "genealogical" criticisms of scholars such as Friedrich Nietzsche and Michel Foucault, who undermined the encyclopedic project in a way that rendered it intellectually and morally untenable. But MacIntyre argues that all is not lost, and that moral enquiry ought rather to be conceived as the conversation of "craft-traditions," communities of discourse and practice who, in the context of pursuing shared ends well, develop standards of excellence and modes of interpretation that evolve as the communities confront internal and external challenges to their best self-articulations. MacIntyre argues that a "tradition-constituted" understanding of moral enquiry can protect it from the fatal vulnerabilities of encyclopedia and from the corrosive critique of genealogy.

In this essay I will argue that MacIntyre's typology provides a useful way to understand the weaknesses and strengths of the DSM. I will argue that insofar as the DSM is described by its creators and defenders along the model of MacIntyre's "encyclopedia," it is vulnerable to the many "genealogical" critiques that have been levied against it. But there is a better way to understand the DSM—not as encyclopedia, but as a tradition-constituted, political document that displays the collective judgment of American psychiatry within a particular cultural and historical context.[2]

2. Two Case Studies

Before engaging in this MacIntyrean exploration of the DSM, two clinical case studies are in order, to which we will return later in the chapter.

Case 1: Thomas

Thomas is a 32-year-old lawyer who presents for psychiatric care stating that he feels like the most miserable person on the earth, and that he would rather die than continue to live as he is feeling. Although he has been able to continue working—barely—his sleep and appetite have been poor and he has been losing weight. He admits that he has thought frequently of suicide for years, even on one occasion writing a suicide note, though denies any current suicide plan or intent. He is preoccupied by feelings of regret and loneliness; current stresses include a sense of disconnection from his wife, from whom he feels emotionally distant, the demands of running a small-town law practice, and a long and cold winter, which he feels generally makes his mood worse. He has not been drinking alcohol but did use cocaine once to medicate himself, though denies doing so presently. He says that he decided to seek care after friends became so concerned about him that they removed knives and razors, as well as firearms, from his home. He states that he has never been hospitalized or previously sought psychiatric treatment, but that he had felt very similarly six years earlier when he was 26, after the sudden death of a close female friend. At that time also he had been preoccupied by thoughts of suicide, but had never attempted to harm himself.

Case 2: John

John is a 22-year-old combat veteran who presents to a primary care physician at the urging of his concerned father. He says that he is haunted by memories of a battle during a recent combat deployment in which many of the men under his command were killed or injured, and that he himself was captured and taken as a prisoner of war. Though he does not give details of his experience as a POW, he says that it was brutal. He is now separated from the military and back in his hometown, but finds it intolerable. He feels constantly on edge and is tormented by recurring thoughts of combat. He also feels lost and angry: angry at those, including his father, who supported the war in its early days and yet now can't seem to listen to the brutal reality of his experience; angry at those who expect him to be the same as he had been before war, as if that were possible. He says that he would not be seeking care were it not for his father, who has noted his insomnia and erratic sleep patterns, his habit of leaving the house at night and walking the streets, and even of leaving home and sleeping in abandoned buildings when he wants to be alone. He is even thinking of returning to combat, with the idea that at least he knows who he is as a soldier; as a civilian, he's not so sure.

If Thomas and John were to present to most mental health care settings in the United States, it is likely that their treatment would be approached in a relatively standardized way. In the case of Thomas, the interviewing clinician would probe in detail about his suicide risk and about whether or not he required inpatient hospitalization. In one of his first appointments, Thomas would likely be offered antidepressant medication, would be referred for individual or group psychotherapy, and would very likely be diagnosed with Major Depressive Disorder, Severe, Recurrent Episode (296.33). John, on the other hand, would almost certainly be diagnosed with Post-Traumatic Stress Disorder (309.81). He would very possibly be directed to the Veterans Affairs (VA) healthcare system or to another clinic with specialized knowledge about combat trauma, and would eventually be offered specialized treatments for combat-related PTSD. He would likely be offered antidepressant/anxiolytic medication such as sertraline or fluoxetine, and, if he was fortunate, would be offered evidence-based trauma-focused psychotherapies such as Prolonged Exposure Therapy or Cognitive Processing Therapy. Both Thomas and John, were they to present in these ways and agree to recommended treatment, would very likely improve as a result. They would feel better over time. They would be in less pain. They would be happier, and better able to attain future goals and to cope with ongoing stresses of life.

3. The DSM and the Construction of Thomas and John

Thomas and John, as described here, are both relatively straightforward examples of how many patients present to mental health care settings and how that care is organized. And it is clear that the DSM pervades every aspect of their care. Nearly everything in these cases, from the way that these patients' "symptoms" are formulated, to the way that their diagnoses are applied and described, to the way that clinical research is conducted (and specific therapies thereby offered to them), to the way that systems of mental health care are organized, are all formed by the post-1980 DSM (beginning with *DSM-III*). How did the DSM come to bear so much power?

It is important to note that the DSM has not always been as important or powerful as it is today. The first edition of the DSM, *DSM-I*, emerged in 1952 to meet the needs of returning World War II combat veterans who were seeking outpatient psychiatric care (Committee on Nomenclature and Statistics of the American Psychiatric Association, 1952). At the time, American psychiatry was heavily oriented toward inpatient treatment facilities and, as such, lacked appropriate diagnostic language to meet the needs of large numbers of psychiatric outpatients. To address this, the American Psychiatric Association (APA) Committee on Nomenclature and Statistics developed a small coding manual, the *Diagnostic and Statistical Manual for Mental Disorders*, which drew on a previous inpatient coding document and was based heavily on the work of Adolf Meyer (Grob 1991). *DSM-II* appeared in 1968, and, like the version before it, it was a small book with sparse detail, consisting mainly of diagnostic labels and, for some diagnoses, paragraph-length descriptions. Neither *DSM-I* nor *DSM-II* were seen as practice-shaping documents in their time.

Both the small professional stature and the small physical size of the DSM began to change in the 1960s and 1970s, as American psychiatry dealt with internal and external challenges that seemed to threaten the status of psychiatry as a valid medical specialty. Thomas Szasz's *The Myth of Mental Illness*, along with other texts and voices (such as those of Michel Foucault) within the so-called "antipsychiatry" movement, challenged that psychiatric language and treatments were fronts for various modes of social power (Szasz 1974; Foucault 2006). The US-UK Diagnostic Study showed that when provided with identical case descriptions, psychiatrists in the United States were more likely to diagnose patients with schizophrenia, while those in the United Kingdom were more likely to diagnose patients with manic depression, suggesting that psychiatric diagnosis was not cross-culturally valid (Kendell et al. 1971). The "Rosenhan experiments," published in *Science* in 1973, documented the experience of a group of research confederates masquerading as psychiatric patients who, having falsely claimed on initial presentation to a hospital that they were hearing hallucinations like the word "thud," but denying all such experience thereafter, were held in 12 different psychiatric hospitals for an average of 19 days and usually left with diagnoses of schizophrenia (Rosenhan 1973). And most prominent and damaging was the very public debate about the status of homosexuality as a diagnosis in *DSM-II*, which resulted in its removal from the document in 1973 (Bayer 1981).

All of this gave rise to unease within the leadership of American psychiatry at the time. The APA therefore convened another task force, this time chaired by Robert Spitzer, to re-envision psychiatric diagnosis and to revise the DSM. The fruit of this effort was the publication of *DSM-III* in 1980 (American Psychiatric Association 1980). *DSM-III*, informed by the principles of operationalism, introduced the criteria sets familiar to modern clinicians—and with them specific diagnostic labels such as "post-traumatic stress disorder," "bipolar disorder," and "major depressive disorder." *DSM-III* aimed primarily not for *valid* diagnoses but, rather, for reliable diagnostic criteria sets by which different clinicians trained in different places—maybe even in different theoretical schools—could see similar patients and respond in similar ways or, at least, use the same diagnostic language. Those who crafted *DSM-III* also strove to be "atheoretical with regard to etiology" (7). They sought to organize diagnoses, that is, not around how mental disorders are caused, but simply on how they manifest in experience and behavior (Decker 2013). All of the subsequent DSM editions since 1980 can be understood as modifications—sometimes very minor modifications—of *DSM-III*. The DSM that we use today is still, in a sense, very much *DSM-III*, so much so that we might call all of the DSM versions since 1980 (*DSM-III*, *DSM-III-R*, *DSM-IV*, *DSM-IV-TR*, and *DSM-5*) the "DSM project." Having been vested with the standardization of psychiatry's core diagnostic language—and, therefore, with the ability to shape psychiatry's research paradigms, reimbursement mechanisms, models of care delivery, educational and training programs, and mechanisms of professional advancement—*DSM-III* and its successive editions became, by most accounts, the most influential psychiatric texts of the past century, more than capable of constructing the way that Thomas and John would be treated upon entering most mental health care systems.

The socially conferred power of the DSM, however, has not been uncontested, as evident in the controversies that exploded during the revision process leading to the publication of *DSM-5*. Though the *DSM-5* review process started in the late 1990s and gathered steam with the appointment of a formal task force in 2006, the *DSM-5* revision process was ensnared in controversy in 2009 when Robert Spitzer, the principal architect of *DSM-III*, and later, Allen Frances, the principal architect of *DSM-IV*, wrote scathing and vitriolic articles in the newsletter *Psychiatric Times* criticizing the structure of the revision process. Spitzer was most concerned about what he perceived to be the secrecy of the revision process, particularly because the task force was not releasing minutes from initial planning meetings (Spitzer 2009). Frances, also concerned about secrecy, weighed in at a higher rhetorical pitch, arguing that in its current structure the *DSM*-5 revision process would lead to diagnostic inflation and to inappropriate medicalization of ordinary life (Frances 2009).

The APA and the DSM-5 Task Force quickly responded to the concerns of both Spitzer and Frances with a very sharp defense of the *DSM-5* planning process, calling it "the most open and inclusive ever," and praising it as "scientific" (Schatzberg, Scully, and Kupfer 2009). This initial response concluded with an *ad hominem* attack on Frances suggesting that Frances' criticism of the Task Force was motivated by his own desire to protect publication royalties from *DSM-IV* and related texts. The Task Force response gave way to a rhetorical war that kept publishers busy for several years—especially those at *Psychiatric Times*—and that quieted only with the publication of *DSM-5* in 2013. One of the results of that debate was the appointment of a scientific review committee chaired by Kenneth Kendler that reported directly to the APA Board of Trustees in order to provide an institutional monitor for the *DSM-5* revision process that was formally separate from the DSM-5 Task Force (Kendler 2013).

Three lines of criticism have emerged in the context of this animated debate about *DSM-5* and in other clinical and philosophical critiques of the DSM. First, many critics have voiced concern about "diagnostic inflation"—the tendency of psychiatric diagnoses to cover broader categories of human experience in successive editions of the DSM—and, correlatively, the medicalization of ordinary life. Although this is a core of Frances' argument against *DSM-5* (Frances 2013a, 2013b), it also finds nuanced articulation in the work of Allan Horwitz and Jerome Wakefield (2007), who argue that the construct of Major Depressive Disorder in every edition since *DSM-III* inappropriately lumps biologically mediated depression ("melancholia") and sadness that is the normal human response to painful events ("normal sadness") into one category, rendering them difficult to distinguish and placing psychiatry in the awkward position of claiming *both* that major depression is a serious and life-threatening medical condition *and* that it affects up to 20 percent of the population at some point.

Second, critics such as Carl Elliott have charged that the DSM, including *DSM-5*, masks professional or commercial interests that threaten its scientific and moral integrity. Elliott has observed, for example, that social phobia (now social anxiety disorder) gained prominence as a diagnosis in the 1990s only after the development of antidepressant/anxiolytic drugs marketed for social phobia, and that the increased rates of diagnosis were correlated with heavy marketing from the pharmaceutical industry (Elliott 2003). In a different mode, other critics, including Frances, have argued that there is conflict of interest inherent in the APA's dependence on the DSM for publishing revenue (Frances 2013a, 2013b: 218–20).

Third, prominent research psychiatrists have charged that the modern DSM—*DSM-III* and beyond—has been a barrier rather than a conduit to groundbreaking research into mental illness. National Institute of Mental Health director Thomas Insel attracted press attention in May 2013, just prior to the publication of *DSM-5*, that NIMH would not organize its research paradigms around *DSM-5*. Insel noted that "symptom-based diagnosis, once common in other areas of medicine, has been largely replaced in the past half century as we have understood that symptoms alone rarely indicate the best choice of treatment," and strongly suggested that a new NIMH-sponsored diagnostic research program, the Research Domain Criteria (RDoC), would eventually produce a diagnostic classification system superior to the DSM (Insel 2014).

4. Is the DSM an Encyclopedia? The Pursuit of a Valid Psychiatric Nosology

The question, then, remains: Why has the DSM been conferred so much power to shape the way that mental health problems are understood and mental health treatments are organized? Why do people care so much about it? Why does this document—a document that is really just a medical coding text—engender so much energy, debate, and fear?

MacIntyre's engagement with nineteenth- and twentieth-century moral philosophy provides helpful insight into these questions. This might seem counterintuitive, given that MacIntyre's work does not directly address psychiatry and that we are not accustomed to thinking of psychiatry as a form of moral enquiry. But—I argue—psychiatry *is* a form of moral enquiry, and the DSM functions in our culture as a kind of moral document that, by designating certain forms of experience and behavior as disorder, displays personal and cultural judgments about the shape of a life well lived. To be sure, the DSM does not contain an account of how one ought to live or of exactly what a well-lived life looks like, nor do I wish to argue that the architects of the DSM understand the document in this way. Yet, in defining normative parameters outside of which medical intervention and medical technology are "clinically indicated," the DSM demarcates certain outer limits of the good life and, therefore, displays certain conceptions about how one ought to live, if one is influenced by prevailing cultural judgments (as most are).[3] This claim that the DSM is a moral document that displays certain parameters of the good life is, of course, contrary to the self-understanding of many mental health clinicians, who try very hard to not make any categorical claims about how one ought to live. But the DSM does this by displaying certain limits, even though, it is important to note, it does not and cannot explicitly name their source.

Although I will not fully defend it here, I suggest that just as American psychiatry conferred *clinical* power on the DSM at a time when it needed a standardized language to bolster psychiatry's legitimacy as a medical specialty, so also the American public of the past three decades has conferred *moral* power on the DSM by expecting it to serve as a unifying, if minimalistic, language for understanding what it means to live well. That, I suggest, is the root of its cultural prominence. In a culture in which political, religious, racial/ethnic, and familial affiliations are increasingly tentative, the DSM provides a comforting moral framework, which, by specifying only *pathological* forms of life, leaves room for multiple interpretations of the well-lived life and therefore attracts broad cultural consensus. It is not hard, in a pluralistic culture, to unite in opposition to the common enemies of "mental disorders" such as depression, bipolar disorder, or PTSD. And correlatively, it is this status of the DSM as a moral document that feeds the anger and energy of those who feel oppressed by its language, as was prominently the case for the "gay liberation" activists of the early 1970s (Bayer 1981).

The problem with understanding the DSM as a moral document is that it opens the DSM to moral critique—which is evident in the work of many DSM critics and, at the same time, unwelcome among some who seek to defend the DSM as a scientific document and, in doing so, to garner the widest possible cultural acceptance of the DSM. But underlying this resistance to moral critique in many cases is an understanding of the role of the DSM as what MacIntyre terms "encyclopedia." For MacIntyre, encyclopedia refers both to a particular paradigmatic text—in his account, the Ninth Edition of the *Encylopaedia Britannica*, itself an indirect heir of *L'Encyclopedie* of Diderot—and to an approach to moral enquiry formally displayed in that text. Encyclopedia conceives of moral enquiry as a form of science, MacIntyre argues, and science (in the late nineteenth-century context) rests on four intercalated assumptions about the progressive acquisition of knowledge. First, there are *facts* that are open to examination. Second, methodical analysis of the facts gives rise to "unifying synthetic conceptions," which so order the facts as to show them to be exemplifying more general laws. Third, uniform methods are used to achieve these unifying synthetic conceptions. Fourth, the systematic application of these methods to facts engenders the progressive elucidation of increasingly comprehensive unifying conceptions and fundamental laws. In an encyclopedic approach, one starts with uninterpreted facts, applies consistent method to those facts in order to achieve unifying synthetic conceptions, and then continuously applies these consistent methods until fundamental laws are eventually defined, which can then organize the facts and which can be compiled in a text or texts—the encyclopedia—that enable a progressively comprehensive knowledge of truth (MacIntyre 1990: 19–20).

This typological account of encyclopedia may indeed have been characteristic of the Ninth Edition of the *Encyclopaedia Britannica*—but is it characteristic of the DSM? Does the DSM present itself in this way? The answer is complex. It is clear that the text of the DSM does not describe itself as an encyclopedia of psychiatric knowledge in the way described above. Nor is the DSM described in this way by most of its principal architects. Since *DSM-III*, the DSM has explicitly avoided claims that it provides a foundational account of mental disorder; it generally rather accounts for itself in pragmatic terms, as in *DSM-IV*'s self-description as a "helpful guide to clinical practice" (American Psychiatric Association 1994: xv).

This restrained humility in the text, however, has not precluded those who use the DSM from interpreting it as encyclopedia, in the way that MacIntyre describes. Just beneath much social discourse about the DSM is the assumption that the DSM project, taken as a whole, is progressively explicating the fundamental nature of mental disorder. This is perhaps most evident in the way that the Platonic idiom of "carving nature at its joints" repeatedly surfaced in discourse and debate about *DSM-5* (for example, see Regier et al. 2009). The overall goal of the DSM project—not realized, to be sure, in *DSM-5*, but perhaps in some future edition—is a psychiatric nosological classification that carves nature at its joints, that gets to the core of fundamental psychopathology. A sophisticated articulation of this aspiration is evident in a recent paper by Kenneth Kendler, the chair of the DSM-5 Scientific Review Committee. Kendler suggests not only that the DSM project as a whole should be characterized by "epistemic iteration," but that this philosophical model guided the work of the Scientific Review Committee and was attractive to the psychiatric leaders tasked with the oversight of the *DSM-5* revision process:

> Epistemic iteration should lead through successive stages of scientific research toward better and better approximations of reality in 'a spiral of improvement', each subsequent stage producing more accurate estimates than the stage that came before. … I felt that this model could be usefully applied to psychiatric nosology and represent a potential framework for the future of DSM. But how might we try to ensure that each edition of the DSM produced better and especially more valid diagnoses? The response would be to put all proposals through a rigorous scientific review. This vision for the [Scientific Review Committee] was supported by [then-APA President] Dr [Carol] Bernstein and the APA leadership.
>
> *(Kendler 2013: 1796)*

Kendler never claims that *DSM-5* is a valid classification of nosology in this sense, but he does embrace the possibility that a fully valid psychiatric classification can be obtained through a disciplined, iterative process of scientific discovery and refinement—a close approximation to MacIntyre's model of encyclopedia.

5. Genealogy Against Encyclopedia: What the DSM Critics have Right

Conceiving of the DSM as encyclopedia is attractive for anyone who wishes to understand the DSM as an objective, value-neutral, scientific document capable of unifying diverse clinicians and publics against the common enemy of "mental disorder." Unfortunately, however, this approach is untenable for the same reason that, in MacIntyre's narration, the epistemological optimism of the Ninth Edition of the *Encylopaedia Britannica* became untenable over the course of the century following its publication.

Encyclopedic approaches to moral enquiry, MacIntyre argues, slowly suffocated over the course of the nineteenth and twentieth centuries under the withering assault of what MacIntyre typologically describes as "geneaology." As was the case for encyclopedia, for MacIntyre genealogy is both embodied in a particular text—in this case, Nietzsche's *Genealogy of Morals*—and also a characteristic set of critiques made against texts that assume an encyclopedic approach to knowledge (particularly, in

MacIntyre's case, to ethics). MacIntyre (1990: 32–57) argues that there are four principal modes of genealogical critique; I will present them and, rather than giving MacIntyre's own examples of these critiques in the context of the history of moral philosophy, will suggest how each of these four modes of genealogical critique manifests within published criticism of the DSM.

First are *psychogenetic critiques*, which argue that "what is taken to be fixed and binding about truth … is an unrecognized motivation serving an unacknowledged purpose" (35). Psychogenetic critics charge that sometimes people who serve as moral authorities are motivated in ways that they don't fully understand, and what they say is to be discounted by these unrecognized motivations. The most crude critiques of *DSM-5*, and conversely of *DSM-5*'s critics, have taken this form, as when the DSM-5 Task Force charged that Allen Frances' initial critique of the Task Force's work was motivated by a desire to maintain his stream of *DSM-IV*-related royalties (Schatzberg, Scully, and Kupfer 2009). But there are more subtle and sophisticated psychogenetic critiques also, levied both against individuals and against organizations. In the context of his historical account of the DSM-5 Scientific Review Committee, for example, Kendler (2013) states that the expert consensus model of the DSM-5 working groups created a possible bias toward diagnostic change because for hard-working volunteer workgroup members, "it is a natural source of pride to 'make a difference,' to 'put their mark' on the document," or, more rarely, because workgroup members saw potential career advantages in the inclusion of a particular new category into the DSM-5 classification (1795). This psychogenetic bias toward change has little to do with the validity or reliability of the DSM diagnostic constructs, and much to do with the professional structures of academic psychiatry.

Second, genealogists undercut encyclopedia with *epistemological* critiques, which argue, contrary to the universalizing aspirations of encyclopedia, that knowledge is always perspectival and therefore contextual. Epistemological critique of the DSM project most often shows up in debates about which DSM disorders, if any, should be seen as "culture-bound" (Mezzich, Parron, and Kleinman 1996). Such critique, in subtle form, also is evident when anthropologists such as Allan Young (1995), writing about PTSD, challenge the common conception (reinforced in the work of prominent trauma theorists such as Judith Herman and Bessel van der Kolk) that PTSD is a nearly universal human response to trauma that has only in the past several decades been elucidated by the use of careful clinical observation. Young challenges this essentialist account of PTSD, arguing that "the disorder [of PTSD] is not timeless, nor does it possess an intrinsic unity. Rather, it is glued together by the practices, technologies, and narratives with which it is diagnosed, studied, treated, and represented and by the various interests, institutions, and moral arguments that mobilized these efforts and resources."

Third, genealogists engage in *historical* critique, arguably the most common mode of criticism lobbied against the DSM. The essence of historical critique, applied to the DSM project, is that the DSM evolved historically within a particular sociopolitical context and serves to maintain the power interests of the individuals and organizations (particularly the APA, but also psychiatrists as a whole) that continue to sustain it. Although this critique continues to appear in the contemporary work of Gary

Greenberg (2013) and others, the basic point was conceded by Robert Spitzer soon after the publication of *DSM-III*, who writes with characteristic forthrightness that *DSM-III* resulted because American psychiatry was trying to make itself more legitimate within the pantheon of American medicine, and that *DSM-III* was a means to that end (Spitzer 1985). As such, the interests of psychiatry are very much tied to the DSM project. Although the DSM is ostensibly a resource for anyone with interest in mental health treatment, from patients/consumers to clinicians of all theoretical persuasions, it remains very much a *psychiatric* document, reflecting the interests and priorities of American psychiatrists, and, specifically, of the APA. The importance of the DSM to psychiatric professional influence and power is evident, in part, in the way that successive DSM task forces have been careful not to alienate other mental health professional disciplines in a way that would jeopardize broad use and acceptance of the DSM among mental health clinicians as a whole. When the American Psychological Association strenuously objected to a proposed *DSM-III* definition of "mental disorder" that defined mental disorders as *medical* disorders, Spitzer promptly dropped the term "medical disorder" from the definition (Spitzer, Williams, and Skodol 1980; Spitzer and Williams 1982).

Fourth and finally, for MacIntyre genealogists undercut encyclopedia with *literary* critique. Literary critique, as MacIntyre describes it, entails the rejection of standard argumentative forms, exemplified by Nietzsche's contemptuous disregard for the philosophical conventions of his day. In the debates about the DSM, literary critiques emerge from critics who charge that the categorical and criteria-based language of the DSM obscures important forms of clinical knowledge and stands as a barrier to good psychiatric care. Such critique comes, for example, from people who argue that categorical descriptions of symptoms have contributed to the decline of psychotherapeutic proficiency among psychiatrists (e.g., Carlat 2010).

MacIntyre's charge in *Three Rival Versions of Moral Enquiry* is that the cumulative effect of the genealogical critiques of Nietzsche, Foucault, and others eventually discredited encyclopedic approaches to ethics and moral enquiry, such that encyclopedia is no longer tenable within moral philosophy or moral theory. Most contemporary readers of the (now digital-only) *Encyclopaedia Britannica*, or for that matter of contemporary texts in ethics, do not expect to find a progressively refined encyclopedic display of moral truth. In that sense, although large reference works called "encyclopedias" continue to exist, encyclopedia as a mode of moral knowing is a thing of the past. But what about the DSM? Have psychogenetic, epistemological, historical, and literary genealogical critiques undermined the DSM and rendered it untenable also?

On the face of it, the answer is clearly "no." Psychiatrists like me still use the DSM, organize our diagnostic and treatment plans around the DSM, educate students and residents to render DSM diagnoses, and bill third-party payers using DSM (and ICD) codes. For these practical tasks, lacking anything better, we continue to need the DSM and can't imagine what things would be like without the DSM. But that does not mean that the accumulated genealogical critiques of the type mentioned above have failed. They have not, it is true, led (yet) to the *destruction* of the DSM project, but they have exerted a cumulative corrosive effect that is displayed in widespread cynicism about the DSM among clinicians, even those who are not philosophically self-aware. Psychiatric residents and medical students are taught the DSM, therefore, but are often taught by teachers who find the DSM lacking and themselves don't value the DSM's approach to standardized diagnostic language. This cynicism, like all cynicism in education, is readily apparent to students, and can easily lead to disillusionment about psychiatry as a whole. And even when teachers themselves are not cynical, students can recoil at the degree of power that the DSM wields within American psychiatry. I remember, in my first clinical exposure to psychiatry as a second-year medical student, being required to memorize many of the *DSM-IV* diagnostic criteria and then to apply these constructs within a structured diagnostic interview. This was a useful exercise—I learned *DSM-IV*, and therefore could get by in any psychiatric clinical setting—but it was clinically unsatisfying and intellectually stultifying, so much so that I resolved at that time not to go into psychiatry. This experience is not uncommon among medical students, psychiatric trainees, and practicing psychiatrists.

The bad news for the DSM project is that if the DSM is understood and interpreted as encyclopedia in MacIntyre's sense—that is, as a method-governed, iterative process of progressively more refined nosology that strives eventually to carve the nature of psychopathology at its joints—then modern-day genealogical arguments will continue to undermine it and, therefore, to corrode the utility and relevance of the DSM to clinicians and consumers. The accumulated criticisms that those charged with the revision of the DSM are driven by unrecognized and unnamed self-interest, that the DSM categories take shape in particular sociopolitical contexts, that the criteria-driven form of the DSM effaces more narrative approaches to psychiatric diagnosis and nosology, and, above all, that the DSM originated to protect the professional turf of American psychiatry and continues to serve that role—none of these criticisms will ever go away precisely because they are, at least in part, correct.

The good news for the DSM, though, is that as those charged with writing the introductory text of each edition of the DSM, including *DSM-5*, have recognized the DSM does not have to be interpreted as encyclopedia; indeed, given the salience of criticisms against it, it *should* not be interpreted this way. If not as encyclopedia, though, how ought the DSM to be constructively interpreted? For one possibility, we turn to MacIntyre's account of tradition, which he intends as an alternative to encyclopedia capable of resisting the corrosive effects of genealogy.

6. Tradition Against Genealogy (and Encyclopedia): A Political-Scientific Account of the DSM

MacIntyre's account of tradition in *Three Rival Versions of Moral Enquiry* holds that moral theory—or, in our case, psychiatric nosology—doesn't emerge in a political vacuum. Nor does it usually emerge from an individual work of genius, nor from isolated theoreticians, nor from disciplined application of theoretical method alone. All of these things—individual geniuses, revolutionary groups of theorists, method-driven approaches—might be part of the history of any mode of moral enquiry, but never account for its emergence entirely. Rather, formal moral enquiry—or, again in our case, psychiatric diagnosis—always arises in the context of particular communities responding in particular ways to particular challenges across time. MacIntyre renders no sharp distinction between the content of a theory and the political context that gives rise to it, because all moral theory emerges out of originating and sustaining communities and continues to serve the interests of those communities. Nor, for MacIntyre, is there a sharp distinction between fact and value, since "facts" are always reflective of the commitments of those that discern them, elucidate them, and settle on them.[4] MacIntyre describes tradition as a "historically extended, socially embodied argument," and argues by use of multiple historical examples that traditions develop and function in variable but predictable ways (MacIntyre 1984: 222). Paradigmatically, argues MacIntyre, traditions begin with a text or texts—which might be a person or a personal office—that are conferred with authority and accepted without question. Eventually, however, in a second stage, these authoritative texts and voices are put to the question, either by internal dissension in the originating community, through changing circumstances, or through external challenges, such that weaknesses and inadequacies in the text (or voice) are exposed. When an authoritative text is questioned in a way that threatens its credibility, the community must either reject the authoritative text, and possibly dissolve as a community, or find a way to preserve the text or voice as authority while also responding adequately to the challenge. If the community does so successfully, this is a crucial third stage, in which the previously settled truths of the community are reformulated and re-evaluated, leading to "new formulations and evaluations designed to remedy inadequacies and overcome limitations" (MacIntyre 1988: 355). For MacIntyre this process can, and must, occur repeatedly in the development of any moral tradition, as traditions put each other to the question and continue to encounter new contexts that threaten previously settled accounts of authority and truth. MacIntyre argues that as traditions mature they develop institutions (e.g., universities, political institutions, commercial institutions), intellectual and moral virtues (standards of excellence about what it means to live well, commensurate with the norms of the tradition), and moral theories. But theories do not originate the tradition; they simply name the tradition's response to challenge in particular contexts (MacIntyre 1988: 349–69).

The historical development of clinical psychiatry, and particularly of psychodynamic psychotherapy, provides one historical example of the formation of tradition inside a psychiatric context. There is, on one hand, a discernible historical and conceptual thread which connects Sigmund Freud, Melanie Klein, and John Bowlby and Mary Ainsworth, the founders of modern attachment theory. And yet the nature and significance of drive, which appears in each of their theories, is substantially different for Freud, Klein, and Bowlby, as Klein reformulated Freud's original theories, and Bowlby reformulated Klein's theories, in order to meet the needs of particular intellectual challenges and particular social and political contexts (Karen 1998). Traditions in MacIntyre's sense are fluid, contextual, and responsive to the needs of their originating and sustaining communities.

MacIntyre argues that, as an account of moral enquiry, tradition is superior to both encyclopedia and genealogy. Tradition is superior to encyclopedia because, unlike encyclopedia, it is open and forthright about the historical nature of moral reasoning—or, more specifically in the present context, diagnostic reasoning. Unlike encyclopedia, tradition can account for its own historical and political contingency. Genealogical critique, when it comes, may seem threatening to encyclopedia as well as tradition; but already aware of its sociopolitical and historical location, tradition can respond and adapt. Faced with genealogical critique, tradition invites the genealogist in to look around, to explore, and to discuss. Genealogical critiques, therefore, can be treated not as existential threats but as opportunities to explore, with the aim of achieving greater self-knowledge within the community. Furthermore, for MacIntyre tradition is superior to genealogy, because genealogical critique eventually corrodes not only encyclopedic approaches to knowledge but, eventually, also the self capable of posing such critique. Unlike genealogy, therefore, MacIntyre argues that tradition always has a way to account for the existence of the self, because the self is grounded in the history and practice of a traditioned community (MacIntyre 1990: 54–55).

How might MacIntyre's account of traditioned moral enquiry, which is admittedly typological, inform a responsible reception and interpretation of *DSM-5* and the DSM project as a whole? Just as MacIntyre argues that tradition can rescue coherent moral enquiry from the corrosive effects of genealogy, I suggest that tradition can rescue the coherence of the DSM from the genealogical critiques that perennially surround it. Tradition provides a way to describe what the DSM does well. But what would an account of the DSM from the perspective of tradition look like?

In many ways, from the perspective of MacIntyre's model of tradition, not much would need to change. The DSM could continue to describe itself—and be understood—as a "helpful guide to clinical practice." It could continue to be understood as a reflection of the collective judgments of American psychiatry, or at least of dominant voices within American psychiatry, in a particular cultural and historical context. And it could continue to be understood, honored, and used as a scientific document, an empirically supported compendium that gathers together, in clinically useful and accessible form, an enormous body of empirical research. In the context of MacIntyre's model of tradition, those charged with revising the DSM could still even aspire to "carve nature at its joints," though with the acknowledgement that the concept of nature itself emerges within the language and practice of particular communities, and is therefore a political concept. If psychiatry wants to carve nature at its joints—especially when thinking about human nature—we need some account of what human nature is, which of course cannot be separated from the communities within which subjective and political selfhood emerges.

What would have to fall away in a "traditioned" account of the DSM is any pretension—again, a pretension not generally found in the text of the DSM itself, but rather in the way that the DSM is described by some of its creators and received by clinicians and their patients—that the DSM is an apolitical, timeless, "objective" classification of mental illness. Nor may it be understood as a triumph of progressive scientific method that is growing nearer and nearer to a foundational psychopathology. The DSM is, indeed, a useful scientific document. But it is also a political document, reflective of the practices, commitments, and needs of its originating and sustaining communities—particularly those of American psychiatry and the American Psychiatric Association.

Understanding the DSM as a political-scientific document should helpfully frame psychiatry's response to foundational criticisms of the DSM. If the DSM is understood in the mode of encyclopedia, foundational criticisms are lethal threats to be ignored or discredited. But if the DSM is understood as a product of tradition, foundational criticisms can be understood, and even welcomed, as challenges that will ensure the tradition's robust survival in the long run—especially if they are right. The charge of Frances and others, for example, that the APA's ownership of the DSM franchise presents an inherent conflict of interest should prompt, from the perspective of tradition, not defensiveness but soul-searching. What would it mean for the APA to examine how such a conflict of interest might display itself? How might the APA's reliance on publication revenue from the DSM affect the way that DSM task forces and workgroups are organized and, therefore, how diagnostic constructs in psychiatry develop and form? There is no objective or politically neutral way to frame these kinds of questions, since they are both empirical *and* political questions involving both fact and value—not one or the other. But from the perspective of tradition, it is clear that the DSM is likely to display both the virtues and also the vulnerabilities of the community that originated it and sustains it—which is, for the most part, American psychiatry—and the communities that continue to use it and to confer it with social, political, and clinical value.

7. Is the DSM Helpful for Thomas and John?

This leads us back to Thomas and John—who, it turns out, are both people well known to history. "Thomas" is Abraham Lincoln, who was well known in his time to have been "melancholic" both prior to and during his tenure in the White House. Joshua Wolf Shenk documents that, at least twice in his early political career, Lincoln experienced sustained periods of unhappiness and despair that in the post-*DSM-III* era would almost certainly have been diagnosed as major depressive episodes. In 1835, after his first depressive episode and the death of a close friend, Lincoln contemplated suicide and may have even written a suicide note, which was later published anonymously in a local newspaper. His friends were so worried about him that they watched him continuously and took his firearms and knives away from him. He even stayed with a local Justice of the Peace and his wife in Springfield for several weeks, during which he was unable to function. In 1841, while serving as an attorney and legislator in Springfield, Illinois, Lincoln experienced a second and more severe depressive episode, also in the context of significant professional stress and the moving away of a close male friend and bedmate, Joshua Speed, who had married and moved to Kentucky. During this second episode, he sought the care of a local physician; while the details of his treatment are unclear, it is likely that he was treated with "biological" treatments current at the time, such as bloodletting. Lincoln wrote a letter during that time in which he referred to himself as "the most miserable man alive." Other writings from the same period are quite dark, conveying much of what is now labeled as "depression" (Shenk 2005a, 2005b).

Would *DSM-5* have been helpful for Lincoln had it existed in 1841? Possibly so. He could have been straightforwardly diagnosed with major depressive disorder, and spared unhelpful biological treatments (or offered others), and offered a course of cognitive-behavioral therapy, after which he would have been better able to resume his political career. He could have possibly avoided the brooding disposition that plagued him until the end of his tragically foreshortened life. But there may have been costs to this; costs that are hard to recognize in a clinical culture so pervasively shaped by the DSM. In his book *Lincoln's Melancholy*, Shenk readily argues that Lincoln was melancholic and likely depressed. But Shenk argues that melancholy in the early nineteenth century was not simply a pathological diagnosis; it retained something of the romantic and morally salient resonance that it had enjoyed since at least the time of Robert Burton's *Anatomy of Melancholy*. Melancholy was understood in the nineteenth century not as something to be medicated away but, at least sometimes, as a source of moral wisdom and clear insight into the tragic realities of the world. (This appraisal of melancholy echoes what is now known as "depressive realism.") Melancholy, Shenk argues, was Lincoln's bane and misery; but it was also a source of energy and wisdom that rendered him capable of the leadership he demonstrated in the 1850s and 1860s. Shenk notes that

> Lincoln did suffer from what we now call depression, as modern clinicians, using the standard diagnostic criteria, uniformly agree. But this diagnosis is only the beginning of a story about how Lincoln wrestled with mental demons, and where it led him. Diagnosis, after all, seeks to assess a patient at just a moment in time, with the aim of treatment. But Lincoln's melancholy is part of a whole life story; exploring it can help us see that life more clearly, and discern its lessons. In a sense, what needs "treatment" is our own narrow ideas—of depression as an exclusively medical ailment that must be, and will be, squashed; of therapy as a thing dispensed only by professionals and measured only by a reduction of pain; and finally, of mental trials as a flaw in character and a disqualification for leadership.
>
> *(Shenk 2005b)*

This leads to John, whose formal name is Giovanni di Pietro di Bernardone, but better known by his nickname, Francesco. We know him as St. Francis of Assisi. Before he became "St. Francis of Assisi," however, Francesco was a young man, the son of a prominent merchant in the town of Assisi, who was a commander in a local but brutal battle with the militia of the neighboring principality of Perugia. Francis saw many of his fellow soldiers die, and he was taken captive and spent a year as a prisoner of war in a Perugian dungeon. He emerged a scarred man. He came back to his hometown disoriented and disillusioned. He was described as wandering the streets at night and sleeping in abandoned buildings. He actually did attempt to return to combat, but gave away his armor prior to reaching the front, and so returned home again. He even sought the care of a physician, who was supportive. But Francis's story doesn't end there. Francis came to understand himself, through a series of spiritual experiences, as called to follow not the lord that he followed into battle, but a different lord—in this case, Jesus. Francis then gathered together with other combat veterans—some from Assisi and some from Perugia and other area towns. These veterans, with a few civilian comrades, banded together under a different rule; one of poverty and obedience and chastity. They called themselves the Lesser Brothers, or Friars Minor, giving rise to what is more commonly known as the Franciscan movement that continues to shape not only Western Christian belief and practice but also Western culture as a whole. But it all started with a combat veteran and former POW struggling to navigate a world that had become troubling and alienating after the experience of war (Matsler 2013). Again, would *DSM-5*, with its clinical construct of post-traumatic stress disorder, have been helpful for Francis?

It is in its use, rather than in its essence, that the DSM shows its value—or not. Although it is certainly true that not everyone with major depressive disorder or PTSD could become an Abraham Lincoln or a Francis of Assisi, I have offered their examples to illustrate that psychiatric diagnosis is a moral enterprise that does not simply name experience and behavior, but also constructs the way that unwanted experience and behavior are interpreted and engaged by the afflicted person and by others. Those charged with creating and applying language to describe unwanted experience or behavior, and to use that language to walk with those who are suffering, therefore bear a heavy moral burden. Clinicians ought always to use language in a way that is empowering and that promotes agency and freedom. At its best, the DSM categories do promote agency and freedom when wisely and judiciously applied. Most mental health clinicians have at times recognized that a certain DSM category seems to hit the mark in accounting for a patient's presentation—that it seems to fit, and that this fit points the way to useful and agency-building therapeutic approaches. When a previously inchoate and confusing set of experiences can be accurately described as a "manic episode," as "obsessive-compulsive disorder," or as "schizophrenia," and when this language serves to empower the patient, then the categories of the DSM are very helpful. In these cases, the DSM's ability to harness a vast range of research and clinical observation into useful form is invaluable. It brings the honorable and rich tradition of psychiatry to the service of someone who is suffering.

But this is not always so. Sometimes the categories of the DSM do not empower, but only constrict imagination and constrain agency. If the construct of major depressive disorder, for example, renders it impossible for contemporary Americans to see melancholy as a possible source of wisdom, or the construct of PTSD renders it less likely that Americans will regard post-combat suffering as a possible wellspring of prophetic witness and social critique, then the DSM is getting in the way. And when it gets in the way, it is not defensible.

The secret of using DSM well is to use it for what it is: a contingent collection of psychiatric diagnostic language, intended to inform certain equally contingent practices, that reflects influential American psychiatrists' best understanding about mental illness at a particular time and in a particular cultural context. We cannot expect it to be a timeless encyclopedia that carves nature at its joints. Instead, we need to celebrate it as the contingent, tentative, political, and scientific document that it is—and nothing more.

Acknowledgments

This paper was delivered in a different form at the Medical Center Hour of the University of Virginia School of Medicine on February 26, 2014. I am grateful to Elliott Haught for his editorial assistance.

Notes

1 A note on terminology: When I refer to a specific edition of the DSM, for example, *DSM-5*, I denote the document by italicizing it. When I refer generically to all of the DSM editions, I do not use italics. For reasons discussed later in the paper, I refer to the editions of the DSM starting with *DSM-III* as the "DSM project."

2 I have previously engaged MacIntyre's typology with regard to the DSM in Kinghorn (2011b), but in this chapter seek to connect this argument to clinical practice and to situate it within the contemporary conversation about *DSM-5*.

3 For a more sustained defense of this position, see Chapter 4 of Kinghorn (2011a).

4 MacIntyre (1988: 357) quips that "facts, like telescopes and wigs for gentlemen, were a seventeenth-century invention."

References

American Psychiatric Association (1980) *Diagnostic and Statistical Manual of Mental Disorders*, 3rd ed., Washington, DC: American Psychiatric Association.

——(1994) *Diagnostic and Statistical Manual of Mental Disorders*, 4th ed., Washington, DC: American Psychiatric Association.

——(2013) *Diagnostic and Statistical Manual of Mental Disorders*. 5th ed., Washington, DC: American Psychiatric Association.

——(2013) "American Psychiatric Association Releases DSM-5," News Release, May 17. Available at: http://www.psychiatry.org/advocacy – newsroom/newsroom/news-releases. Accessed February 22, 2015.

Bayer, Ronald (1981) *Homosexuality and American Psychiatry: The Politics of Diagnosis*. Princeton, NJ: Princeton University Press.

Carlat, Daniel J. (2010) *Unhinged: The Trouble with Psychiatry—A Doctor's Revelations about a Profession in Crisis*. New York: Free Press.

Committee on Nomenclature and Statistics of the American Psychiatric Association (1952) *Diagnostic and Statistical Manual for Mental Disorders*. Washington, DC: American Psychiatric Association Mental Hospital Service.

Decker, Hannah (2013) *The Making of DSM-III: A Diagnostic Manual's Conquest of American Psychiatry*. New York: Oxford University Press.

Editorial Board (2013) "Shortcomings of a Psychiatric Bible," *New York Times* May 12, p. SR 10. Available at: http://www.nytimes.com/2013/05/12/opinion/sunday/shortcomings-of-a-psychiatric-bible.html?ref=sunday. Accessed February 22, 2015.

Foucault, Michel (2006) *History of Madness*, trans. Jonathan Murphy. London: Routledge.

Elliott, Carl (2003) *Better than Well: American Medicine Meets the American Dream*. New York: W. W. Norton.

Frances, Allen (2009) "A Warning Sign on the Road to DSM-V: Beware of Its Unintended Consequences," *Psychiatric News*, June 26, 2009. Available at: http://www.psychiatrictimes.com/dsm-5-0/warning-sign-road-dsm-v-beware-its-unintended-consequences. Accessed February 22, 2015.

——(2013a) "DSM-5 – Where Do We Go From Here?" *Psychiatric Times*, May 17, 2013. Available at: http://www.psychiatrictimes.com/blogs/dsm-5/dsm-5-where-do-we-go-here. Accessed February 22, 2015.

——(2013b) *Saving Normal: An Insider's Revolt Against Out-of-Control Psychiatric Diagnosis, DSM-5, Big Pharma, and the Medicalization of Ordinary Life*. New York: William Morrow.

Greenberg, Gary (2013) *The Book of Woe: The DSM and the Unmaking of Psychiatry*. New York: Blue Rider Press.

Grob, Gerald N. (1991) "Origins of *DSM-I*: A Study in Appearance and Reality," *American Journal of Psychiatry* 148: 421–31.

Horwitz, Allan V., and Wakefield, Jerome C. (2007) *The Loss of Sadness: How Psychiatry Transformed Normal Sorrow into Depressive Disorder*. New York: Oxford University Press.

Insel, Thomas (2014) "Transforming Diagnosis," NIMH Director's Blog, April 29, 2013. Available at: http://www.nimh.nih.gov/about/director/2013/transforming-diagnosis.shtml. Accessed July 9, 2014.

Karen, Robert (1998) *Becoming Attached: First Relationships and How They Shape Our Capacity to Love*. New York: Oxford University Press.

Kendell, R. E., Cooper, J. E., Gourlay, A. J., Copeland, R. M., et al. (1971) "Diagnostic Criteria of American and British Psychiatrists," *Archives of General Psychiatry* 25: 123–30.

Kendler, Kenneth S. (2013) "A History of the *DSM-5* Scientific Review Committee," *Psychological Medicine* 43:1793–800.

Kinghorn, Warren (2011a) "Medicating the Eschatological Body: Psychiatric Technology for Christian Wayfarers," Th.D. dissertation, Duke University, available at: http://dukespace.lib.duke.edu/dspace/bitstream/handle/10161/4644/KinghornThDDissertationfinal.pdf. Accessed April 13, 2015.

——(2011b) "Whose Disorder? A Constructive MacIntyrean Critique of Psychiatric Nosology," *Journal of Medicine and Philosophy* 36: 187–205.

MacIntyre, Alasdair (1984) *After Virtue: A Study in Moral Theory*. 2nd ed., Notre Dame, Ind.: University of Notre Dame Press.

——(1988) *Whose Justice? Which Rationality?* Notre Dame, Ind.: University of Notre Dame Press.

——(1990) *Three Rival Versions of Moral Enquiry: Encyclopaedia, Genealogy, and Tradition*. Notre Dame, Ind.: University of Notre Dame Press.

Matsler, Jeff S. (2013) "Post-Traumatic Saint: Examining the Life of Saint Francis of Assisi in Light of His Experiences as a Combat Veteran and Prisoner of War," Th.M. dissertation, Duke University.

Mezzich, Juan E., Parron, Delores L., and Kleinman, Arthur (eds.) (1996) *Culture and Psychiatric Diagnosis: A DSM-IV Perspective*. Washington, DC: American Psychiatric Press.

Regier, Darrel A., Narrow, William E., Kuhl, Emily A., and Kupfer, David J. (2009) "The Conceptual Development of DSM-V," *American Journal of Psychiatry* 166: 645–50.

Rosenhan, D. L. (1973) "On Being Sane in Insane Places," *Science* 179: 250–58.

Schatzberg, Alan F., Scully, James H., and Kupfer, David J. (2009) "Setting the Record Straight: A Response to Frances Commentary on DSM-V," *Psychiatric Times*, July 1, 2009. Available at: http://www.psychiatrictimes.com/dsm-5-0/setting-record-straight-response-frances-commentary-dsm-v. Accessed February 22, 2015.

Shenk, Joshua Wolf (2005a) "Lincoln's Great Depression," *The Atlantic*, October 1, 2005.

——(2005b) *Lincoln's Melancholy: How Depression Challenged a President and Fueled His Greatness*. Boston: Houghton Mifflin.

Spitzer, Robert L. (1985) "DSM-III and the Politics-Science Dichotomy Syndrome: A Response to Thomas E. Schacht's 'DSM-III and the Politics of Truth,'" *American Psychologist* 40: 522–26.

——(2009) "DSM-V Transparency: Fact or Rhetoric?" *Psychiatric Times*, March 6, 2009. Available at: http://www.psychiatrictimes.com/dsm-5-0/dsm-v-transparency-fact-or-rhetoric/page/0/1. Accessed February 22, 2015.

Spitzer, Robert L., and Williams, Janet B. W. (1982) "The Definition and Diagnosis of Mental Disorder." In W. R. Gove (ed.), *Deviance and Mental Illness*. Beverly Hills: Sage Publications, pp. 15–32.

Spitzer, Robert L., Williams, Janet B. W., and Skodol, A. E. (1980) "DSM-III: The Major Achievements and an Overview," *American Journal of Psychiatry* 137: 151–64.

Szasz, Thomas (1974) *The Myth of Mental Illness: Foundations of a Theory of Personal Conduct*, revised edition. New York: Harper & Row.

Tavris, Carol (2013) "How Psychiatry Went Crazy," *Wall Street Journal*, May 17, 2013. Available at: http://online.wsj.com/news/articles/SB1000142412788732371630457848122760113886. Accessed February 22, 2015.

Williams, John (2013) "The Nature of Suffering: Gary Greenberg Talks About 'The Book of Woe,'" *nytimes.com*, May 29, 2013. Available at: http://artsbeat.blogs.nytimes.com/2013/05/29/the-nature-of-suffering-gary-greenberg-talks-about-the-book-of-woe/. Accessed February 22, 2015.

Young, Allan (1995) *The Harmony of Illusions: Inventing Post-Traumatic Stress Disorder*. Princeton, NJ: Princeton University Press.

3b

Commentary on Kinghorn: Evaluating Traditions in Psychiatry

Christian Perring

Warren Kinghorn's topical paper defends the DSM with a provocative argument. There is a lot to like about it, and his moderate conservative defense of DSM is plausible; it does not seem a terrible mistake to continue to use the DSM in clinical practice. However, I am troubled by Kinghorn's claim that seeing the DSM as a socio-political document can rescue it from its many critiques. This is not a warranted conclusion, and Kinghorn's embrace of MacIntyre's distinction between an encyclopedic approach and a traditioned approach, when applied to psychiatry, is problematic. I will argue that a focus on history and current psychiatric practice, understanding psychiatry as a tradition, leads us even more clearly to the conclusion that we should adopt an attitude not just of caution, but of downright suspicion.

The DSM is often referred to as the "psychiatric bible," and although this characterization is facile, it is true in a way that those using the phrase do not consider. That is to say, it is a document often referred to, but is not well understood by many who use it, and not taken to be the literal truth by experts. A good deal of debate revolves around it, but different groups use it to further their own agendas. Thus I am skeptical that the DSM itself carries as much power as Kinghorn ascribes it, and I am dubious of Kinghorn's assertion that it "displays the collective judgment of American psychiatry" (p. 61). While it is undoubtedly a useful document in the sense that its use enables many medical practices in teaching, research and treatment, and these practices both help individuals who are suffering and also keep many people employed, it nevertheless remains true that we should remain aware of the major problems facing the practice of psychiatry in the current moral and political context. As a symbol of modern psychiatry, DSM deserves sustained critique, and rather than defend it, we should highlight the problems it faces and search for alternative approaches that may require sweeping changes to how we help people who are diagnosable with mental illnesses.

Much of Kinghorn's argument is based on criticizing the model of DSM as encyclopedia. But the analogy between DSM and encyclopedias is a stretch, and it is far from clear that the arguments of the DSM critics have depended on making such assumption. Summarizing MacIntyre's ideas in *Three Rival Versions of Moral Enquiry*, Kinghorn writes, "In an encyclopedic approach, one starts with uninterpreted facts, applies consistent method to those facts in order to achieve unifying synthetic conceptions, and then continuously applies these consistent methods until fundamental laws are eventually defined, which can then organize the facts and which can be compiled in a text or texts—the encyclopedia—that enable a progressively comprehensive knowledge of truth" (p. 67). Kinghorn concedes that DSM does not present itself as an encyclopedia and avoids any attempt to causally explain mental disorders, but rather aims to classify and be a guide to clinical practice (and also psychiatric research, which Kinghorn does not mention at this point). But he says that it has been used as an encyclopedia by others. He cites a passage by Kendler in support of this claim, where Kendler explains that a goal of the DSM process with each revision is to get closer to reality (Kendler 2013). However, even if we accept MacIntyre's characterization of an encyclopedia, Kendler's description of his goals does not fit well with MacIntyre's model of encyclopedic knowledge. There is no mention of starting from uninterpreted facts and moving to fundamental laws in Kendler.

Many proponents of DSM want to see it as unbiased and scientific classification, but that does not require seeing it as an encyclopedia. A better comparison could be to a guide to edible plants in North America: We would want the information to be action guiding and accurate, and we would want each successive edition to be more accurate and comprehensive, but there would be no need for such a guide to attempt to describe laws of nature. DSM is similar to an encyclopedia in that it has many different entries, but this seems if not incidental, then not particularly important. Some critics (e.g. Shorter 1997) argue that DSM should be drastically slimmed down to include only the most well-established and severe mental illnesses, and on such an approach it would be a much shorter document, but it would still be a manual. Kinghorn later refines the meaning of "encyclopedia" to "a method-governed, iterative process of progressively more refined nosology that strives eventually to carve the nature of psychopathology at its joints" (p. 71), which does fit DSM moderately well, but this lacks the notion of generalizing from evidence to laws that he earlier specified.

Kinghorn argues that we do better to analogize the psychiatric tradition to the tradition of moral enquiry. The idea that moral enquiry is a good analogy to psychiatric research is implausible on its face, since psychiatry is meant to be understanding the best way to categorize mental disorders, and find their causes and the best treatments, and as such is a scientific examination of the natural world, while moral enquiry is a far more evaluative enterprise. The skills and training of researchers in these different projects are profoundly different. This is not to say that there are no similarities between psychiatric research and moral enquiry, and the links between the two may indeed be illuminating. However, as I will argue, it does not follow that we should end up defending the DSM.

Let us move on to the analogy between genealogical critiques of encyclopedias and the DSM criticisms. Kinghorn, following MacIntyre, lists psychogenetic, epistemological, historical, and literary critiques, and he shows how criticisms of DSM can fall into each of these four categories. He points out that even after many critiques, DSM is still used, if only because it dominates the market and there is no easy alternative. He goes on to say that the critiques have had an effect in leading to a general cynicism about DSM among clinicians. Unfortunately, he does not cite any evidence for this claim apart from personal experience. He does say that the psychiatric critiques are partially correct, although he says little about which parts are correct. But his main point is that despite there being a good reason to be cynical about DSM if we take it to be encyclopedic in MacIntyre's sense, we should not be too concerned, because we can understand DSM in a different way, using a "political-scientific" account (p. 71).

In spelling out this account, Kinghorn takes us through some of the main ideas of MacIntyre's moral and political philosophy, with focus on the idea of moral *tradition*, which is superior to both encyclopedia and genealogy. Kinghorn gives as an example the idea that psychodynamic psychotherapy forms a tradition within psychiatry, and does not say anything about other traditions: Presumably they would be the biological traditions that lead to psychopharmacology, and possibly more sociologically oriented traditions that focus on changing society in order to improve people's mental health. His claim is that there is less reason to be cynical about the DSM if we look at it from the perspective of tradition. He says that we would have to do away with any claims that the DSM is "an apolitical, timeless, 'objective' classification of mental illness" (p. 73), and it would instead need to be seen as both a scientific and a political document, in the sense that it reflects the psychiatric polis, "reflective of the practices, commitments, and needs of its originating and sustaining communities" (p. 73).

In assessing this claim, much depends on the meanings of terms. He is drawing on MacIntyre's notion of tradition, and when we look at MacIntyre's work, his main example is the Thomist tradition. It is a very broad historically based approach that encompasses plenty of internal disagreement and evolution of thought, although MacIntyre never provides a definition of the term (Porter 2003). When we import the idea of tradition to understand DSM and psychiatry, it will help to be clear about how fine-grained the notion of tradition should be, and to what extent it would encompass differing models and theories. We can be sure that modern psychiatry and shamanism would be different traditions, but we will need clarification whether psychoanalytic and biological approaches should both count as part of the same psychiatric tradition, or whether they are different.

Kinghorn also puts weight on the idea of the DSM as a *political* document: It is clearly a broad approach that largely equates social forces with political forces, rather than a narrow definition referring to organized politics. So the claim that DSM is political in this sense is uninformative, and does not distinguish psychiatric classification from other medical or biological classification, in that all are the product of organizational agreement, and much research has highlighted how science is a profoundly social process subject to a variety of forces and biases. Obviously, the DSM is not timeless in the sense of establishing timeless truths, and no one ever thought it was.

So the substantive claim here that Kinghorn's case rests on is that we should not see the DSM as "objective." This could take some unpacking, because "objective" is a term with many possible meanings. Kinghorn embraces that idea that psychiatric classification does not need to be valid, in the sense of its categories corresponding in a strong way with some external reality. It is true that some critiques of DSM have taken it to task for its problems with validity, and one way to defend the DSM is to argue that we do not need to achieve a metaphysical validity. One can, for example, take a pragmatist approach to classification, which, if it does not do away with the idea of validity, at least reconfigures it.[1]

However, Kinghorn basically reduces the issue of objectivity to the question whether the fact that the APA financially depends on revenue from the DSM compromises its objectivity. He makes the claim there is no politically neutral way to frame these questions about objectivity because they involve both fact and value. It seems that we have to assume that MacIntyre's moral and political philosophy is correct in order to accept Kinghorn's argument here. As far as I can make sense of the argument, he is suggesting that seeing psychiatry as a tradition obviates the need for it to be objective in some important sense. It seems that being part of a tradition is reason enough to accept it; there is no rational way to assess the claims of the tradition, and our only choice would be to step out of the tradition and adopt a different one.

This is not the place to assess the overall adequacy of MacIntyre's arguments about moral traditions, although it is clear that his claims are contentious. MacIntyre's body of work has addressed the question of the objectivity of moral judgment with great subtlety, steering a line between cognitivism and non-cognitivism. It is a matter of continuing debate whether he has managed to secure an alternative to absolutist theories, such as those of Kant and Mill, without opening himself up to a charge of relativism. Kinghorn's appeal to MacIntyre's work is intriguing as a way to understand the problems psychiatry faces with its own objectivity.

One of the puzzles in interpreting MacIntyre's work, especially in his work *Three Rival Versions of Moral Enquiry* (1990), is working out how much weight to put on the notion of an encyclopedia itself, especially the particular encyclopedia he discusses in that book, and how much this is a stand-in for the model of absolutist, cross-cultural knowledge claims. One of his central themes is about the incommensurability of different moral perspectives, and the impossibility of assessing a moral approach from an Archimedean perspective. He rejects absolutist claims. Yet when we consider moral knowledge, we can see that an encyclopedia can take a comprehensive approach including many different traditions and views. It is true that we don't expect to find the correct moral theory established and set out as knowledge in an encyclopedia. On the other hand, many would hold on to the idea that our moral knowledge and sensitivity are gradually increasing with time; for example, in medicine, we look back on past practices and condemn the moral abuses that occurred. We look at the immoral treatment of women and minorities that has occurred in the past and we feel secure in condemning it. We have some confidence that we are improving our moral practices, although we may well be extremely aware of how much of moral debate is hard to settle. The year 2014 saw the publication of the fourth edition of the *Encyclopedia of Bioethics*, in 6 volumes, with 3,000 pages (edited by Bruce Jennings). In 2013, Wiley-Blackwell published the first edition of the *Encyclopedia of Ethics*, edited by Hugh LaFollette, spreading over 6,000 pages. There are other similar works also available. These may not exactly fit the definition of encyclopedia used by MacIntyre, but their existence at least suggests that the conception of an encyclopedic approach to ethics is far from dead. Of course, those encyclopedias are very different kinds of documents from the DSM, and do not necessarily count against Kinghorn's suggested approach to the DSM.

A central question in assessing Kinghorn's argument is whether MacIntyre's replacement of encyclopedic approaches to ethics by an approach based on a conception of tradition is a useful model for psychiatry. If his argument is to be plausible, he needs to make his case about objectivity independently with respect to psychiatry. He faces an uphill battle, since while it may be somewhat plausible to argue that there is no neutral ground in debates over morality, it will be much less plausible to say that psychiatric disputes can't be resolved by appeal to neutral scientific practices. While there may be incommensurability between modern psychiatry and shamanism, because they come from such divergent perspectives, the different theories in psychiatry, such as the psychoanalytic and the biological, share many central concepts and ideas, and the debates between them have been vigorous. Indeed, the history of both clinical and research psychology has been driven by the disagreements in theories, and while the different sides may sometimes be exasperated with each other on occasion, it is implausible that the theories are incommensurable.

It is worth discussing the "case histories" Kinghorn offers, which he reveals are disguised versions of the cases of Abraham Lincoln and St. Francis of Assisi. As illustrations, they do not add any weight of evidence to his argument. It is rather puzzling why he uses these examples, apart from simply to keep the reader's interest, because they are both of people in unusual circumstances, and they hardly count as typical cases. Furthermore, diagnosing people from earlier centuries is notoriously fraught with difficulty. Kinghorn explains that he gives these examples "to illustrate that psychiatric diagnosis is a moral enterprise that does not simply name experience and behavior, but also constructs the way that unwanted experience and behavior are interpreted and engaged by the afflicted person and by others" (p. 76).

We can work to unpack the meaning of *construction* here. It can be understood as a very mild claim that diagnosis has an effect on experience, or a very strong claim that it completely determines the experience. Kinghorn concludes that clinicians "ought always" (p. 76) to "use language in a way that is empowering and that promotes agency and freedom." He says that such use makes the categories of DSM very helpful. When PTSD is described in a way that makes it less likely that those with the conditions could be regarded as possible fountains of "prophetic witness," then he says the DSM is a problem.

Kinghorn seems to be suggesting that DSM affects how people experience themselves and how other people view them, and in this his suggestions are reminiscent of various writers. We might consider the research program from Michel Foucault about how the academic, clinical, and medical trades of psychology tend to construct the subject.[2] Maybe the work of Nikolas Rose has been clearest in setting out these ideas in a series of books explicitly on the idea of the construction of the self.[3] In a similar vein is some of the work of Ian Hacking, maybe with a less pessimistic view about the totalitarian role of the psychological sciences.[4] Recently, Serife Terkin has described the role of the DSM in shaping the self, employing Hacking's ideas of "looping effects."[5] There has been plenty of work on possible links between melancholy, mania, bipolar disorder, creativity and leadership, although there seems to be far less on possible links between PTSD and prophetic powers. There is also plenty of work on stigma, how that makes the lives of mentally ill people worse, and how reducing stigma can improve their lot.[6] However, Kinghorn seems to be making a link between the wording of the DSM and the treatment of people with particular disorders, with an implication that there is a problem. These issues need to be seen in a larger context of stigma, and much more needs to be said to make such a link plausible. We can only understand the effects of the DSM as part of the wider cultural reception of psychiatry and mental disorder, which includes not only psychiatric practices, but also the legal criminal system, disability law, the educational system, and the whole media complex that generally serves as the main way that most of the public get their ideas about mental illness. So Kinghorn's comments here suggest that his notion of psychiatric tradition, which he is already clear includes more than the DSM itself, may also include popular representations of mental illness.

The title of Kinghorn's piece leads us to expect a defense of the DSM, but in the end it turns out his claim is more moderate: that the DSM might be defensible if it does not have stifling effects on people who are diagnosed with mental illness. It also seems that the focus of evaluation is much wider than the text of the DSM itself, but also includes the way it is used in psychiatric training and clinical work, the way it is used by the medical insurance industry, social work, and psychotherapy, or the way it is explained to the wider public in self-help books, websites, TV shows, and the wider media.

This points us towards how a promising evaluation of DSM could proceed. Far from give up on a scientific evaluation, we need to embrace a scientific piecemeal approach, evaluating each diagnosis for reliability and validity, and comparing it with competitors. While there may be disputes about some or even most diagnostic categories and how to evaluate them, the project of making sure that each fits the purpose of classification is important.

As Kinghorn points out, there is tension between different users of classification schemes as to how it should go. This leads me to a tangential point. It seems that the needs of scientific research and clinical treatment are currently diverging, and it may be necessary to have different classification schemes in clinical manuals from those that are used in research. Maybe psychopharmacologists could use different classifications from those who do talk therapy. We might even start to have different classification schemes in health insurance, criminal law, disability policy, and education. This could help evaluation of the categories for each group. It would of course raise difficult questions about how the different classification schemes relate to each other. Right now there are small differences between the DSM and the ICD, and there is a lot of effort to minimize them and play down their significance. But even though there would be undoubted confusion, there could be advantages too, in that each group would come to focus on what was important to them, and would give up on the implicit assumption that one classification scheme can meet the needs of all groups. It may be that this is already done to a greater or lesser extent in different ways of dividing up the disorders, and the editors of DSM might welcome such a move, since they explicitly say that it not designed to be used outside of a medical and clinical context.[7] It is striking that Allen Frances says that one of his greatest regrets about his work on the DSM is that he did not take into account how the document would be used in non-medical contexts.[8] Frances himself seems to have come to decide that the editors' hopes that they should not be responsible for how their document is used outside of their own professional domain is unrealistic, but having a proliferation of different classification schemes would help avoid the promotion of the DSM as the only classification that counts.

Returning to the question of how to evaluate DSM, we need to separate it from the evaluation of different treatments. It certainly has proven difficult to know exactly how successful different medications and forms of talk therapy are, but that does not mean it is impossible. The evaluation of different treatments is of the utmost importance, given that we are spending a large amount of money and resources on these. Many claims have been made for the effectiveness of different treatments, only for them to be thrown into doubt by new data or re-evaluation of old data. It is relatively clear that whatever problems there are in evaluating the ideas of a tradition from within a tradition, which Kinghorn emphasizes, it is straightforward matter to identify malfeasance, dishonesty, and incompetence.[9] We have the resources to test from within the psychiatric tradition which treatments are successful and which are not: the problems are simply getting the system to work without being unduly influenced by the pressures of the free market and individual ambition and greed. It is possible that there may be some genuine difficulties in some cases in finding some neutral way to evaluate some parts of the DSM or some treatments, but we have a long way to go before those problems are conceptually central.[10] We have the ability to test the effectiveness of medications and other forms of treatment, and to assess whether the policies of our mental health care system are improving the health of the population, and we are moving towards achieving such testing.

Kinghorn makes a plausible case that it is reasonable and helpful to see DSM as part of a tradition in MacIntyre's sense, even if he needs to be much clearer how he delineates this tradition from others. I have suggested that we can, to a large extent, engage in atomistic evaluation of each part of that tradition, but we can also examine the tradition as a whole. Recent work by Robert Whitaker does this for the way that we bring people with the most serious mental illnesses into the mental health system.[11] He presents evidence that the mental health system has failed to improve the condition of these individuals in the last 50 years. I take Whitaker's case against psychiatry to be especially troubling because it is well made, but it is part of a nearly constant stream of books and articles raising questions about the effectiveness of modern mental health care. The set of criticisms of DSM that arises with each publication is also a part of this flow of criticism.

The tradition of psychiatric classification centered around the DSM dates back to around the middle of the twentieth century, and its roots go back to the start of the twentieth century. Kinghorn leaves it open exactly what date he puts the start of the tradition he is referring to, and he leaves it somewhat undetermined how much of psychiatric practice he would count as being part of that tradition. It is however clear that he accepts MacIntyre's stipulation that this tradition, as with any, must be associated with virtue and be an ongoing project that progresses. This need for a positive evaluation leaves us to wonder how the psychiatric tradition can accommodate its problematic history. Kinghorn comments that "the DSM is likely to display both the virtues and also the vulnerabilities of the community that originated it and sustains it—which is, for the most part, American psychiatry—and the communities that continue to use it and to confer it with social, political, and clinical value" (p. 74). His mention of "vulnerabilities" is pertinent but does not go far enough: We have to bear in mind that clinical psychology has had a troubled history. The task of achieving a value-neutral account of the development of modern psychiatry is itself up for inspection, but it is at least plausible that the scientific project of psychiatric classification has been closely tied to methods of treatment, the pharmaceutical industry, and there have been many problematic uses of classification.[12] Whatever its overall status, the DSM tradition is certainly checkered.

If we see the DSM as a document firmly enmeshed in a moral, political, and social context, and we consider the troubled, often alarming history that goes with the DSM, together with the difficulty that psychiatry has of showing it really provides beneficial treatment in most cases, we should hesitate before endorsing a defense of DSM. While acknowledging that we currently have few systematic alternatives to using the DSM available to us, we can at least withhold judgment and be ready for better evidence that we should endorse the DSM. Kinghorn ends by suggesting we should celebrate the DSM—but, even on the terms he adopts, this is not the appropriate reaction. We can admire and respect the sincerity and good will of so many who work in the psychiatric and mental health professions who use the DSM and do the research that supports research around it, and we may even hold a grudging respect for the tenacity of the DSM itself. However, we should maintain a critical and skeptical stance towards it, given its historical context.

Notes

1 See for example Peter Zachar (2000, 2014).
2 Foucault (1961/2006).
3 Rose (1989, 1998); Rose and Abi-Rached (2013).
4 Hacking (1995).
5 Terkin (2011).
6 See for example Hinshaw (2006).
7 APA (2000).
8 Frances (2011).
9 See for example Goldacre (2013).
10 According to the summary of the views of MacIntyre by Porter, it does not take much for there to be no neutral ground from which to evaluate two competing traditions: Even if there can be genuine communication between them, they are still forced to operate from

within a tradition if there are "at least some disagreements that cannot be resolved by appeals to mutually agreeable standards of reasonableness and excellence because the disagreements have to do, at least in part, with those very standards themselves" (Porter 2003: 38–69). These are difficult general claims to evaluate, but with regard to different theoretical stances within psychiatry, there is so much overlap and common ground between them that we would need strong particular arguments regarding those theories to make a case that they can't be evaluated in a way that would be agreeable to both sides.

11 Whittaker (2010).

12 A selection of relevant books includes Shorter (2008); Healy (2013); Horwitz and Wakefield (2007).

References

American Psychiatric Association. 2000. *Diagnostic and Statistical Manual of Mental Disorders*, 4th Edition, Text Revision (DSM-IV-TR). Washington DC: American Psychiatric Association.

Foucault, Michel. 1961/2006. *History of Madness*. New York: Routledge.

Frances, Allen. 2011. "DSM-5 Writing Mistakes Will Cause Great Confusion." *Huffington Post*. June 6. Updated: 08/11/2013. Accessed 9/21/2014. http://www.huffingtonpost.com/allen-frances/dsm5-writing-mistakes-wil_b_3419747.html

Goldacre, Ben. 2013. *How Drug Companies Mislead Doctors and Harm Patients*. London: Faber & Faber.

Hacking, Ian. 1995. *Rewriting the Soul: Multiple Personality and the Sciences of Memory*. Princeton: Princeton University Press.

Healy, David. 2013. *Pharmageddon*. Los Angeles: University of California Press.

Hinshaw, Stephen. 2006. *The Mark of Shame: Stigma of Mental Illness and an Agenda for Change*. New York: Oxford University Press.

Horwitz, Allan V., and Wakefield, Jerome C. 2007. *The Loss of Sadness: How Psychiatry Transformed Normal Sorrow into Depressive Disorder*. New York: Oxford University Press.

Jennings, Bruce (ed.). 2014. *Encyclopedia of Bioethics*. Fourth Edition. New York: Macmillan.

Kendler, Kenneth S. 2013. "A History of the DSM-5 Scientific Review Committee," *Psychological Medicine* 43: 1793–800.

MacIntyre, Alasdair. 1990. *Three Rival Versions of Moral Enquiry: Encyclopaedia, Genealogy, and Tradition*. Notre Dame, Ind.: University of Notre Dame Press.

LaFollette, Hugh (ed.). 2013. *Encyclopedia of Ethics*. New York: Wiley.

Porter, Jean. 2003. "Tradition in the Recent Work of Alasdair MacIntyre." In *Alasdair MacIntyre*, edited by Mark C. Murphy, 38–69. New York: Cambridge University Press.

Rose, Nikolas. 1989. *Governing the Soul: The Shaping of the Private Self*. London: Routledge.

——1998. *Inventing Our Selves: Psychology, Power and Personhood*. New York: Cambridge University Press.

Rose, Nikolas, and J.M. Abi-Rached. 2013. *Neuro: The New Brain Sciences and the Management of the Mind*. Princeton, NJ: Princeton University Press.

Shorter, Edward. 1997. *A History of Psychiatry: From the Era of the Asylum to the Age of Prozac*. New York: John Wiley & Sons.

——2008. *Before Prozac: The Troubled History of Mood Disorders in Psychiatry*. New York: Oxford University Press.

Terkin, Serife. 2011. "Self-Concept Through the Diagnostic Looking Glass: Narratives and Mental Disorder." *Philosophical Psychology* 24, no. 3: 357–80.

Whittaker, Robert. 2010. *Anatomy of an Epidemic: Magic Bullets, Psychiatric Drugs, and the Astonishing Rise of Mental Illness in America*. New York: Broadway Books.

Zachar, Peter. 2000. "Psychiatric Disorders Are Not Natural Kinds." *Philosophy, Psychiatry, & Psychology* 7 (3): 167–82.

——2014. *A Metaphysics of Psychopathology*. Cambridge: MIT Press.

4a

Free Will, Moral Responsibility, and Mental Illness

Benjamin Kozuch and Michael McKenna

1. Introduction

What is the relationship between mental illness and moral agency? The default assumption is that mental illness undermines a distinctive form of moral agency: morally responsible agency. More precisely, it is thought that when a person's mental illness plays a significant role in the causes of her moral wrongdoing, her illness provides reason to excuse her.[1] Or, when it does not excuse, it provides grounds for mitigation. As such, in the absence of competing reasons, either judgments of moral blameworthiness are unjustified, or their force is diminished by virtue of the mitigating influence of the illness. Moreover, in a wide range of cases, it seems that this is explained in terms of the illness's impairing of an agent's freedom. In this essay, we wish to scrutinize this pervasive assumption, as well as the freedom-impairing explanation associated with it. While we do not intend to reject it, we do wish to qualify it considerably and in the process come to a deeper understanding of it. The relation between mental illness and moral excuse is simply far more delicate than it is sometimes taken to be.[2]

Of course, this common association between mental illness and excuse is not without exception. It is widely agreed that some mental illnesses do not undermine or diminish a presumption of moral responsibility. Pedophilia, for instance, is a sexual disorder according to DSM IV, but the condition is not recognized as grounds for excusing from criminal culpability (Edwards 2009: 106). This is despite the fact that a clinician's response to a pedophile would be and ought to be to interpret the behavior through the lens of pathology, addressing the person as a patient in need of treatment. In short, the aptness of the "sickness" role in such cases is not assumed to foreclose treatment as a morally responsible agent.

Nevertheless, there is a compelling association between the influence of mental illness on behavior and reason not to blame, to punish, or more generally to regard as morally responsible. It is, for instance, a familiar piece of politically correct liberal doctrine to insist that an enlightened approach to the problem of substance abuse should be to decriminalize consumption and instead focus upon problems of addiction. While this may be the most defensible policy to adopt, if it is, we wish to argue that it is not simply because behavior issuing from a mental illness—in this case, drug use caused by addiction—is incompatible with moral responsibility for that behavior. The compelling association masks a constellation of considerations that need teasing apart in order to take proper measure of how mental illness defeats or diminishes moral responsibility and when it genuinely does do so.

Looking to legal practice is helpful in certain respects. Criminal culpability is not easily defeated by credible claims of mental illness (e.g., see Brink 2013). Hence, as regards legal responsibility, actual legal practice strongly suggests that the default assumption we wish to scrutinize is indeed not widely accepted.[3] There are, however, two problems with looking to legal practice for wisdom here.

First, legal responsibility is simply different from moral responsibility; the normative and pragmatic pressures in the realm of law vary from those pertaining to morality more generally (e.g., see Hart 1961). Admittedly, we ourselves uncritically elided this distinction in these introductory remarks. For instance, our ground for claiming above that pedophilia is not typically taken to excuse is largely based on legal practice. Likewise, we have remarked upon the tension between addiction and moral responsibility in terms of decriminalization, which is about legal responsibility, not moral responsibility. But these observations are innocent enough as a set of preliminary remarks. There is at least an aspirational expectation that our legal practices track our considered moral convictions, and hence that our grounds for legal responsibility arise out of our commitment to moral responsibility.[4] Nevertheless, the two practices, practical pressures and norms differ, and we are here concerned with the more inclusive phenomenon of moral responsibility.[5]

Second, and more importantly, looking to legal practices and accepted norms is unreliable, since they might be misguided or poorly motivated. (Recall the now debunked separate-but-equal Jim Crow laws.) It is, for instance, likely that one reason why pedophilia does not typically excuse is because the sexual molestation of children is so abhorrent and evinces such strong reactions of contempt and disgust. Visceral reaction is thus liable to swamp countervailing considerations, should there in fact be any (not that we think there are). Hence, it is unlikely that legal practice would ever bend much in the direction of excusing, regardless of any discoveries about the causes of pedophilia—even if it could be shown that pedophiles suffer from a mental illness involving literally irresistible urges.

In this essay, we will examine the relation between mental illness and moral responsibility by drawing upon two resources. First, we will examine philosophical work on the related topics of free will and moral responsibility. Along the way, we'll pay special attention to how free and responsible agency is related to underlying principles accounting for various pleas designed to show that a person is not morally responsible for something she is alleged to have done. In doing so, we will argue that it is misguided to think that when mental illness undermines moral responsibility, it does so simply by showing that a person's moral competency is defeated. Second, we will turn to a loose collection of mental illnesses that are not all that fashionable in the literature on free will and moral responsibility. These include generalized anxiety disorder, clinical depression, and attention-deficit disorder. In focusing on these sorts of mental illnesses, we will focus mostly upon mild cases. We will not attend to cases on a spectrum in which persons with these illnesses are so massively impaired that they cannot function well at all in their daily lives. Rather, we will attend to cases that are, in certain respects, at the borderlines. By focusing on these cases, we intend to argue that those laboring with these conditions retain their status as morally responsible agents and are not excused for their objectionable behavior—even when their illness plays a nontrivial causal role in it. Or at the very least we hope to show that such cases are perfectly intelligible. We hope that by tending to them we can get clearer on the conditions under which mental illness does and does not provide an excuse for an act of wrongdoing.

2. Free Will and Moral Responsibility

We begin this section with a plea to those unfamiliar with contemporary philosophical work on free will. We ask readers to set aside the impressions they may have acquired about free will from popular sources, and even recent discussions in some much-publicized scientific literature in the neurosciences.[6] Despite how it is often understood in arenas outside of philosophy, the meaning of the term "free will" does not necessarily presuppose substance dualism, or any sort of supernatural powers or abilities.[7] Nor can one infer, simply by grasping the meaning of the term, that free will is opposed to the prospect of a fully naturalistic, scientifically credible explanation of mental life and intentional action. To be clear, we are not claiming that free will does not require substance dualism. Perhaps careful philosophical inquiry will show that it does. Nor are we claiming that free will is compatible with a naturalistic account of human behavior. Maybe careful examination will show that it is not. All we are saying is that if any of these things are true, this cannot simply be read off the meaning of the term—as if it could simply be looked up in a dictionary. It is, as philosophers sometimes put it, an open question just what free will is and whether human persons possess it. In any event, what we are especially concerned to make clear, for the purposes of the present essay, is that on a wide variety of philosophically respectable approaches free will is consistent with a scientific explanation of the causes of actions. This is not a patently incoherent thesis. Hence, one can at least attempt to understand free will in a manner suited for a science of human behavior, including the sciences of psychology and psychiatry. We shall thus proceed by assuming that free will is a respectable notion, and that human persons really do possess it.[8] But we only mean to commit to this thesis as an operating assumption, one that naturally could be discredited.[9]

How should one understand free will? Although controversial, many philosophers understand free will in terms of the conditions for moral responsibility.[10] In this essay, we shall adopt this strategy. Here is a relatively common proposal: "Free will is the unique ability of persons to exercise all of the control necessary for moral responsibility" (McKenna 2013). A free act, as we shall understand it, is simply an act that issues from an exercise of the free will ability. This proposal is meant to be neutral between more refined theories of free will. Naturally, the hard philosophical work involves giving an adequate theory of the pertinent sort of control. Here there is room for a considerable amount of philosophical dispute. For now, we can skirt these issues and simply take it that free will skepticism is false and that at least some persons on some occasions—indeed, most psychologically healthy persons on most occasions—possess free will. That is, they possess the ability to control their conduct in the strongest manner necessary for moral responsibility.

Now consider moral responsibility. We will restrict attention to responsibility for moral wrongdoing and focus just upon a sense of "responsibility for" captured by the notion of accountability (e.g., Shoemaker 2011; Watson 1996). To explain: When an agent is accountable for her moral wrongdoing—when she is blameworthy—she can justifiably be held to account for what she has done.[11] How so? It would be appropriate to blame her overtly by directing one's moral anger, resentment, or indignation toward her.[12] It might (depending upon context) be appropriate to make demands upon her to explain herself, or apologize, or correct her behavior and make efforts to repair the moral landscape. It is, furthermore, reasonable to assume that her being morally responsible in the accountability sense for her wrongdoing and thus being blameworthy is a precondition for her being an apt target of punishment.

In the preceding paragraph, we fixed upon moral responsibility for something—for wrongdoing. It will also be useful to clarify the distinct notion of morally responsible agency. Morally responsible agency is a matter of a person's status as an agent. A morally responsible agent is one who is sufficiently competent—who has what it takes—to be accountable for her behavior were she to do something of moral import. Small children are not morally responsible agents, but most mature, sane, fully developed adult persons are. Perhaps an example of a borderline case is the character Lenny from Steinbeck's *Of Mice and Men*, a man-child of sorts, whom readers are liable to see as at least mildly mentally retarded and thus not really a fair candidate for holding to account (at least fully) for his moral failings.

3. A Taxonomy of Pleas: Exemptions, Excuses, and Justifications

We turn now to an examination of the various kinds of pleas meant to show that a person is not blameworthy. Since our focus is upon how and when mental illness defeats moral responsibility, it will be instructive to consider in more general terms the different grounds that our norms and practices treat as reasons to withdraw judgments of blameworthiness.

To begin, note that a person who is not a morally responsible agent might nevertheless be a moral agent, one capable of doing morally wrong. Such a person would not be blameworthy for wrongdoing simply because she is not a morally responsible agent.[13] Why? Only morally responsible agents are candidates for being accountable for what they do when they engage in wrongdoing. Certain sorts of mental illness are often thought to absolve the sufferer of any responsibility for her actions because the illness so thoroughly impairs a person that it undermines her having the capacities requisite for responsible agency (Strawson 1962; Elliott 1996:

Chap. 7). Extreme forms of mental retardation or schizophrenia are clear cases. The term of art used to capture such excuses is *exemption*.

Non-exempting excuses, hereafter referred to as "excuses," function by showing that one who is a morally responsible agent did in fact do wrong, but special circumstances exonerate her from being responsible for acting as she did. Pleas such as "she did not know" or "she could not help it" call attention to some reason showing why an agent is not blameworthy for her wrongdoing.

Exemptions and excuses are to be distinguished from justifications. Pleas such as "it was the only way to save him" or "she has a right to do that if she pleases" are meant to show not that a person who did wrong does not deserve blame, but rather that the person did no wrong in acting as she did. There is no wrong for which she is to blame, and so she is not blameworthy.

There is also a further way to qualify both exemptions and excuses by way of mitigation. A mitigating exemption or excuse appeals to grounds for partial but not full exculpation; it invokes grounds to show that an agent is less blameworthy than she might otherwise be. In the case of excuses, for instance, imagine the two examples offered above but modified as follows: "it was difficult for her to know, given the situation" or "although she could have helped it, it would have been very difficult for her to do so." Similar remarks might apply for certain exempting considerations. A person might be mildly rather than severely mentally retarded and so be merely on the borderline of competent agency of the sort required for moral responsibility. Likewise, an adolescent just emerging from childhood might be just beginning to become a morally responsible agent and so accountable only to a small degree and in only some moral domains but not others.

What can we learn about the preceding taxonomy as it bears on pleas involving mental illness? It might initially be thought that when mental illness defeats moral responsibility it only does so by way of exemption, and many philosophers' discussions of the relationship imply as much (Strawson 1962; Scanlon 2000: Chap. 6). But careful consideration suggests otherwise. Here we come to a point at which we can begin to explain how the blanket assumption (that mental illness undermines morally responsible agency) masks important complexity worth teasing apart.

A person suffering from a mental illness might not be so impaired that she is incapacitated for morally responsible agency (Elliott 1996; Bjorklund 2004; Kennett 2007). She might be perfectly capable of being held to account for her conduct in some domain of activity and yet, nevertheless, her illness might, on a particular occasion, impede her ability to exercise her conduct in that very domain of activity. Consider, for example, a person, Jane, with generalized anxiety disorder, who is able to manage her illness well enough to function in most social contexts and comport herself reasonably well with others, though perhaps it is onerous to do so. Now imagine some special occasion in which Jane's anxiety gives rise to a level of irascibility leading her to explode and say something cruel to a coworker. Suppose it counts as morally wrong to say what she said in that environment. And suppose as well that in this case her anxiety and her agitation rendered it true in that moment that "she could not help it." If Jane literally could not help acting as she did, then she has a legitimate excuse for her wrongdoing. She has an excuse in which her mental illness plays a significant causal role. It would be a distortion to regard her as incapacitated for morally responsible agency. She would after all still be able to comply with lots of other expectations, and perhaps even keep her emotions in check in subsequent interactions of the very same sort that gave rise to her outburst. So an appeal to her mental illness should not be thought of as an exemption, but rather a "localized" excuse.

The above point is not merely an academic one of taxonomy. Whether we can carve out a space in which one with a mental illness is excused for an action while still being a morally responsible agent has important practical and moral implications: Clearly, we want to be able to sometimes absolve someone with mental illness for an act of wrongdoing, given that mental illness sometimes makes people behave in ways that appear beyond their control. However, using exemption to absolve an agent comes with its own costs. It involves adopting, toward the mentally ill person, what P. F. Strawson (1962) referred to as the "objective attitude," treating the mentally ill person not as someone who is to be reasoned with, but rather as a "force to be dealt with" (Scanlon 2000: 280). To exempt someone because of mental illness, it would seem, is to deny that the person is a participant in the system of morality within which adult humans normally participate. As has been pointed out (Bjorklund 2004; Kennett 2007), this risks robbing the person of both their dignity and autonomy, and stands to undermine their effectiveness as moral agents, perhaps running contrary to therapeutic goals. It appears important, then, that we be able to understand how a mental illness can remove blameworthiness for an action without also taking the person's capacity for moral responsibility.[14]

Another implication of this concerns what might be called "moral residue." What is moral residue? To illustrate, suppose you promise to pick up your friend at the airport but through no fault of your own your car breaks down on the way. As a result, you cannot follow through—you cannot help it. You are excused for failing to fulfill your promise, and so you are not morally responsible and blameworthy for your wrongdoing. While this is all true, insofar as now your friend is in a pickle, you still owe it to her to aid in the untoward residue of your (admittedly excused) moral failure. Perhaps you should at least walk to her apartment and let the dog out, or call someone to help make arrangements for another way to get her home, and so on. The point is, you are still morally accountable for the fallout, and you would be to blame for other wrongs were you just to ignore the entire affair, as if the failure to meet your friend were just a natural disaster that might be unfortunate but is not your business in the least.

So, when mental illness excuses but does not exempt a person from moral responsibility, there is of course a sense in which the person is not morally responsible and blameworthy for her wrongdoing. But there is another sense in which the mentally ill person remains morally responsible: First, she persists in being a morally responsible agent, and, second, depending upon context, she might remain accountable for further moral burdens incurred as an upshot of her (blamelessly) doing morally wrong. For instance, Jane in the scenario mentioned above would likely owe her coworker an apology and an explanation. She might bear the burden of taking steps to avoid certain conversations or correct any misimpressions caused by the hurtful things she said. Now, if she were simply not a sufficiently competent moral agent, she would not bear these burdens and would not be to blame for failing to comply with them. Hence, Jane's mental illness and the excuse it provides leaves much for which she continues to be responsible; this would not be the case if her illness exempted her altogether.

What about justifications? Might a mental illness serve as a warranted plea for blamelessness by way of justifying an action and so showing why behavior that otherwise would be morally wrong is not? Perhaps. We don't want to rule this out as a possibility. One might make the following case for the thesis that sometimes mental illness can function as a justification: As a general point about the moral landscape, many of the moral obligations, duties, burdens, and responsibilities we incur are only meant to apply to us at all in certain contexts. If you owe your fellow neighbors a certain degree of good will and due regard, as well as a degree of kindness and civility in daily life, you do not necessarily owe it to anyone at all if you have a splitting headache, or if your family has recently been killed in a horrific accident. To be clear, on the proposal we are now entertaining, it is not that in such cases you are excused from a moral burden you have. It's that it is unreasonable in such contexts to presume that this ought to be a burden on you at all. Perhaps this point can be extended to all sorts of mental illnesses. If Josephine and Joe, husband and wife, owe each other as spouses a certain degree of kindness and affection in their daily lives, a level of intimacy that allows their home life to be a source of comfort to them, Josephine is not under any such obligation if she suffers from a significant albeit not completely debilitating episode of depression and simply can find little joy in much of anything. Here, Joe would be unreasonable to presume his wife owes him her kindness and good cheer while the darkening clouds are gathering for her.

Here too there are important moral and practical implications that flow from these observations and so distinguish the way mental illness might count as a justification rather than an excuse or an exemption. In particular, in this case, Joe has no cause to regard Josephine as if she is not a morally responsible agent at all. It's not that he need regard her as exempted. More importantly, Joe and Josephine would misunderstand their moral relationship if either thought that there was any moral residue due to Josephine's doing Joe wrong. As Josephine does not wrong Joe at all, there are no further burdens she incurs for any (blameless) wrongdoing.[15]

Others have argued for a similar thesis. Elliott (1996: Chap. 3) has argued that volitional disorders such as kleptomania or voyeurism can justify an action normally considered wrong (e.g., shoplifting) if the action was the lesser of two evils. The person with Tourette syndrome, then, is justified in barking an insult at someone if inhibiting the insult causes her greater distress than whatever distress would be caused to the recipient of the insult, were the Tourettic individual to indulge the tic.[16] But even in a seemingly favorable cases like this, we think it is questionable whether there would be moral wrongdoing and no moral residue (the Tourettic individual might rightfully be considered to owe an apology to the person insulted), and perhaps this indicates such a case is more naturally interpreted as an instance where the action was excused, rather than justified.[17] Overall, the issue of whether a mental illness can justify an action normally considered wrong looks to us to be unsettled (see also

Brady 1997); as nothing we argue for below hinges on this, we are happy enough to leave it this way.

In closing this section, recall the initial default assumption we proposed to scrutinize: mental illness undermines morally responsible agency. We hope we have now made clear that of course sometimes mental illness undermines judgments of moral responsibility by exempting. In these cases, it clearly does undermine an important form of competent moral agency. But this is not always so. Mental illness sometimes undermines judgments of moral responsibility simply by excusing a person from wrongdoing while in no way showing that her agency is impaired in such a way that she is rendered incompetent. Other times, perhaps mental illness undermines judgments of moral responsibility simply by showing that a person did not after all act in a way that is morally objectionable.[18]

4. Kinds of Excuses and the Conditions for Blameworthiness

We turn now to the conditions for blameworthiness. Attending to these, we can then examine in more detail the various ways that a mental illness might undermine a person's moral responsibility for wrongdoing. Before doing so, we need to offer one further refinement to the taxonomy set out in the preceding section. Recall that in explaining excuses, we mentioned two sorts of pleas: "she did not know" and "she could not help it." Note that the first type of plea is designed to defeat a presumption of knowledge or understanding, while the second is designed to defeat a presumption of freedom or control. As it happens, these two types of pleas are just instances of numerous pleas for excuse that seem to fall into one or another of these categories. Consider, "My vision was clouded, and I thought it was she I saw," or, "I was sure she told me to get the bottle of pills from the right-hand side of the cabinet," and so on, all of them being variations on a did-not-know plea. Now consider, "I was pushed," or, "You startled me and made me jump, and that's why I hit the lever," and so on, all of them being variations on a could-not-help-it plea. That there are these two types of pleas suggest that there are distinct necessary conditions for being morally responsible (and blameworthy) for something.[19] These different types show that one or the other of the necessary conditions is not satisfied.[20] Hence, we can identify an epistemic (or knowledge) condition for moral responsibility, and also a freedom (or control) condition. As should now be clear, free will, as we defined it in section 2 above, just is the ability that enables a person to satisfy the control condition for moral responsibility when she is responsible for something or other (either by way of being blameworthy or praiseworthy).

Momentarily we will present a proposal offering the conditions necessary and sufficient for moral blameworthiness. Before doing so, we pause to build on the point just made regarding kinds of excuses—those pointing to an epistemic failure and those pointing to a freedom failure. Drawing upon these as conditions for being morally responsible for something, we can also infer the general abilities or capacities a person must have to be a morally responsible agent. She must have the ability to act freely by being able to adequately control her conduct, and she must have the ability to understand morality, as well as the further practical details pertaining to moral considerations. Hence, knowing that these are the general kinds of abilities a person needs to be a morally responsible agent, we can also see how different mental illnesses are liable to be grounds for different sorts of exemptions. Some mental illnesses, such as schizophrenia, cause failures of understanding, and so defeat the possibility of morally responsible agency not so much by undermining a person's freedom but by undermining her understanding and moral knowledge of the world. Other mental illnesses, however, leave a person's perceptions and understanding intact but impair a person's ability to control her behavior and do what she has reason to think she should. This seems to capture more accurately how mental illness exempts in the case of impulse-control disorders or maybe extreme forms of addiction.[21]

Drawing upon the preceding taxonomy, here is an account of moral responsibility and blameworthiness for an action, principle MB, cast in terms of necessary and sufficient conditions:

MB: A person, P, is morally blameworthy for an action, A, just in case:

(a) A-ing is morally wrong;
(b) P knows that in A-ing she is doing morally wrong;
(c) P acts freely in A-ing.

This principle, MB, is a caricature of what a fully defensible account of moral blameworthiness amounts to. It ignores important details, but these needn't detain us here. With one qualification we shall take up presently, MB is an adequate approximation for the purposes of this essay.[22]

As for that qualification, MB does not make room for "tracing" cases. A very simple example is a case of drunk driving in which at an earlier time a person freely and knowingly gets drunk and then later drives home with no understanding of what she is doing and no ability to control herself or her car. When she kills someone, she is morally (and legally) responsible, but at the time she did wrong, she did not know what she was doing and was not acting freely. Nevertheless, we can ground her culpability by tracing the roots of her drunken behavior to prior directly free conduct. Here, it seems that both the knowledge and the freedom conditions in MB need qualifying so as to allow for tracing an exercise we shall forgo.

A different sort of case that is more relevant to our topic is recreational drug use that later leads to addiction, where addiction is understood by DSM IV as a mental illness. Suppose that recreational drug use is morally wrong (not that we think it is), and suppose that extreme addiction genuinely does render an addict unfree with respect to her drug consumption. A tracing principle can be used to argue that someone who is presently an addict is nevertheless morally responsible and blameworthy now for acting as she does even if now she is not free with respect to her drug use. Of course, this would be so only if one could genuinely trace to an earlier time in which the (now) addict was a morally responsible agent who freely and knowingly embarked on a pattern of reckless drug use, with some understanding that by doing so she might later make herself an addict with little ability to control her cravings for the drug.

In light of MB, we can now identify all of the following distinct ways in which mental illness might defeat a person's blameworthiness for a (putative) wrong act:

1. Her status as a morally responsible agent is undermined by compromising her ability to control her conduct, and so a could-not-help-it exemption applies (MBc is defeated).
2. As a morally responsible agent, she is not able to exercise her ability to control her conduct, and so a could-not-help-it excuse applies (MBc is defeated).
3. Her status as a morally responsible agent is undermined by compromising her ability to understand the moral status of her actions, and so a did-not-know exemption applies (MBb is defeated).
4. As a morally responsible agent, she is not able to exercise her ability to understand the moral significance of her actions, and so a did-not-know excuse applies (MBb is defeated).
5. She did not actually do anything morally wrong, and so a justification applies (MBa is defeated).

Further refinements could be made to variations on points 1 through 4 to account for different sorts of mitigation. We'll not spell each of these out here. Moreover, there can be mixed cases, wherein, for example, a mental illness might exempt by compromising both control and understanding.

5. Working with a Reasons-Responsive Theory of Freedom

Thus far, we have been working to tease apart the different ways mental illness might defeat or diminish a person's moral responsibility and blameworthiness for something. But we have yet to focus our attention directly on (alleged) cases in which an agent is morally responsible and blameworthy despite the fact that her mental illness does play a nontrivial causal role in her wrongdoing. Are there such cases, and how can we make sense of them? To focus our discussion, we restrict attention to the control or freedom condition. It is common to associate compromises of moral responsibility due to mental illness as arising from impairments of freedom. So it will be most instructive to attend just to conditions that are allegedly freedom-impairing. What we are especially interested in considering are cases in which mental illness plays a causal role in an agent's exercising her ability to control her conduct but in which she nevertheless is morally responsible and blameworthy for acting as she does. Hence, no could-not-help-it excuse or exemption (from categories 1 and 2 in the previous section) would apply. In the cases we wish to consider, if there are any, the causal contribution of mental illness would not even provide grounds for mitigation.

To proceed, we devote this section to sketching a theory of free will in terms of responsiveness to reasons.[23] While reasons-responsive theories are not universally accepted as the means by which to theorize about free will and free agency, they are widely accepted. The fundamental insight used to explain freedom in terms of reasons-responsiveness is basically this: When an agent acts freely, she acts from causal sources that are sensitive to reasons. To put it a bit more precisely, she acts from causal sources that are expressive of her sensitivity to reasons.[24] Why is this an appealing way to ground freedom? What seems to distinguish persons from other creatures that are non-persons is their ability to relate to the world rationally. Recall Aristotle's thesis: man is a rational animal. Reasons-responsive theories capture a distinctive sort of freedom, one that helps to distinguish persons from non-persons, and one that seems to be featured in the sorts of moral demands and expectations involved in holding people morally accountable for how they conduct themselves.

A simple example will help illustrate how a reasons-responsive theory of free will works, and it will at the same time help expose the main explanatory burden for such theories. Take Ann and Beth, who both have occasion to wash their hands. Both have just fallen in some mud. Because both have dirty hands, both have reason to wash their hands. But there is a difference. Unlike Ann, Beth suffers from a strong form of Obsessive-Compulsive Disorder, which manifests itself for her with constant hand-washing. While Beth washes her hands for good reason (because they are muddy), she would wash them just as well if she happened to see a bit of trash fall off a garbage truck outside from the comfort of her spotless apartment, or if someone even uttered the word "germ" in her presence. There are, as it happens, a wildly large number of considerations in which Beth would wash her hands despite not having any good reason to do so. This shows that when Beth washes her hands, the cause of her doing so does not express her being suitably sensitive to reasons in this domain of her life. She thus does not wash her hands freely, or, as some might put it, of her own free will. But assuming Ann does not suffer from any similar impediment to her agency, she does wash her hands freely. Moreover, unlike Beth, if Ann were given good reasons not to wash her (now) dirty hands even though she had just fallen in the mud, she would be able to refrain from doing so. Imagine, for instance, that Ann heard a large crash around the corner and was given reason to believe that someone had been hurt. Ann, unlike Beth, would respond to that reason as one that rightly defeated her need for clean hands just then, and she would go running. Beth, on the other hand, is a slave to her need to wash her hands, and so would not respond likewise.

Thus far, the case of Ann and Beth handily explains how a reasons-responsive theory works. How does it also expose the theory's main explanatory burden? Consider Beth again. It might seem that Beth is not at all reasons-responsive. But this need not be so. She might simply not be suitably reasons-responsive. Why? Suppose there are some reasons such that, were they present, she would not wash her muddy hands. Suppose that if she washed her hands, her daughter would immediately be disemboweled, or that New York City would instantaneously disintegrate. More realistically, suppose that if a fire was raging through the house and she'd be incinerated were she to stay to wash her hands, she'd not wash her hands then but instead flee.[25] Turn now to Ann. We've suggested that Ann is suitably reasons-responsive insofar as we have described her as acting freely in washing her hands. But does this mean Ann is perfectly reasons-responsive? Must it be, for her to act freely, that she would respond to every good reason to wash her hands and ignore every bad reason to do so? Suppose in some non-actual but possible scenario she learned that if she washed her hands exactly at that moment, she'd violate some local taboo that would offend her hosts.

Suppose that this really does count, even by her own standards, as a good moral reason not to wash her hands just then. But suppose that Ann would still wash her hands. This is a reason she'd just ignore. (Sometimes, not often, Ann is a bit of a jerk and just does things she knows she really ought not to do.) Would this possibility—which we are supposing is not the actual context of her action—show that she does not wash her hands freely when she actually washes them due to falling in the mud? Bear in mind that she is still sensitive enough to reasons to respond aptly to a very rich range of other reasons. It seems not. It seems we should regard Ann as washing her hands freely in the actual situation.

So Beth does not wash her hands freely even though she is at least a little bit reasons-responsive, and Ann does wash her hands freely even though she is less than optimally reasons-responsive. Clearly, what is needed is a way to specify a suitable or adequate degree of responsiveness to reason that captures what it is for a person to be able to navigate the space of potential reasons in her environment reliably enough to function as a competent moral agent in the world. The hard work for all reasons-responsive theorists of free will is to capture that range in an elegant and compelling fashion, one that seems to explain intuitively the distinction between moral (and in other contexts, say, legal) responsibility.[26] This is not something we will develop here. We simply leave it as an intuitively plausible thesis that free and morally responsible agents are suitably reasons-responsive to a degree that displays (roughly) their (moral, social, legal, practical) sanity.

6. Refining a Reasons-Responsive Theory and the Etiology of Action

As might be expected, our plan is to consider carefully the way particular manifestations of mental illnesses are liable to influence different agents' responsiveness to reasons. Reasons-responsiveness comes in degrees, and it allows for a threshold above which an agent might act freely even if less (or differently) responsive than she would be in the absence of the illness. Hence, it seems to be an open empirical question whether in fact a person's having a mental illness that causally influences her exercise of free will is after all excused for occasions in which she engages in wrongdoing.[27] To help see in a finer-grained way just how mental illness might influence a person's responsiveness to reasons, it will be helpful to attend in more detail to the different elements involved in being responsive to reasons. It will also be useful to attend to further details in the etiology of some paradigmatic cases of action that naturally flow from an exercise of a person's deliberative, rational capacities.

As for the needed refinements, here we draw upon Fischer and Ravizza (1998: 41–46 and 69–76) in distinguishing between a receptivity component of reasons-responsiveness and a reactivity component. Reasons-receptivity concerns an agent's ability to be receptive to—that is to be able to recognize—the reasons that an agent has to act as she does or to act other than as she does. (In our example of Ann and Beth above, these would be candidate reasons not to wash one's hands, as well as candidate reasons to persist in washing one's hands.) Reasons-reactivity concerns an agent's ability to react to the good reasons she recognizes by acting upon them. An adequate theory of reasons-responsiveness needs to be able to account for a suitable degree of reasons-receptivity. An agent must be able to recognize a considerable range of good reasons for acting as she does or instead acting otherwise. But she need not be able to recognize every such good reason. If this were required, no one but perfectly rational gods would be adequately reasons-responsive, and so free and morally responsible. Furthermore, an adequate theory of reasons-responsiveness needs to account for a suitable degree of reasons-reactivity (McKenna 2005). An agent must be able to react to a considerable range of the good reasons she is able to recognize by choosing and acting on the basis of such reasons. But she need not be reactive to the full spectrum of reasons she is able to recognize. If this were required, then no one who ever fails to do what she judges best to do would be reasons-responsive and so free and morally responsible.

As Fischer and Ravizza point out, failures of suitable receptivity can be associated with "delusional psychosis" (1998: 41). Whereas lack of suitable reactivity "afflicts certain compulsives or phobic neurotics" (42). Their examples of mental illness are offered as grounds for exemption. We are presently interested in different sorts of cases (ones in which exemptions do not apply), but it is especially helpful to see how refining reasons-responsiveness helps to expose the way different mental illnesses can potentially compromise different aspects of free agency.

For ease of discussion in the next section, we offer the following toy model of an agent, X, who, as a suitably reasons-responsive agent, satisfies a suitable degree of reasons-receptivity and reasons-reactivity with respect to an action, A. Treat "Rx1," "Rx2" and so on through "Rxn" as names that pick out reasons for X doing other than A or instead for X persisting in doing A. Suppose this model captures X's receptivity to reasons with respect to X's act of A-ing. Now treat Rx1 through Rxm as the smaller class of reasons falling within Rx1 through Rxn to which X is also reactive with respect to doing A.

Note that any particular person's reasons-responsive "profile" will permit features that are unique to her. If some other agent, Y, were also reasons-responsive, and to roughly the same degree as our agent X, the reasons picked for her in relation to a similar act of A-ing, reasons such as Ry1 through Ry2, and so on, while naturally overlapping somewhat with X's reasons-responsive profile, would capture a different, but equally rich and stable class of reasons. For ease of reference below, call the above the Agent X Model of reasons-responsiveness. Call relevant variations the Agent Y Model, the Agent Z Model, and so on.

Before applying the resources of a reasons-responsive theory to our present concern—the prospects for acting freely even when mental illness is involved—we offer a few further distinctions useful in the theory of action. These are distinctions regarding the etiology of certain paradigmatic actions, actions issuing from exemplar exercises of well-functioning agency. In the cases we have in mind, the causal story unfolds roughly as follows:

> An agent is faced with *uncertainty about what to do*, perhaps regarding something that is morally loaded, although that need not be so. She then engages in a *process of deliberation* wherein she weighs reasons. As this transpires, *reasons occur to her*, and in this respect, she cannot simply "will" them to occur. While she can make some effort, say by doing some research or consulting with others,

and so on, what reasons occur to her is the product of a process that is not fully within her control. As the saying goes, thoughts sometimes simply "spring to mind," and at other times they do not. During this process, by applying her ability to *think critically*, she forms a *judgment about what it is best to do*—and we can think of this as a *conclusion to a piece of practical reasoning*. In coming to this conclusion, she drew upon values to which she was committed, *values* regarding what she thinks is good and right. And she also relied upon *principles for weighing reasons* that aid her in assessing things such as the reliability of others' testimony and the like. In doing all of this, she reasoned rather well as a relatively sane, intelligent person. But in coming to her conclusion, her *motivational set* is not completely cooperative. She has *desires and preferences*, fears and countervailing values that *oppose her settled course of action*. In certain respects, then, she does not want to act as she has decided she should, and she feels the pull of this. As such, she is *tempted to act weakly* by forming an intention to do, say, the cowardly or the self-indulgent thing rather than the thing she now judges she really should do. But she *exercises strength of will* by exerting effort to tend to the important elements of her reasons to do what she judges best. By doing so, she successfully *forms an intention* to do the right thing by *choosing* and thereby *setting her will* to act rightly. And even though doing it makes her tremble with fear, she is able to *exert control* over her body to follow through with *the plan which is her intention*. She acts as she judges best.

Consider the above case as of a kind of exemplar exercise of practical agency for imperfect beings like us.[28] We have identified with italics several salient action-theoretic elements in the etiology of these types of actions.[29]

Of course, not all actions issuing from competent agents have the sort of causal history these actions have. Indeed, most do not. People often act well from habit, make choices on a whim, and so on. But these exemplar sorts of actions allow one to use a magnifying glass to think about all of the elements that might go into exercises of relatively healthy human agency. This in turn can help us think about where normal agency can be short-circuited and so go wrong. Moreover, it is easy to see how these action-theoretic elements "interface" with the distinct elements of reasons-responsiveness as we have set it out. Think of cases like Tourette syndrome, where the causal pathways between formed intention and action are apparently dysfunctional. Or consider cases of severe clinical depression, in which a person's motivational system might be so depleted that she simply is incapable of acting as she judges best. In these sorts of cases, it appears we would have distinctive reasons-reactive failures. Something similar might be true about addiction, should a person's motivational states simply flood her resources for exercising self-control. But other mental illnesses, such as extreme attention-deficit disorder, might powerfully handicap a person for sustaining a process of deliberation while making an effort to settle on what is best to do. Or once that is formed, it might impede her from retaining that judgment in the process of translating it to decision and intention formation. Moreover, in yet other cases, a person's anxiety might instead so flood her cognition that she would not be able to evaluate potential reasons in light of her values and principles so as even to identify what genuine reasons she has for how she ought to act. Here we would have compromises or failures of reasons-receptivity.

7. Zeroing in on an Interesting Thesis: Examining Mundane Cases of Mild Mental Illness

Are there cases in which a person is morally responsible and blameworthy for free actions causally influenced by mental illness? For the question to be at all interesting, we need to set aside cases in which any blameworthiness is due to some tracing consideration. Naturally, if a fully competent person engaged in an activity at an earlier time knowing she would be liable to make herself ill and then as a result act wrongly, she could be morally responsible for these wrong acts by being morally responsible for embarking on such a course of action to begin with. We also note before proceeding that the causal influence needs to be proximal and nontrivial. How so? Imagine that years ago an episode of mental illness led Jill to check into a mental hospital. When there she both recovered and met her criminal future husband, Jack, who turned her toward a life of crime. Years later, while mentally healthy, she robs a bank. Now, in some sense, her mental illness was a cause of her robbing the bank. Had she not been mentally ill, she'd have not met Jack. And had she not met Jack, she'd have not become a criminal and then not robbed a bank. But her mental illness was not a proximal cause, and it was also a trivial cause. It might pass a "but-for" test of counterfactual dependence, and might strictly be a cause, but it does not fix upon explanatorily salient features in the ongoing mental life that is proximally causally engaged in her deliberations, intention formations, and the like. Finally, we set aside a further "indirect" way that a person could be blameworthy for actions resulting from mental illness. If she is capable of seeking help that would cure her, and she knows this and fails to seek the help, she might also be morally responsible and blameworthy for any foreseeable wrongdoing that might be caused by her actions. So, to proceed, we intend to consider cases in which the causation of the mental illness is "direct" and there is no question about prior culpable, negligent history leading to her current illness or resultant behavior.

We shall focus on cases of mental illness not often considered in the literature on free will and moral responsibility. Philosophers currently working in these areas, when attending to issues of mental illness, tend to fix on dramatic cases. In these cases, the illness massively impairs an agent's competency. Featured mental illnesses include psychopathology, autism, and mental retardation, and are fairly far along on a spectrum.[30] They are frequently used to test the boundaries for moral responsibility (e.g., see Shoemaker 2015). Rather than tend to these cases, we are interested in rather pedestrian cases.[31] There are, presumably, numerous people living among us, carrying on their lives well enough, who suffer from some mild form of mental illness[32] such as depression, anxiety disorder, or attention-deficit disorder.[33] Do we have reason to think that often they are frequently not morally responsible for what they do? Or is at least mitigation in play? If so, there is ground for limited skepticism about moral responsibility. If many people are mildly mentally ill, and if their illness plays a significant causal role in many of their actions much of the time, then many people are not morally responsible for much of what they do. Or, if they are, they are less responsible than one might otherwise think. Is this true?

8. Freedom, Moral Responsibility, and Mild Depression

Consider simple cases of depression. Along with feeling fatigue, individuals with depression tend to have diminished motivation to engage in typical activities they otherwise find pleasurable. They are as well liable to feel irritable or sad and assess themselves as worthless. Moreover, their negative assessments are not limited to themselves; their assessment of their environment is apt to be "meaner and grayer" (Church 2003: 175). As a result, they are liable to see their options and others in a negative light. Depression thus poses several risks to exemplary exercises of agency of the sort we sketched in the preceding section. It is liable to affect her motivation, and so her ability to form intentions that align with what she judges best to do. It is also likely to affect her deliberations, since her ability to assess others and her environment, as well as her own needs, will be colored by her negative outlook. Hence, it will also affect her ability to judge what it is best to do. As such, it is liable to affect both one's reasons-receptivity and her reasons-reactivity.

Now consider the case of Jenny, who suffers from mild depression. Jenny decides not to pick up her friend at the airport as she promised simply because she does not want to deal with managing the task. Grant that doing so is morally wrong. Should we conclude that Jenny's illness excuses or exempts her? Insofar as we assume her illness is mild, we assume that she is not incapacitated due to her illness and so is able to exercise control over much of her life most of the time. So no exemption applies. But if her illness figured in the causes of her decision not to pick up her friend, does it excuse?

Suppose Jenny's illness played a causal role in the motivational states at the time, rendering her less inclined to do what she knows she should—which is slog through rush hour traffic to pick up her friend as promised.[34] Imagine as well that when reflecting upon whether she should, her illness also affected her assessment of the value of her friend and so the desirability of doing right by her. As a result, in modeling Jenny's spectrum of receptivity, the value of Jenny's friend would not count as one of the reasons to which Jenny would be receptive. Or, if she were receptive to it, she would weigh it as less significant in relation to the rest of the reasons available to her for deliberation. As for modeling her level of reactivity, she would not be reactive to a range of reasons that would involve her having to do something like brave the stress of rush hour traffic. Finally, suppose these causal influences would pass a test of counterfactual dependence: Were Jenny not mentally ill, she would weigh the value of her friendship differently and would not withdraw in the face of the nasty traffic: She'd make the drive and do as she promised.

An initial reaction to the case as we have set it out here is likely to be that Jenny is excused since, were she not ill, she would follow through and avoid wrongdoing. But not so fast. Consider Sarah. She is a morally responsible agent who suffers from no mental illness at all. Sarah is roughly just about as receptive and reactive to reasons as Jenny is, given Jenny's current condition. Of course, Sarah's reasons-responsive profile is unique to her. So she is not receptive and reactive to the same complete spectrum of reasons to which Jenny is—she is not in this respect Jenny's psychological duplicate. But she is roughly the same. While Jenny's illness is partially what explains why she values her friend only to a certain limited degree, Sarah values similar friends to similar degrees as a result of causes that do not include mental illness. Sarah has simply acquired a sour outlook upon many of her friends as an upshot of a different sort of history. Were Sarah to decide not to pick up one of her friends as promised in similar circumstances, she would do so from a similar reasons-responsive spectrum, but one not causally influenced by mental illness. Note also that there are surely some counterfactuals involving details of Sarah and her past which are such that, were she to have had some sort of different history in some way, then she too would pick up her friend as promised in a similar situation.

With the cases of Jenny and Sarah before us, we now deploy our toy Agent X, Agent Y, etc. models to each agent. We also include a Mentally-Healthy-Jenny model along with the actual mentally ill Jenny. Of course, Mentally-Healthy-Jenny would be receptive and reactive to the further reasons that mentally ill Jenny would not, and so when acting in a similar context, she would have a wider and richer degree of reasons-responsiveness. To make perspicuous just how reasons-responsive each agent is, and how it is that each is a morally responsible agent (not an exempted one) we also include the model of a person, Tina, who is sufficiently impaired due to depression to be exempted were she in a similar situation. Figure 4a.1 shows each of the modeled agents:

Mentally-Healthy-Jenny

Receptivity: RH1, RH2...RHs

Reactivity: RH1, RH2...RHr

Jenny

Receptivity: RJ1, RJ2.......................................RJn

Reactivity: RJ1, RJ2...................................RJm

Sarah

Receptivity: RS1, RS2.......................................RSn

Reactivity: RS1, RS2...................................RSm

Tina

Receptivity: RT1, RT2.........RTd

Reactivity: RT1, RT2......RTc

Figure 4a.1

With these models in hand, we offer the following argument for the conclusion that Jenny acts freely and is blameworthy for her wrongdoing: By hypothesis, unlike Tina, Sarah is a morally responsible agent who acts freely and is blameworthy for her wrongdoing. And, unlike Tina, she displays a sufficiently rich pattern of reasons-responsiveness to ground her freedom. But if Sarah is morally responsible and blameworthy for her freely doing morally wrong, and if her degree of responsiveness to reasons is no different than Jenny's, then Jenny is also equally morally responsible and blameworthy for her freely doing morally wrong.[35]

A critic might protest that it is fallacious to regard Jenny as equally free and responsible as Sarah. After all, what caused Jenny's relative degree of freedom as in contrast with a Mentally-Healthy-Jenny was her mental illness. Were it not for her illness, Jenny, qua Mentally-Healthy-Jenny, would have done right, not wrong. Jenny's illness counts as a difference for why, between Sarah and her, Jenny is excused and Sarah is not. But here we would counter that the initial motivation for regarding mental illness as a grounds for excusing is that it impeded an agent's exercise of her freedom to a degree that undermines responsibility. However, in this case, there is no such impediment for Jenny if Sarah is not impeded—and we have simply stipulated as a feature of the case that Sarah is not impeded. So, we would counter this critic by pointing out that it now seems that she is simply assuming that mental illness is *itself* a basis for excuse even when it does not in itself count as an impediment that would be grounds to excuse any agent from lacking a pertinent degree of freedom.

At this point, our critic might respond by pointing out that Jenny's freedom is impeded at least by comparison with that of a Mentally-Healthy-Jenny. That is not true for Sarah. Of course, this is correct. But it is irrelevant. Most fully morally responsible agents most of the time act in suboptimal conditions which are such that, if things were different in some way, then they would have performed better. (Sometimes their blood sugar is low and they are not as mentally crisp as they otherwise would be.) Regardless, when they act above some threshold (such as that of Tina's) they make themselves liable to be held to account by fair standards. If Jenny was just as free as Sarah was, Jenny was just as able as Sarah to act well rather than badly. She was just as much responding objectionably to the poor reasons as Sarah would have been had Sarah been similarly situated. Furthermore, as we noted above, surely there are details about Sarah's situation and history that make it true that if they had been slightly different, then Sarah too might instead act differently were she in a similar situation. Indeed, this is true for pretty much every agent in most every context in which they act. Should all of these agents also then be excused, or should some mitigating factor also apply to them? If not, why? Is it because mental illness is somehow a special basis for excusing above and beyond the degree to which it affects freedom? If so, it is our critic's burden to state what the special basis is, since it was originally assumed that mental illness in these contexts excuses by impairing freedom.[36]

Naturally, the preceding treatment is not unique to depression. We could just as well have executed our argument by working with a case of generalized anxiety disorder or instead with attention deficit disorder. Both in their mild forms are bound to causally influence the execution of the sorts of exemplary acts of deliberative agency we highlighted in section 6. And both are bound to do so in ways that are liable to have some bearing on an agent's reasons-responsiveness and so her degree of freedom. People with anxiety disorder find it difficult to control persistent worries. Of course this will affect their ability to assess reasons presented to them, as their consciousness will frequently be drawn to the worrisome facets of their environments in ways that could "crowd out" attending to other matters. Also, the impulse to act in ways that would alleviate the worry will have an effect on their motivational systems. As for attention-deficit disorder, as we already noted above, this can affect a person's ability to attend to the reasons she has for judging what is best to do, and also for retaining those judgments when committing on a plan and forming intentions to act as she judges best. With these sorts of illnesses as well, in their mild form, it seems a live possibility that the casual influence these conditions might have on an agent could affect her in a way that does not undermine her freedom and responsibility for acting as she does.

We closed the previous section by raising the prospects for a limited kind of skepticism about moral responsibility: If many people are mildly mentally ill, and if their illness plays a significant causal role in many of their actions much of the time, then many people are not morally responsible for much of what they do. Or, if they are, they are less responsible than one might otherwise think. Is this true? In this section, by focusing just on the freedom condition for moral responsibility, we have attempted to resist this skeptical worry. We have tried to make credible a causal story according to which mental illness might influence a morally responsible agent's freedom without impeding it and so without excusing her—or for that matter without even providing grounds for mitigation. We believe we have cast doubt on this skeptical thesis. But can we in good conscience answer our question by confidently asserting that the answer is no—by asserting that the skeptical thesis is false? Of course not. Our effort to resist this skeptical challenge is by way of a just-so story that we believe is consistent with how the actual causal facts might be. But in the end, this is an empirical question to be settled by the sciences of psychology and psychiatry. It might simply be that the way a condition like depression, even in its mild form, "gums up" the causal machinery of deliberative rational agency is simply inconsistent with the contention that an agent like Jenny really could be similar in relevant ways to an agent like Sarah. Our job as philosophers is to help clarify what is at issue, not to pronounce on how agents like Jenny or others suffering from mild mental illness might really be causally shaped.

9. Conclusion

We began this paper by promising to scrutinize the pervasive assumption that mental illness undermines morally responsible agency. It is for this reason that mental illness is allegedly assumed to defeat an agent's culpability for moral wrongdoing. As stated, we do not wish to reject outright this assumption as a default presupposition. As an initial point of inquiry, learning that a person is mentally ill provides a defeasible reason to consider the possibility that the person's competency as a morally responsible agent is defeated or compromised in some way. But in our estimation, this assumption should function as no more than a presumptive starting point for further inspection.

In this paper, we have advanced two main theses. First, we have argued that when a plea of mental illness does carry exculpatory force, it does not always do so by demonstrating that a person is not a morally responsible agent. That is, it does not always exempt. Sometimes it excuses, and it may even sometimes justify. If so, important moral consequences follow insofar as the mentally ill person can still be regarded as competent moral agent. As well, she may bear responsibility arising from the moral residue of her (excused) moral wrongdoing.

Second, we have challenged the presumption that mental illness is always at odds with moral responsibility and blameworthiness for wrongdoing. We have attempted to make credible the thesis that sometimes a person's mental illness might play a nontrivial causal role in her actions and yet she could still be morally responsible and blameworthy for acting as she does. We fully acknowledged that our second thesis is at the mercy of the empirical details of how mental illness really functions—of the underlying dirty details in the etiology. But we do hope to have clarified how it might be that those with mild mental illness could persist in being morally responsible for what they do. To this extent, we mean to have countered the skeptical worry that if many people suffer from at least mild mental illness, and if their illness has a direct effect on much of what they do, then many people are not morally responsible for a wide swath of their behavior.

We close with one final observation: The default assumption we set out to scrutinize comes with a considerable risk. It is a costly and disturbing affair for one to come to see one's own behavior as the product of an illness. But what seems especially disturbing about it is the further dubious presupposition that this is at odds with retaining an understanding of one's self as a morally competent person who remains accountable for herself. Both of our main theses are meant to help make clear that the mere presumption that one is mentally ill, and that her behavior sometimes flows from her illness, does not provide decisive grounds for one to conceive of herself merely as a patient and not as a competent, accountable person, one who retains her dignity in the face of the burdens that plague her.

Acknowledgments

For helpful advice on various issues developed in this paper, we would like to thank Ishtiyaque Haji, Terry Horgan, Alfred Mele, Shaun Nichols, David Shoemaker, Danielle Steffey, and Mark Timmons. We would also like to thank the editors, Gary Gala and Daniel Moseley, for kindly inviting us to contribute to this volume.

Notes

1 For the moment, we use "excuse" to include what might more accurately be expressed by "exemption." Exempting excuses show that a person is so impaired that she is incapable of being a morally responsible agent. Other excuses show that one who is a morally responsible agent is not blameworthy for some bit of wrongdoing.

2 We also take it as an assumption that there is such a thing as mental illness. Surprisingly, this is something that has at times been emphatically denied (e.g., Szasz 1960). See Graham (2013: Chap. 4), for an extended defense of the reality of mental illness.

3 According to a U.S. Department of Justice Bureau of Justice Statistics study, 56 percent of jail and prison inmates have a mental health problem (James and Glaze 2006).

4 Moreover, it is likely that there is a deeper explanation for the similarities between moral and legal responsibility. According to David O. Brink (2013), they share a similar architecture, and the normative grounds for each are rooted in the notion of fair opportunity. While Brink's diagnosis of the underlying normative rationale is perhaps contestable, the fact that moral and legal responsibility share a similar architecture is not. Nevertheless, Brink also takes care to point out and explain the differences between the two sets of norms and practices.

5 For an especially interesting discussion of the relationship between mental illness and moral responsibility, see the exchange between Craig Edwards (2009) and Jerome C. Wakefield (2009). While their contributions are most illuminating, one shortcoming is that both uncritically accept that our current legal practices and norms are reliable grounds for theorizing about the relation between mental illness and moral responsibility.

6 For a debunking of recent attempts by neuroscientists to show that no one has free will, see Mele (forthcoming).

7 Substance dualism is the thesis that the mental is not physical but instead constituted from nonphysical substance that interacts with the physical. Most contemporary philosophers reject substance dualism.

8 We note, moreover, that, as various philosophers have argued, even if it were proven that no one had free will and that free will turned out to be irreconcilable with naturalistically respectable accounts of human nature (whether deterministic or indeterministic), the assumption that we have free will is something about which we should not (Strawson 1962; Smilansky 2001) or could not (Strawson 1962; Nichols 2007) disabuse ourselves.

9 We felt it important to begin this section with the preceding paragraph, since we intend our contribution to this volume to be interdisciplinary. We offer an essay not just to philosophers but also those whose training is primarily in psychiatry. So we want to take care to avoid the misimpression that our focus upon free will is fundamentally at odds with the respectable scientific presuppositions of psychiatric research and practice.

10 For example, see Fischer (1994), Fischer and Ravizza (1998), Haji (1998), McKenna (2013), Mele (2006), and Pereboom (2001).

11 One can also be morally responsible for doing what is morally right or exemplary, and so can be morally praiseworthy. But our focus here is the relation between moral responsibility, mental illness, and excuse—where excuse offers a reason not to hold responsible for wrongdoing.

12 There is considerable controversy over how to explain the sense of appropriateness involved regarding the relation between blameworthiness and blame. Some claim that it is best understood in terms of desert (e.g., Pereboom 2001). Some argue that it can be understood in terms of fairness (e.g., Wallace 1994). We can set that dispute aside here. For an assessment of the controversy, see McKenna (2012).

13 The analog in the law is criminal insanity. The criminally insane are persons who do criminal wrong (and so are, in a sense, legal agents, beings capable of violating laws), but are not legally responsible agents and so cannot be held legally accountable for their conduct.

14 Bjorklund (2004) has doubted whether a mental illness can ever do more than fleetingly take a person's capability for moral responsibility. In a similar vein, Wear (1980) has argued that there can only ever be a diminishing of one's moral responsibility, it never being the case that it is entirely absent.

15 This is not to say that Josephine would not acquire any distinct moral obligations or burdens at all as regards her relationship with Joe. To the extent that Joe is left emotionally

alone and she cannot help him as she usually does, Josephine might owe it to Joe to tend to him as soon as she can. She might owe him a debt of gratitude for his being understanding, and so on. But she would not owe him anything as a result of having wronged him.

16 For non-Tourettic individuals, it would be the equivalent of an itch so overwhelming that you would be willing to scratch it vigorously even in delicate company.

17 Some think it is questionable whether the Tourettic individual would even be excused in such a situation (see Schroeder 2005).

18 What about mitigation? Just as mental illness might fully exonerate from responsibility by exempting or excusing, so too it might diminish responsibility by partially exempting or partially excusing. We'll not pursue this further here, as its extension from the previous discussion seems easily accessible.

19 The distinction between these two types of pleas has its roots in Aristotle's conditions for voluntariness (Nicomachean Ethics 1190b30–1111b5). Contemporary philosophers have taken it on for theorizing, not about voluntariness, but instead about moral responsibility, sometimes appealing to it (as we are) in an account of how mental illness can absolve one of wrongdoing (Elliott 1996; Bjorklund 2004). An application of the distinction can be found in P.F. Strawson's seminal paper "Freedom and Resentment" (1962), wherein Strawson also distinguishes between excuses and exemptions (without using the labels) and in doing so distinguishes epistemic excusing considerations from control excusing considerations. See also Fischer and Ravizza (1998: 12–14).

20 While this distinction between epistemic and control conditions has been often appealed to in understanding how mental illness might excuse (see Elliott 1996; Bjorklund 2004), it is not necessarily a clean one, and marking it is in some respects an artifice. It nonetheless appears theoretically useful, since some features of responsible agency are clearly merely epistemic, and others are clearly about an agent's control. That is adequate for our purposes here. For a careful treatment of this issue, see Mele (2010).

21 These two conditions for morally responsible agency have their parallel conditions for criminal responsibility and the conditions for criminal insanity, according to the American Law Institute's Model Penal Code (2.09).

22 Briefly, to note just two problems with MB: First, the knowledge condition (b) is too stringent because it does not allow for culpable ignorance. Moreover, it requires that an act for which one is morally blameworthy be morally wrong. But it seems that one could be morally blameworthy for acts that are not morally wrong but morally objectionable in some different way (bad or vicious, for example). For a more refined account of moral blameworthiness, see McKenna (2012).

23 Reasons-responsive theorists include Brink and Nelkin (2013), Dennett (1984), Fischer (1994), Fischer and Ravizza (1998), Duggan and Gert (1979), Haji (1998), McKenna (2013), Nelkin (2011), Sartorio (forthcoming), and Wolf (1990), among numerous others. For an account of mental illness characterized partially in terms of impairments to reasons-responsiveness, see Graham (2013).

24 What is meant by a reason? What is at issue here are practical reasons as in contrast with theoretical ones, where practical reasons are just reasons aimed at settling the question of what to do. As for what such reasons are, we wish to remain neutral as between different theories. For present purposes they can be understood as justifying considerations counting in favor of a course of action. Bear in mind, however, that even a brute desire to do something can give rise to a consideration in favor of so acting insofar as satisfying a desire is something that can count in favor of acting.

25 See Mele's case of the agoraphobic (1992: 87).

26 Certainly, the most detailed and impressive development of this strategy can be found in Fischer and Ravizza (1998). For other ways of developing such a theory, see Brink and Nelkin (2013), and McKenna (2013).

27 The view of freedom we shall ultimately settle on shares some illuminating similarities with Allen E. Buchanan and Dan W. Brock's compelling account of competence in decision

making (Buchanan and Brock 1990). While we develop our view by very different means, the results are similar.

28 Why for imperfect beings? For several reasons. For example, a perfect being would not need to exercise strength of will in the face of temptation since her motivations would always effortlessly align with what she judges best. Moreover, all of the best reasons would effortlessly present themselves to her.

29 In sketching these action-theoretic elements, we are relying upon a very rough approximation to the elements of stable, self-controlled action figuring in Mele's work. See for example Mele (1995).

30 On the topic of psychopath, see Haji (2010), Levy (2007), Maibom (2008), and Vargas and Nichols (2007). On the topic of autism, see Kennett (2002). And, finally, on the topic of mental retardation, see Shoemaker (2011).

31 But see Bjorklund (2004) and Schroeder (2005) for discussion of some of the less sensational kinds of mental illnesses.

32 This assumption is at odds with one of the criteria listed in DSM IV for illnesses such as "Major Depressive Episode." In particular, in the cases we have in mind, it would be misleading to describe a subject as experiencing "clinically significant distress or impairment in social, occupational, or other important areas of functioning" (APA 1994: 356). We are imagining cases that permit mild or even moderate impairment rather than significant. Here we set aside the difficult conceptual question as to how one can characterize "mild" cases as mental illness at all in the absence of significant impairment. We shall simply assume we are entitled to expressions like "suffers from a mild form of depression" in contexts that leave subjects functional in most of their daily lives.

33 According to a 2012 SAMHSA survey, 18.2 percent of the US population suffers from a clinically diagnosable mental illness (2013).

34 Timothy Schroeder (2005) insightfully explores an interesting case that is in certain respects similar to the one we develop here.

35 To our knowledge, the only philosophers who have ever explored depression in terms of reasons-responsiveness are Justin Coates and Philip Swenson (2012). Our discussion tracks theirs in certain respects, and we have profited considerably from studying their excellent paper. Despite that, it seems that perhaps our view is at odds with theirs, although it is not clear, since they do not explicitly consider a case in which two agents are equally reasons-responsive when one's responsiveness is influenced by mental illness and the other's is not.

36 At this point our critic does have one viable avenue worth pursuing. She can argue that freedom and moral responsibility are essentially historical properties. Two agents qualitatively identical in terms of their nonhistorical features (like Jenny and Sarah) might differ in terms of their freedom and responsibility properties due to historical differences in how they came to have those features. (For example, see Fischer and Ravizza 1998; Haji 1998; and Mele 1995.) We cannot pursue this here, as space does not permit it. Nor do we wish to foreclose the viability of an historical theory of freedom and responsibility. But we would note that the details of a credible historical theory need not be incompatible with our diagnosis of Jenny. That is to say, Jenny's illness and the way it causally influences her conduct might be of a sort that would not conflict with what would be involved in satisfying the conditions of an historical theory according to which she would still act freely and be morally responsible.

References

American Law Institute. Model Penal Code, §2.09.

American Psychiatric Association. 1994. *Diagnostic and Statistical Manual of Mental Disorders, 4th ed*. Washington, DC: APA.

Aristotle. 1985. *Nicomachean Ethics*. trans. Terrence Irwin. Indianapolis: Hackett.

Bjorklund, P. 2004. "'There but for the Grace of God': Moral Responsibility and Mental Illness." *Nursing Philosophy* 5(3): 188–200.

Brady, J. B. 1997. Carl Elliott, "The Rules of Insanity: Moral Responsibility and the Mentally Ill." *The Journal of Value Inquiry* 31(4): 579–81.

Brink, David. 2013. "Responsibility, Incompetence, and Psychopathy." The Lindley Lectures, University of Kansas.

Brink, David O., and Nelkin, Dana K. 2013. "Fairness and the Architecture of Responsibility." In David Shoemaker (ed.), *Oxford Studies in Agency and Responsibility*, Vol. 1. New York: Oxford University Press, pp. 284–314.

Buchanan, Allen E., and Brock, Dan W. 1990. *Deciding for Others: The Ethics of Surrogate Decision Making*. Cambridge, UK: Cambridge University Press.

Church, Jennifer. 2003. "Depression, Depth, and the Imagination." In J. Phillip and J. Morely (eds), *Imagination and Its Pathologies*. Cambridge, MA: MIT Press.

Coates, D. Justin, and Swenson, Philip. 2012. "Reasons-Responsiveness and Degrees of Responsibility." *Philosophical Studies* 165: 629–45.

Dennett, Daniel. 1984. *Elbow Room: Varieties of Free Will Worth Wanting*. Cambridge, Mass: MIT Press.

Duggan, Tim, and Gert, Bernard. 1979. "Free Will as the Ability to Will." *Nous* 13: 197–217.

Edwards, Craig. 2009. "Changing Functions, Moral Responsibility, and Mental Illness." *Philosophy, Psychiatry, & Psychology* 16(1): 105–7.

Elliott, C. 1996. *The Rules of Insanity: Moral Responsibility and the Mentally Ill*. Albany, NY: SUNY Press.

Fischer, John Martin. 1994. *The Metaphysics of Free Will*. Oxford: Blackwell Publishers.

——, and Mark Ravizza. 1998. *Responsibility and Control: An Essay on Moral Responsibility*. Cambridge: Cambridge University Press.

Graham, George. 2013. *The Disordered Mind*. New York: Routledge Press.

Haji, Ishtiyaque. 1998. *Moral Appraisability*. New York: Oxford University Press.

——. 2010. "Psychopathy, Ethical Perception, and Moral Culpability." *Neuroethics* 3: 135–50.

Hart, H. L. A. 1961. *The Concept of Law*. Oxford: Clarendon Press.

James, Doris J., and Glaze, Lauren E. 2006. *Mental Health Problems of Prison and Jail Inmates*. Bureau of Justice Statistics Special Report No. NCJ 213600. Washington, DC: U.S. Department of Justice, Office of Justice Programs, Bureau of Justice Statistics.

Kennett, J. 2002. "Autism, Empathy, and Moral Agency." *Philosophical Quarterly* 52: 340–57.

——2007. "Mental disorder, Moral Agency, and the Self." In B. Steinbock (ed.), *The Oxford Handbook on Bioethics*. Oxford Handbooks Online.

Levy, Neil. 2007. "The Responsibility of the Psychopath Revisited." *Philosophy, Psychology, and Psychiatry* 14: 129–38.

Maibom, Heidi. 2008. "The Mad, the Bad, and the Psychopath," *Neuroethics* 1: 167–84.

McKenna, Michael. 2005. "Reasons Reactivity and Incompatibilist Intuitions." *Philosophical Explorations* 8(2): 131–43.

——. 2012. *Conversation and Responsibility*. New York: Oxford University Press.

——. 2013. "Reasons-Responsiveness, Agents, and Mechanisms." In David Shoemaker (ed.), *Oxford Studies in Agency and Responsibility*, Vol. 1. New York: Oxford University Press, pp. 151–84.

Mele, Alfred. Forthcoming. *Free: Why Science Hasn't Disproved Free Will*. New York: Oxford University Press.

——. 1992. *Springs of Action*. New York: Oxford University Press.

——. 1995. *Autonomous Agents*. New York: Oxford University Press.

——. 2006. *Free Will and Luck*. New York: Oxford University Press.

——. 2010. "Moral Responsibility for Actions: Epistemic and Freedom Conditions." *Philosophical Explorations* 13: 101–11.

Nelkin, Dana. 2011. *Making Sense of Freedom and Responsibility*. New York: Oxford University Press.

Nichols, S. 2007. "After Incompatibilism: A Naturalistic Defense of the Reactive Attitudes." *Philosophical Perspectives* 21(1): 405–28.

Pereboom, Derk. 2001. *Living Without Free Will*. Cambridge: Cambridge University Press.

Sartorio, Carolina. Forthcoming. *Causation and Free Will*. Oxford: Oxford University Press.

Substance Abuse and Mental Health Services Administration. 2013. *Results from the 2012 National Survey on Drug Use and Health: Mental Health Findings*. NSDUH Series H-47, HHS Publication No. (SMA) 13–4805. Rockville, MD. Available at: http://archive.samhsa.gov/data/NSDUH/2k12MH_FindingsandDetTables/2K12MHF/NSDUHmhfr2012.htm. Accessed April 28, 2015.

Scanlon, T. 2000. *What we Owe to Each Other*. Cambridge, MA: Belknap Press of Harvard University Press.

Schroeder, Timothy. 2005. "Moral Responsibility and Tourette Syndrome." *Philosophy and Phenomenological Research* 71: 106–23.

Shoemaker, David. 2011. "Attributability, Answerability, and Accountability: Toward a Wider Theory of Moral Responsibility." *Ethics* 121: 602–32.

——. 2015. *Responsibility from the Margins*. Oxford: Oxford University Press.

Smilansky, S. 2001, June. "Free Will: From Nature to Illusion." *Proceedings of the Aristotelian Society* (Hardback) 101(1): 71–95.

Strawson, P. F. 1962. "Freedom and Resentment." *Proceedings of the British Academy* 48: 187–211.

Szasz, T. S. 1960. "The Myth of Mental Illness." *American Psychologist*, 15(2): 113.

Vargas, Manuel, and Nichols, Shaun. 2007. "Psychopaths and Moral Knowledge." *Philosophy, Psychology, and Psychiatry* 14(2): 157–62.

Wakefield, Jerome C. 2009. "Mental Disorder and Moral Responsibility: Disorders of Personhood as Harmful Dysfunctions, with Special Reference to Alcoholism." *Philosophy, Psychiatry, and Psychology* 16(1): 91–99.

Wallace, R. Jay. 1994. *Responsibility and the Moral Sentiments*. Cambridge, MA: Harvard University Press.

Watson, Gary. 1996. "Two Faces of Responsibility." *Philosophical Topics* 24(2): 227–48.

Wear, S. 1980. "Mental Illness and Moral Status." *Journal of Medicine and Philosophy* 5(4): 292–312.

Wolf, Susan. 1990. *Freedom Within Reason*. Oxford: Oxford University Press.

4b

Commentary on Kozuch and McKenna: Mental Illness, Moral Responsibility, and Expression of the Self

Chandra Sripada

In their superbly argued piece, Kozuch and McKenna observe that philosophers, "when attending to issues of mental illness, tend to fix on dramatic cases" (p. 103). They are right; there is indeed a tendency in the field to convey an impression of mental illness as something extraordinary, exotic, and rare. The reality is quite different. Mental illness is remarkably common. Most forms are mild or moderate in severity. Symptoms are often episodic with extended intervals of high functioning in between. The manifestations of mental illness are often localized to a specific context allowing typical functioning in most other situations.[1] Indeed, the idea that there is any clear boundary between mental illness and mental health has been coming under increasing attack. Mounting evidence suggests that at the level of behavior, neural mechanisms, and genes, there are only dense continua of variation, with no sharp gaps that mark off order from disorder.[2]

P. F. Strawson said that we sometimes take an "objective attitude" towards persons who are severely impaired or incapacitated (Strawson 1962). They are not to be reasoned with as much as managed, handled, trained, or treated. However, whatever role the objective attitude might appropriately play in the "dramatic cases," for the ordinary cases that are by far more common, this approach seems out of place. This attitude is simply too blunt and pessimistic; it fails to respect the substantial quantities of agency that in the ordinary cases are certainly preserved.

Kozuch and McKenna's focus is on developing a more refined account of moral responsibility for individuals with mental illness; one that is applicable to mild and moderate forms of disorder. They write, "There are, presumably, numerous people living among us, carrying on their lives well enough, who suffer from some mild form of mental illness such as depression, anxiety disorder, or attention-deficit disorder" (p. 103). They set out to produce an account of moral responsibility that allows that such agents are at least some of the time, if not most of the time, fully morally responsible for what they do. To be sure, however, in certain specific circumstances their conduct might still be excused.

I am in solid agreement with Kozuch and McKenna that there is a need to develop this sort of more-refined approach to moral responsibility. Disagreements emerge, however, when we turn to the actual content of their proposed account. A thumbnail summary of their approach goes like this: They begin by observing that most all excuses fall into just two categories—"I didn't know" and "I couldn't help it." This observation suggests that moral responsibility involves at least two distinct conditions that correspond to these two categories of excuse, an *epistemic* condition and a *control* condition, respectively. They focus on the control condition; they analyze the kind of control required for moral responsibility in terms of reasons-responsiveness. They then provide a detailed analysis of the case of Jenny, who has mild depression. They argue that she is morally responsible for what she does because, though the illness plays a causal role in the etiology of her actions, she nonetheless exhibits sufficient levels of reasons-responsiveness.

My disagreement with this proposal arises at the very first stage with their claim that "I couldn't help it" is properly understood as an excuse that pertains to a putative control condition for moral responsibility. In what follows, I want to make two points. First, I argue that when a person invokes "I couldn't help it" as an excuse, what the person says not only conveys that she lacks control over what she does, it also conveys a further piece of information. It says, very roughly, the person's *self*, the part of her that specifies what she cares about and where she stands on matters of value, opposes her action, and thus her self is not at all *expressed* in what she does.[3] I argue it is this further thing that is conveyed—the failure of self-expression and not the failure of control—that actually serves as the basis for excuse. Second, I look in detail at their case of Jenny and argue that this case allows for a quite different interpretation. In my favored interpretation, it is preservation of self-expression rather than preservation of control that explains why Jenny, despite her having depression, remains morally responsible for what she does.

1. The "I Couldn't Help It" Excuse

Consider the following claim:

> CHI: A person is not responsible for doing what he did if he couldn't help doing what he did.

We should all agree that CHI seems at first pass to be plausible. But if we delve further into *why* the principle seems correct, interesting things emerge.

I believe that CHI draws its support from focusing on cases in which a person is forced to do something against his will, for example, cases of physical coercion or irresistible desires. Consider the following vivid case due to the philosopher Harry Frankfurt.

Unwilling Addict

> [The man] hates his addiction and always struggles desperately, although to no avail, against its thrust. He tries everything that he thinks might enable him to overcome his desires for the drug. But these desires are too powerful for him to withstand and invariably, in the end, they conquer him. He is an unwilling addict, helplessly violated by his own desires.
>
> *(Frankfurt 1971: 12)*

Intuitively, the Unwilling Addict is not morally responsible for what he does. When we search for a reason to explain this, the fact that the Unwilling Addict "couldn't help it" looms large in our minds. That is, since he lacks control over what he does, he is not morally responsible for what he does, or so it seems.

But before we settle on this conclusion, consider an additional case. Frankfurt also presents a matched case of the *Willing Addict*, whose desire for the drug "has the same physiological basis and same irresistible thrust" as the Unwilling Addict. However, he does not at all oppose his drug-directed desire:

> [H]e is altogether delighted with his condition. He is a willing addict, who would not have things any other way. If the grip of his addiction should somehow weaken, he would do whatever he could to reinstate it; if his desire for the drug should begin to fade, he would take steps to renew its intensity.
>
> *(Frankfurt 1971: 19)*

Frankfurt argued that the Willing Addict *is* morally responsible for his drug-directed action. I believe this conclusion is correct; if we are careful to interpret the case appropriately, then there is good reason to believe that the Willing Addict is in fact morally responsible for what he does. If this is right, then we have a result that contradicts CHI. The Willing Addict both couldn't help doing what he did and is morally responsible for what he did. I embrace this upshot. I think CHI is indeed false as stated. Moreover, I want to provide a more detailed explanation for *why* CHI, even though false, nonetheless initially seemed so plausible.

However, before I get to all this, I want to spend more time to make the case that the Willing Addict is in fact morally responsible for his drug-directed actions.[4] In order to reach this conclusion, we have to interpret the case appropriately. This takes some work, not in least part because the case is quite underdescribed. So let me fill in a few more details.

First, we must put aside interpretations of the Willing Addict case that invoke what Kozuch and McKenna call "tracing considerations" (p. 103). The Willing Addict would no doubt be morally responsible for using the drug if at some prior time he knowingly and intentionally got himself addicted in the first place. For that matter, the Unwilling Addict would certainly be morally responsible as well. Interpreting these cases in terms of tracing considerations is thus uninteresting. This interpretation sheds no light on the nature of the "I couldn't help it" excuse because the addict's current state "traces back" to a time when they *could* help it. The more interesting claim is that a Willing Addict-type agent *who is not at all culpable for getting himself addicted in the first place* is morally responsible for what he does. It is this version of the case that I will be assuming in what follows.

The Willing Addict is stipulated to have an *irresistible desire* to use the drug. In order to interpret the case correctly, we must get clearer on what this means. While there are presumably a number of different ways in which a desire might be irresistible, let me offer a quick sketch of *one* specific way in which an irresistible desire could occur.

My sketch draws heavily on the picture set out by Kozuch and McKenna of how "well-functioning agency" unfolds (p. 101). Agents, when faced with the question of what to do, engage in deliberation. During this process, they assess the worth of various candidate courses of action in light of their values and their cares. Deliberation concludes in a practical judgment of what overall is the thing to do. Agents also have various other motivational states: desires, preferences, emotions, and so forth. These can potentially oppose their practical judgments. When such opposition exists, agents can exercise strength of will (i.e., willpower) to resist the wayward motives. If the strength of a person's faculty of resistance is greater than the strength of the opposed motive, then the opposed motive can be reigned in, and the person's practical judgment can prevail. This picture naturally suggests how a desire could be irresistible: A person has an irresistible desire when the strength of her faculty of resistance is exceeded by the strength of her opposed desire.

Based on the preceding picture, here is how I understand the unfolding psychological events that lead to the Willing Addict's action:

The Willing Addict feels a desire to use the narcotic.
He deliberates on whether he should in fact use the narcotic. Based on his values and cares, he arrives at the practical judgment that he surely should.
He throws the weight of this practical judgment behind the desire to use the narcotic making this desire yet stronger.
He uses the narcotic.

Now, were the Willing Addict to throw the weight of his practical judgment in the other direction and resist the desire for the drug, he would fail. The desire to use the drug is stronger, perhaps just infinitesimally so, than the strength of his faculty of resistance. The Willing Addict's desire to use the drug is thus irresistible.

Of course the Willing Addict doesn't throw the weight of his deliberative judgment against the desire for the narcotic. This is not because he knows that he will fail at resisting; that is, he is not a "defeated addict." Rather, it is strictly because he has no interest whatsoever in resisting his drug-directed desire. He loves his desires for the drug and doesn't at all want to restrain them.

I believe when we reflect on this case, we think the Willing Addict is morally responsible for his drug-directed actions. Why should it matter that his powers of resistance are ever so slightly weaker than the desire he acts on? What matters is that the cares and values that constitute his genuine practical point of view, that is, the attitudes that constitute his self, via their role in shaping his practical judgment, motivationally support what he in fact does.

Another way we can appreciate this point is to imagine the following. Suppose, unbeknownst to him, the Willing Addict's powers of resistance were augmented by just a tiny amount, just enough so they now exceed the strength of the desire for the narcotic. In my view, nothing would change with regard to whether or not he is morally responsible for what he does. This is because both before and after the augmentation the causal etiology of his action is precisely the same; it consists in the unfolding of the sequence of steps 1–4 listed above. Endowing the Willing Addict with the power to resist a desire that he has no interest whatsoever in resisting, and indeed that he instead actively supports and whose strength he in fact enhanced, does not affect whether he is morally responsible for what he does.

The preceding discussion suggests that CHI is false: The Willing Addict couldn't help doing what he did but he is still morally responsible for what he did. Now, Kozuch and McKenna use CHI as a starting-off point to develop their control-based view of moral responsibility. But if CHI is false, it suggests that their control-based approach could be off on the wrong track from the very beginning.

If control is not the basis of moral responsibility, then what is? Our discussion of the Unwilling Addict and Willing Addict cases suggests the answer. The only respect in which the two addicts differ appears to be in terms of expression of their respective selves. The Unwilling Addict's self is not expressed in his action (indeed, his self strongly opposes what he does), while the Willing Addict's self is very much expressed in his action. These cases thus provide evidence that it is self-expression, and not control, that really matters for moral responsibility.

Earlier I said that "I couldn't help it" does in fact *seem* plausible as an excuse, at least at first pass. We are now in a position to delve deeper into why this is the case. When a person who has done something wrong sincerely avows "I couldn't help it," he is telling us more than what his statement strictly says. He is conveying that he did what he did *only because* he couldn't help it. And a person's doing something only because he couldn't help it is another way of saying something roughly like this: "I opposed what I did, but there was a force that made me do it despite my whole-hearted opposition. It is only because of this force that I did it, and what I did thus does not express my self."[5]

The phenomenon here—in which what a statement conveys goes well beyond what it strictly says—is an instance of what philosophers and linguists call *pragmatic implicature*. Suppose I announce that I ate half of the pie. Given the implicit norms that govern conversation, it would be appropriate for listeners to infer that I *only* ate half the pie, and I did *not* eat the whole pie. Now this doesn't follow as a matter of semantic entailment. What I utter, as a matter strictly of the meaning of my words alone, is consistent with my having eaten the entire pie—any person who eats an entire pie also eats half of it. Yet saying what I said conveys more than what is strictly said, and this extra element is the pragmatic component implied by my message. Similarly, someone's saying "I couldn't help it" pragmatically implies that he did it *only because* he couldn't help it, which as I've just argued is simply another way of saying what he did does not express his self.

If all this is correct, then the "I couldn't help it" excuse is not an excuse based on control at all. Rather, it is an excuse rooted in the self-expression approach to moral responsibility.

2. The Context-Sensitivity of Mental Illness

One of Kozuch and McKenna's most interesting claims is that a person can be morally responsible for an action even if mental illness plays a causal role in the etiology of the action. I think this claim is correct and it represents an important insight. Kozuch and McKenna support this claim in the context of a detailed analysis of the case of Jenny, a woman with mild depression. I want to examine Kozuch and McKenna's reasoning more closely. I will suggest that this case, which is put forward to illustrate their reasons-responsive account of moral responsibility, might be better understood in terms of the self-expression account of moral responsibility that I favor.

The case of interest concerns Jenny, who breaks a promise and fails to pick up a friend at the airport. Jenny suffers from mild depression and, as a result of the effects of the illness on her judgment and motivation, she displays a pattern of reasons-responsiveness that is more constricted than it would otherwise be. This constriction is sufficient for it to be the case that were the depression absent, she would pick her friend up from the airport. So in this sense, her depression causally influences her failing to pick up her friend.

The constriction in reasons-responsiveness due to the depression is, nonetheless, relatively slight; indeed, the extent of her reasons-responsiveness is quite similar to Sarah, a person who is psychologically healthy. Summarizing a bit, Kozuch and McKenna reason as follows: Sarah would surely be morally responsible and blameworthy were she to fail to pick her friend up from the airport. Given that Jenny displays a pattern of reasons-responsiveness that is roughly similar to Sarah's, then Jenny is morally responsible and blameworthy as well.

As I see it, the problem with this reasoning is that it seems to conflict with a plausible thesis about mental illness that Kozuch and McKenna themselves appear to accept. Mental illnesses, especially milder varieties, often create obstacles to the proper execution of one's agency only in certain highly limited circumstances and not in other closely related circumstances. Kozuch and McKenna write, "A person suffering from a mental illness … might be perfectly capable of being held to account for her conduct in some domain of activity and yet, nevertheless, her illness might, on a particular occasion, impede her ability to exercise her conduct in that very domain of activity" (p. 93). Call this idea that mental illness can produce highly local barriers to one's agency the *context specificity of mental illness thesis*, or CSMIT for short.

I want to now present two alternative versions of the Jenny case that illustrate why CSMIT creates problems for Kozuch and McKenna's reasons-responsiveness-based approach.

Consider a version of the Jenny case, call it Jenny-A, in which she is stipulated to care deeply about her friend; she has no ill will whatsoever towards her friend. When she fails to pick up her friend from the airport, no part at all of her self is expressed in what she does. It is rather a combination of the depression and situational factors that explain why she failed to keep her promise to her friend. Furthermore, let me stipulate that Jenny-A's pattern of reasons-responsiveness remains just as it is described by Kozuch and McKenna: There are a fair many counterfactual situations somewhat different from the actual one where, were there sufficient reason to pick up her friend, she would do so.

Is the Jenny-A case as I described it genuinely possible? That is, can it really be the case that a person is prevented from expressing her self in the actual situation, and yet the person maintains a moderate extent of reasons-responsiveness, such that in various alternative situations where there is sufficient reason to do otherwise she does so? I believe that this is indeed possible. Moreover, CSMIT appears to back this up. CSMIT says that mental illness can impose a highly narrow, context-specific barrier to a person's agency in the actual context, while such barriers are mostly absent in roughly similar counterfactual contexts, so CSMIT appears to allow that Jenny-A's pattern of reasons-responsiveness can indeed occur.

Given that the Jenny-A case appears coherent, let us evaluate the case further in terms of whether Jenny is blameworthy for failing to pick up her friend. I am inclined to say that, so long as we heed the stipulation that in the actual situation Jenny's action expresses no ill will whatsoever, then she is not blameworthy for what she does.[6] That is, it seems to me that once we know for certain that there is no ill will at all expressed in what she does, facts about what Jenny would do in counterfactual situations that differ somewhat from the actual one aren't relevant to whether she is blameworthy.

Now consider another version of the Jenny case, call it Jenny-B. In this version of the case, she *does* harbor substantial ill will towards her friend (or perhaps, given her ill will, "friend" would be better). Moreover, given the way her agency unfolds in the actual sequence of events, her self *is* expressed in her failing to pick up her friend. She is glad, indeed wholeheartedly so, that her friend is stranded. Additionally, let me stipulate that Jenny-B's pattern of reasons-responsiveness is very sharply constricted: In alternative situations where there is sufficient reason to pick up her friend (it would have to be selfish reasons to pick up the friend since by hypothesis she harbors ill will towards this person), she would *not* pick up her friend—the mental illness would manifest in these alternative situations by throwing up barriers to the proper execution of her agency.

Once again, it seems that CSMIT allows that the situation described in the Jenny-B case is possible. Indeed, her reasons-responsiveness profile resembles that of the Willing Addict in that her mental illness permits expression of her self in the actual circumstances but raises barriers to her agency in a range of counterfactual circumstances.

When we evaluate the Jenny-B case in terms of whether she is blameworthy for what she did, it seems to me that what matters is that her ill will towards her friend is clearly expressed in what she actually did. Because of this, she is blameworthy for what she did. Once again, facts about what she would do in counterfactual situations that differ somewhat from the actual one aren't relevant to whether she is blameworthy.

The pattern we see emerging in the preceding cases seems to be this: If we are given only limited facts about the reasons-responsiveness of agents, as is the case for the agents presented in Kozuch and McKenna's discussion, we are inclined to infer that a person with a suitably wide pattern of reasons-responsiveness (such as Jenny or Sarah) is morally responsible for what she does, while a person with a very narrow range of reasons-responsiveness (such as their case of Tina, who has very severe depression) is not morally responsible for what she does. But if we are directly given the facts about whether expression of the person's self (and in particular, facts about expression of ill will harbored by the person's self) successfully occurred, then facts about patterns of reasons-responsiveness in various counterfactual situations no longer seem to matter—these facts seem to be *superseded*.

I contend that the best explanation of these observations is that we tend to use patterns of reasons-responsiveness across a range of counterfactual situations as *evidence* for whether expression of the self has occurred in the actual situation. All we are told about Jenny, Sarah, and Tina is how reasons-responsive they are—just a little, somewhat, or very much. Given the information we have, we do the best we can in making inferences about moral responsibility. These inferences, however, are defeasible. If we are directly supplied the facts about self-expression, these initial inferences might very well be overturned. This is precisely what happens with the Jenny-A and Jenny-B cases. Jenny-A has wide reasons-responsiveness but is still not blameworthy for what she does because no ill will on the part of her self is expressed in what she does. On the other hand, Jenny-B has minimal reasons-responsiveness, yet she is blameworthy for what she does because the ill will harbored by her self is expressed in her action.

3. Conclusion

Kozuch and McKenna's project is an important one. They aim to develop a more refined account of moral responsibility for individuals with mental illness, one that is applicable to mild and moderate forms of mental disorder. They adopt a control-based approach that analyzes the relevant form of control needed for moral responsibility in terms of reasons-responsiveness. I have provided some initial reasons to believe an approach based on self-expression might well be more promising.

Notes

1 These were some of the findings from the landmark 1994 National Comorbidity Study, which has since undergone several rounds of updates. See Kessler *et al.* (1994).
2 See for example Meyer-Lindenberg and Weinberger (2006) and Robbins *et al.* (2012).
3 In my "Self-Expression: A Deep Self Theory of Moral Responsibility" (Sripada under review-a), I provide detailed accounts of a person's self and the conditions under which the self is expressed in action. For the purposes of this commentary, an intuitive understanding of these notions will suffice.
4 I present a comprehensive case for why the Willing Addict is morally responsible for his drug-directed actions in my "Frankfurt's Unwilling and Willing Addicts" (Sripada under review-b). The arguments that follow summarize certain select arguments from that manuscript.
5 Readers may recognize that the argument being advanced here closely parallels the argument offered in the closing section of Frankfurt's "Alternate Possibilities and Moral Responsibility" (Frankfurt 1969).
6 I am assuming here a broadly Strawsonian "quality of will" account of the conditions of blameworthiness. My favored version of such an account says a person is blameworthy for an action if and only if the attitudes of her self that are expressed in the action are morally objectionable. For a lucid and sophisticated discussion of quality of will accounts of blameworthiness, see McKenna (2011: chap. 3).

References

Frankfurt, Harry. 1969. "Alternate Possibilities and Moral Responsibility." *The Journal of Philosophy* 66 (23): 829–39. doi:10.2307/2023833.

——. 1971. "Freedom of the Will and the Concept of a Person." *The Journal of Philosophy* 68 (1): 5–20. doi:10.2307/2024717.

Kessler, R. C., McGonagle, K. A., Zhao, S., Nelson, C. B., Hughes, M., Eshleman, S., Wittchen, H. U., Kendler, K. S. 1994. "Lifetime and 12-Month Prevalence of DSM-III-R Psychiatric Disorders in the United States: Results from the National Comorbidity Survey." *Archives of General Psychiatry* 51 (1): 8–19. doi:10.1001/archpsyc. 1994. 03950010008002.

McKenna, Michael. 2011. *Conversation & Responsibility*. New York: Oxford University Press.

Meyer-Lindenberg, Andreas, and Daniel R. Weinberger. 2006. "Intermediate Phenotypes and Genetic Mechanisms of Psychiatric Disorders." *Nature Reviews Neuroscience* 7 (10): 818–27. doi:10.1038/nrn1993.

Robbins, Trevor W., Claire M. Gillan, Dana G. Smith, Sanne de Wit, and Karen D. Ersche. 2012. "Neurocognitive Endophenotypes of Impulsivity and Compulsivity: Towards Dimensional Psychiatry." *Trends in Cognitive Sciences*, Special Issue: Cognition in Neuropsychiatric Disorders, 16 (1): 81–91. doi:10.1016/j.tics.2011.11.009.

Sripada, Chandra. under review-a. "Self-Expression: A Deep Self Theory of Moral Responsibility."

——. under review-b. "Frankfurt's Unwilling and Willing Addicts."

Strawson, Peter. 1962. "Freedom and Resentment." *Proceedings of the British Academy* 48: 187–211.

Part 2

Ethical Dimensions of Psychiatric Treatment

5a

Coercion in Psychiatric Treatment and Its Justifications

George Szmukler

1. Introduction

Coercive interventions in psychiatry have troubled me since my medical student days. Indeed, Sidney Bloch, who was at the time a senior trainee, and I wrote an article for the Melbourne University Magazine on the subject, in which we tried to work out our ideas on psychiatry and social control. Fortunately, I don't have a copy to examine how well we did. After graduating and completing my years of residency in general medicine and surgery, these concerns initially acted as a deterrent to training in psychiatry. In the end, the fact that this specialty was by far the most interesting determined my career choice.

Subsequently, I have had no regrets about my decision, though coercion has continued to worry me. It quickly became evident to me that compelling patients to have treatment against their wishes was the most unpleasant aspect of practice, while for patients it was often the most humiliating. I had the good fortune to have Professor Gerald Russell as a mentor, and he helped me to obtain a research grant from the Department of Health to investigate the subject of my preoccupation. Thus my doctoral dissertation was on "Compulsory Admissions to Psychiatric Hospitals in a London Borough." My study investigated the circumstances of a compulsory admission of 150 consecutive patients from the Borough of Camden in 1977–78. Every fifth informal patient was a control. Being an empirical study, my focus was on the processes that led to admission. The most striking finding was that compulsory admissions were a recurrent event for the majority of patients I saw and that there was a clear failure to engage patients in treatment following discharge. The implications I drew were that outpatient services needed to be redesigned so that the frequency of crises would reduce, and that the management of crises, when they did occur, needed some new ideas, introducing specialist crisis teams being one. Too often it was left to the police to initiate the admission (Szmukler et al. 1981; Szmukler 1981).

At the time of my study, the Mental Health Act 1959 for England and Wales was in force. Involuntary admission was based on the person having a "mental disorder" (i.e. "mental illness, arrested or incomplete development of mind, psychopathic disorder and any other disorder or disability of mind") of a nature or degree warranting detention in a hospital "in the interests of the person's own health or safety or with a view to the protection of others." A police officer, finding a person in a public place who appeared to be suffering from a mental disorder and in "immediate need of care and control" could take the person to a "place of safety" "in the interests of that person or for the protection of others" (HMSO 1959). Although I discussed the ethical aspects of compulsion, this was framed in terms of the debate current at the time – the difficulty of reconciling a legal framework protecting rights with a medical framework offering treatment. There were calls for stronger legal controls and for a stronger focus on "dangerousness." I am sorry to say that I, in common with almost everyone at the time, entirely missed the way in which mental health legislation discriminates against persons with a mental illness. A critical area of discourse eluded us.

I did not uncover this blind-spot until the early 1990s. Attention at that time, especially in the English-speaking countries, had turned to a new idea – the introduction of involuntary outpatient treatment (or Community Treatment Orders). As the focus of mental health care was shifting so decidedly from hospital to community, it was argued, why should involuntary treatment be restricted to hospital inpatients only? This led me to think again about the fundamental justifications for compulsory treatment. Two major influences affected me around that time. The first was an enlightening volume by Campbell and Heginbotham, "Mental Illness, Prejudice, Discrimination and the Law" (1991). The second was the English Law Commission's investigation into the proposal for a "mental capacity" statute that would bring clarity and coherence to the common law on the non-consensual treatment of patients in general. The former showed very persuasively that mental health legislation was unfairly discriminatory against persons with a mental illness and gave expression to two culturally embedded stereotypes of mental illness: that affected persons were incompetent or not fully "persons"; and that these persons were dangerous. The Law Commission's deliberations brought home the interesting fact that involuntary treatment of persons with mental illness was governed by an entirely different set of rules to those governing the involuntary treatment of general medical or surgical patients. A further aspect was especially troubling. The main driver for involuntary community treatment, in England at least, seemed to be the idea that community care was failing and that the public needed protection from dangerous, "non treatment-compliant mental patients," who were now at large on our streets. Homicides by persons who had been in contact with mental health services received huge media coverage, while the government mandated independent inquiries following every such case – their reports, and the press conferences associated with each of them, adding further to the publicity. This, despite the evidence showing that homicides by those with mental illness were not increasing, and indeed, since homicide rates in the population as a whole were steadily rising, mental illness-related homicides accounted for a decreasing proportion of total homicides (Taylor and Gunn 1999; Large et al. 2008).

2. Coercion

Before looking at justifications that can be offered for imposing involuntary treatment, it is worth asking the question: What do we mean by "coercion"? When forced treatment was restricted to hospital inpatients, we tended to think about coercion as being involuntary treatment under a legal order. With the emphasis now on treatment in the community, and especially with service innovations such as involuntary outpatient treatment (IOT), or assertive community treatment (ACT) (involving measures, such as home visits, even uninvited, to prevent patients from dropping out of treatment), the scope for treatment pressures on reluctant patients has expanded.

Paul Appelbaum and I (Szmukler and Appelbaum 2001; Szmukler and Appelbaum 2008) have presented a spectrum of "treatment pressures" based on differences that we hold are morally relevant. A line can be drawn at a point when such pressures can be termed "coercion." The hierarchy is as follows: (1) persuasion; (2) interpersonal leverage; (3) inducements or offers; (4) threats; (5) compulsion. Following Wertheimer (1987), we argue that "coercion" occurs when pressures are exerted at the level of "threats" or "compulsion."

Persuasion involves an appeal to reason, an appraisal of the benefits and risks of treatment for the particular patient based on evidence. The process does not go beyond a debate. In *interpersonal leverage*, the relationship established between clinician and patient is key. In services such as ACT, this relationship becomes more intimate than in traditional outpatient clinics. Key-workers may engage with patients to help with quotidian requirements, such as budgeting, shopping, and cleaning. They may help in accessing a range of non-healthcare services. The patient may consequently develop a significant degree of emotional dependency and may then wish to please someone who has proved helpful.

The next level of pressure arises with the introduction of conditional "if/then" propositions. *If* the patient accepts treatment A, *then* the clinician will do X; or *if* the patient does not accept treatment A, the clinician will do Y. At this point, application of the term *coercion* is likely to be considered. Wertheimer argues that *threats* coerce but *offers* (or *inducements*) generally do not:

> The crux of the distinction between threats and offers is that A makes a threat when B will be worse off than in some relevant base-line position if B does not accept A's proposal, but that A makes an offer when B will be no worse off than in some relevant base-line position if B does not accept A's proposal.

What properly fixes the "baseline"? Wertheimer argues for a "moral baseline" and gives an example. A comes upon B who is drowning. A proposes to rescue B on condition that B pays A a large sum of money. There are no other potential rescuers. Has A made a threat or an offer? The answer depends on where we set the baseline.

Under a moral test, the key issue is whether A is *morally required* (ought) to rescue B (or whether B has a *right* to be rescued by A). If A is morally required to rescue B, then B's baseline includes a right to be saved by A. A's proposal is therefore a threat. On the other hand, if A is not morally required to rescue B, then A's proposal is an offer. A *threat* thus anticipates making the recipient worse off according to the proposed moral baseline, while an *offer* – even if declined – typically does not. Baselines other than "moral" have been proposed. For example, a "legal" baseline has been proposed by Bonnie and Monahan (2005). This is more easily defined than a "moral" baseline, but has the disadvantage of relativity, being dependent on the law in a particular place.

There are two kinds of act that resemble coercion, but they do not meet the definition above. The first is *exploitation* (Wertheimer 1996, 2001; Rhodes 2000). Exploitation involves an offer that nevertheless takes *unfair advantage* of a person in a difficult predicament. Rhodes considers the example of a homeless person in a cold climate who is offered a warm apartment but at a very high rent. The threat is a "background threat," and not of the landlord's doing. The key issue is the moral baseline. On Wertheimer's account, exploitation, while often morally questionable, is not "coercive." Is it the person's "right" in this example to be offered a room at a "fair" rent? Most would say it is not. Further, exploitative offers, in some sense, expand possibilities for the recipient; if the offer is not accepted, the person is no worse off than he would have been if the offer had not been made. Both the exploiter and the person exploited can derive advantage from an exploitative offer (a warm room for the former, and a larger income for the latter). The harm lies in taking *unfair advantage* of a person who is at a disadvantage. The second is an *unwelcome* prediction. If a clinician were to say to a patient that stopping medication will result in involuntary admission to hospital, a distinction can be drawn between this being an *unwelcome prediction* – a statement of fact, over which the clinician has no control – or a threat. Much depends on the factual basis of the prediction; the past history may indicate repeated similar instances that have resulted in a compulsory admission. Whether the clinician will be an instigator of the event is also relevant. A prediction of an unwelcome event, based on sound evidence, would not be considered as "coercive." However, a clear line between them may be difficult to draw in practice.

The Problem with Inducements

Inducements can be problematic. An example is a proposal to pay non-compliant patients with a psychosis to accept treatment (Claassen et al. 2007). As an offer it is therefore not "coercive." Yet the results of a survey of clinicians in the UK revealed a widely held intuition that the practice is unethical (Claassen 2007). There may be a number of explanations for this. First, the transaction involves an exchange of "goods" involving what might be seen as "incommensurable values" – that is, values that cannot be measured on a single metric, one good being in a higher, and thus separate, domain than the other. Selling a child is a stark example. Such an exchange corrupts or degrades the higher value. In paying patients to take medication, money could be seen as being exchanged for an aspect of respect for the person – that is, there is a failure to respect a patient's decision about what is in his or her best interests (assuming the patient has capacity).[1] The person's agency is threatened with being undermined. There is also a denigration of the treatment: it becomes a commodity rather than having a value in fostering human flourishing. Second, there may be a possibility of exploitation. It is the patient's vulnerability, psychological or material – often both, that would induce an acceptance of the offer. As noted above, in exploitation one party gains unfairly at the expense of the one who is exploited (even though the exploitee may still derive some gain) (Mayer 2007). Who gains here? A significant motive for monetary inducements may be to reduce costs to the health service by preventing relapse and rehospitalization. Third, there is an issue concerning the fairness of paying non-treatment-adherent patients but not treatment-adherent patients. There is also a range of other problems – for example, ensuring treatment adherence actually occurs, and how possible it would be in practice for payment to be terminated (for a more detailed discussion of the issues, see Szmukler 2009).

There are other problems with inducements that may appear on the surface to be less troubling, for example, offering a ticket to a football match or introducing the patient to a second-hand-furniture store whose owner is sympathetic to people with a mental illness. Fairness is one. Why should not all patients have such benefits or assistance? Again there is a lack of regard for the patient's sense of agency and a potential devaluation of the treatment. The reason for accepting treatment may be not because it has value related to human flourishing but because of a value measured on a metric appropriate to commodities.

Having reflected further on the problematic aspects of inducements in mental health care, I am now inclined to place them outside the hierarchy of treatment pressures and to conclude that they have little or no place in treatment. In most everyday settings, offers may be less coercive than threats. Many will be quick to point out that exposure to financial incentives are commonplace in many spheres of life in our market-orientated society. However, the particular context of mental health care requires special recognition. Our patients commonly experience a lack of respect from many sources for their preferences and values, and are marginalized as participants in society. Psychiatric treatments should aim to empower patients and strengthen their sense of personhood and agency, not undermine them. Inducements are likely to be undermining. There is an important argument to be had here.

3. Compulsion

Next in the hierarchy of pressures is *compulsion*, legally authorized. As mentioned above, a number of jurisdictions have introduced *IOT* orders. Three forms can be discerned:

1. As a substitute for involuntary hospital admission: IOT is considered a less restrictive option when alternatives to compulsory treatment have been exhausted.
2. To facilitate earlier discharge from hospital (a form of conditional discharge): The patient is not considered well enough to leave hospital as a voluntary patient, but could do so if compulsion ensured treatment acceptance.

3. To prevent relapse: There is a proven history of relapse secondary to discontinuation of treatment, and relapse is believed to pose a significant risk to the patient or others.

Outpatient commitment orders carry varying powers (Dawson 2005). Some allow recall of the patient for compulsory treatment as an inpatient. Others may permit the conveying of the patient to a clinic where forced treatment can be administered. Still others only permit conveyance to a clinic to be subject to non-coercive treatment pressures. IOT orders also vary in the range of conditions attached to the order (e.g., specification of clinician, clinic, frequency of reviews, treatments, residence) and their duration (Dawson 2005).

Finally, there is the option of *compulsory admission to hospital.*

4. Objective and Subjective "Coercion"

There is a distinction to be made between "objective" and "subjective" coercion. The subjective experience may not follow an "objective" schema such as the one above. Indeed, studies have shown a disjunction between subjective coercion and involuntary status. Patients' perceptions of how fairly they have been treated and the motives of decision makers may be more influential than actual legal status. For a patient, this may be the most important aspect. However, for clinicians seeking a framework for justifying coercive interventions, distinctions of an "objective" kind may prove more helpful. The hierarchy outlined above attempts to meet this aim, but it may also need to take account of a particular patient's preferences and values.

5. Justifications for Coercive Interventions

The Anomalous Position of Mental Disorder

At this time, clinical practice is best established for the extreme end of the coercion spectrum – that is, legally enforced compulsion. Although there have been swings at different epochs between the degree of discretion and power given to doctors versus protections of liberty through legal process, the basis for involuntary treatment in psychiatry has been more or less unchanged since the early to mid-nineteenth century (Szmukler 2014). I suggest this is a good place to start a discussion of justifications since the conventional approach, despite being widely accepted, is, I shall argue, unfairly discriminatory and based on denigrating stereotypes of people with mental illness. Furthermore, if it is inappropriate at the extreme end of coercion, it is likely to prove even more unsuited to the less extreme forms – for example, to decision-making in relation to involuntary outpatient treatment, and, indeed, lesser forms of treatment pressure such as whether an uninvited home visit or contact with a relative against the patient's wishes can be justified.

The vast majority of mental health statutes permit involuntary detention (or civil commitment), usually including involuntary treatment, essentially when two criteria are met: First, that the person is suffering from a mental disorder – variably but generally loosely defined; and second, that there is a risk of some kind to the person or to others. In England and Wales, for example, involuntary admission and treatment (s3 of the Mental Health Act 1983) requires that the person is suffering from a "mental disorder" of a nature or degree that makes it appropriate to have treatment in hospital and that this is "necessary for the health or safety of the patient or for the protection of other people" (HMSO 1983). The second, "risk," criterion varies across different jurisdictions, sometimes being broadly drawn so that a need for treatment weighs substantially, and in other places narrowly drawn, emphasizing dangerousness with an imminent risk of physical harm. When a person meets the necessary criteria, the legislation will usually authorize their certification by medical practitioners, their emergency detention (including transportation to a hospital or place of safety), their compulsory assessment followed by treatment when deemed necessary, which may continue provided the person's involuntary status as a whole is kept under regular, continuing review by a court or tribunal.

What is noteworthy is a comparison with the very different criteria characterizing statutes or case law governing the involuntary treatment of patients in medical specialties other than psychiatry. Examples here include the restraint of patients attempting to leave a ward who are confused post-operatively or due to an adverse drug reaction or serious infection, or whose level of consciousness is impaired following a head injury, epilepsy or stroke. In countries with developed legal systems, there are usually two criteria that are required for restraint or involuntary treatment in such cases. These are, first, that the person lacks decision-making capacity (or competence); and, second, that the treatment is in the person's "best interests" (BI). A patient with a "physical disorder" may refuse treatment even if the disease is life-threatening. UK courts, and other common-law jurisdictions in Western countries, set a very high value on the person's "autonomy" (in the sense of being able to determine what shall be done to one's body). A mentally competent patient has an absolute right to refuse to consent to medical treatment for any reason, even where the decision may lead to death. We accept this decision unless there is reason to believe that the patient's decision-making capacity is impaired.

Decision-making capacity and BI require much more discussion and will be considered in more detail below. For the present argument, the following definitions may suffice. Decision-making capacity involves the patient's ability to understand and retain information about the nature of the treatment, why it is being proposed, and the consequences of accepting it or not, and to use and weigh up that information so as to arrive at a choice. The patient "appreciates" the information, accepting its relevance to his or her predicament. Furthermore, he or she is able to generate and weigh the consequences of accepting or rejecting the proposed treatment for his or her life in the light of what is important for that person. BI, in the way I prefer it to be understood, attempts to determine what the patient might have chosen in this situation if he or she had retained capacity, based on past statements (as in an advance statement) or according to accounts of the person's values and preferences from those who know the patient well. When a future period of incapacity can be anticipated, a patient may also appoint a person to take healthcare decisions on his or her behalf according to stated preferences or principles.

There is thus a huge difference in the approach to involuntary interventions for "mental" versus "physical" disorders. The former is based on the person having a particular "status" – that is, being categorized as having a "mental disorder," and then being deemed to present a risk to the person or to others. Unlike the position of someone with a "physical" disorder, there is no consideration of whether persons with a "mental" disorder are able to make the required treatment decision for themselves – that is, are able to pass an appropriate "functional" test of their decision-making ability. The patient's reasons for rejecting the treatment do not require exploration (as must be done in determining capacity), nor, explicitly, is the question of whether treatment is in the best interests of the patient. The key considerations are the presence of a mental disorder and risks to the patient's "health or safety," presumably from the perspective of the clinician or treatment team (or other representatives of society), not the patient. But we accept that patients with physical disorders, provided they have capacity, can make decisions that may be seriously detrimental to their apparent well-being. For persons with capacity, their personal values are given dominion. Those with mental disorder are not accorded the same privilege.

Why are the Legal Regimes Different?

How can we account for the differences between the two legal regimes? The most likely explanation is that deeply entrenched stereotypes of mental illness are at work. The first is that people with mental illness are, by virtue of being mentally ill, "incompetent"; their deranged minds mean they cannot make competent decisions. Their wishes and values are thus not accorded the same respect as for those without a mental illness. This stereotype is grossly inaccurate. The vast majority of people with a mental illness, even those with a diagnosis of a "serious mental illness," have capacity for all or most decisions, all or most of the time. Even patients in their most distressed or disturbed states and ill enough to be admitted to an acute psychiatric ward retain capacity for treatment decisions in around 50 percent of cases (Owen et al. 2008). Furthermore, even if capacity is more likely to be impaired in persons with a mental illness, there is no good reason why it should not be tested in the individual patient who is rejecting a treatment proposal in an odd manner, as it is for all non-psychiatric patients.

The second stereotype is that people with mental illness are intrinsically dangerous. A consequence of this stereotype is a clear form of discrimination in conventional mental health law. People with mental disorders are unusual in being liable to detention (albeit in hospital) because they are assessed as presenting a *risk* of harm to others, but without having actually committed an offence. This is best illustrated diagrammatically in Figure 5a.1. Those in the larger circle might include, for example, habitual spouse abusers, those with short tempers – especially when intoxicated or provoked – or those who drive recklessly. The smaller circle comprises everyone with a mental disorder. Only those people in the area of overlap between the circles, those with mental disorders who are judged "risky," can be detained under mental health legislation on the basis of risk alone. This constitutes a form of preventive

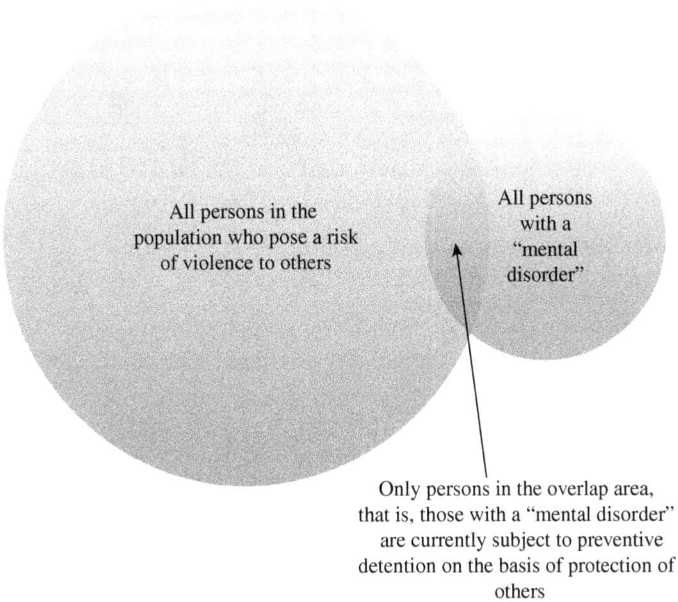

Figure 5a.1 Mental disorder, risk, and protection of others

detention. Such provisions are usually available both under civil and forensic provisions of the legislation.

Imagining that everyone in the larger circle presents an equal level of risk – assuming that this can be accurately judged (which in reality it cannot: see, for example, Large et al. 2011; Szmukler and Rose 2013) – why should the person with a mental disorder in the overlap zone be more liable to be detained on the basis of that risk than the person without a mental disorder? If preventive detention is to be allowed for the mentally disordered solely on account of their risk to others, if we are to avoid discrimination, so should it be for all of us. Thus fairness demands that all those presenting an equal level of risk to others (that is, all those in the larger circle in Figure 5a.1) should be equally liable to detention. This of course amounts to a generic dangerousness or preventive detention provision against which many, including me, will recoil. But the principle of non-discrimination requires that either we have generic legislation applicable to all of us, or that we have no preventive detention for anyone, including those with mental disorder.

On the issue of dangerousness it is worth pointing out that this may be a consequence of having a mental illness in a small minority of patients. The risk, in the absence of alcohol or substance misuse, or of an antisocial personality – that is, someone who already has a propensity to commit antisocial acts – is only modestly raised. People with severe mental disorder perpetrate a small fraction of serious violence in our society, probably around 5 percent (Fazel and Grann 2006). Violence is no more predictable in them than in those without a mental illness, nor is the propensity for violence clearly more "treatable" in them. Psychological interventions to reduce violence, such as "anger management" for violent persons who are not mentally ill, such as spouse abusers, may be more effective than interventions for those who are mentally ill. However, even if violence were much more common in people with a mental illness, the discrimination I have described would still be unjust.

6. Towards Justifications for Coercion that are not Discriminatory: The "Fusion Law" Proposal

The most obvious means of avoiding discrimination against persons with a mental illness is by no longer differentiating between them and other persons. In other words, whatever the provisions that govern coercive interventions, they should be generic and equally applicable to all persons, regardless of the type of diagnosis, whether it be a mental or a physical disorder. A "status" criterion of "mental disorder" or something similar should not operate. (This becomes of special significance, as we shall see, when we come to consider the implications of the UN Convention on the Rights of Persons with Disabilities, 2006.)

What kind of legislative framework would thus be non-discriminatory? Let us look first at the most extreme form of coercion: compulsion. John Dawson and I have proposed what we termed a "Fusion Law" (FL) (Dawson and Szmukler 2006). This would be a single, generic statute, covering everyone, in any medical specialty, in any area of healthcare – and indeed social care, in any setting. There would be no separate mental health or civil commitment legislation. The FL would address persons where there are indications they have an impairment of decision-making in relation to a serious decision. We propose that the basis of such a framework would rest squarely on an impairment of decision-making capacity, or, for reasons I shall discuss later, is probably better termed "decision-making capability" (DMC). In this respect it is founded on similar principles to those underlying the non-consensual treatment of people in general medicine under a "Mental Capacity" Act or "Guardianship" legislation (though certainly not of the type where plenary guardianship is permitted).

In our proposal, involuntary treatment would only be permitted, first, when the patient has an impairment of DMC and, second, if treatment would be in the patient's BI. What is especially important is that the impaired DMC could be of any cause – a head injury, post-epileptic confusion, schizophrenia, confusion due to an adverse drug reaction or infection, Alzheimer's Disease, and so on. Involuntary treatment would cease when DMC had been re-established in a sufficiently stable manner.

Why have we termed the approach "fusion"? The proposal builds on the strengths of the two existing regimes. Existing capacity-based legislation's strength in giving due weight to autonomy is nearly always counterbalanced by a number of weaknesses. These lie in the lack of sufficient attention to emergency treatment, forced treatment and detention in hospital. But these are exactly those areas in which civil commitment schemes are strong; detention and the use of force are clearly authorized and regulated. The lack of clarity in these areas in capacity-based legislation may pose a problem for the treatment of patients with "physical disorders" who object to treatment, as it would for those with mental disorders. Patients who object to treatment but who do not suffer from a "mental disorder" may be treated under civil commitment – inappropriately – because of a reluctance of clinicians to use force unless they can rely on clear statutory authority. Or perhaps they are not treated at all even though treatment would have been in their best interests.

Coercion in the Community

If a patient lacks DMC and treatment is in his or her BI (and can be given effectively and safely), the analysis above suggests no ethical objection to the treatment being given in the community rather than in a hospital. But non-consensual treatment should end when the patient recovers DMC. This is especially important in the use of outpatient commitment to prevent relapse in patients with a history of persistent non-compliance. Such orders may be prolonged for months if not years. Clear criteria for terminating the order are essential. In the FL framework, the criteria for termination of the order would be based on recovery of DMC (or, if impaired DMC continues, the compulsory treatment no longer being in the best interests of the patient).

It should be evident that the DMC-BI principles are also applicable to the justification of interventions in the community that fall short of compulsion – for example, making uninvited home visits or contacting relatives against the patient's wishes, or making threats to do so. If the patient retains or has regained DMC, such interventions would be unjustified. I argued earlier that inducements were difficult to justify in the mental healthcare context where patients had DMC. Perhaps there is scope for inducements where DMC is impaired, where such an intervention would be in the person's BI, and it would cease when DMC is regained. However, I imagine that the agency-undermining effect and the devaluing of the treatment by its monetization would weight heavily in the BI determination.

Implication for the "Protection of Others"

Some people raise the question about what the FL would entail concerning the "protection of others." Two circumstances where there may be a danger to others could be covered by the BI requirement. These are where the BI of the patient are served by measures that involve the protection of others, for example, where a patient is violent to their spouse resulting from delusional jealousy and where what has been a long-term, stable, and valued relationship is threatened with irreversible breakdown. The second instance is where the treatment of the person in their BI incidentally endangers others, for example, on a ward, where until the treatment is effective, the patient is aggressive to others. In cases where the person with a mental illness presents a danger to others, retains DMC, but refuses treatment, even if it might reduce the likelihood of violence, recourse to the criminal justice system would be necessary – as it would be for a person without a mental disorder, even where an intervention exists that might reduce the risk of violence.

Where a person with a mental disorder has committed an offence, especially a serious one, the following principles would apply. First, any mentally impaired offender with DMC who consents to their treatment could be treated in an appropriate facility (while any sentence could continue to run). Second, any offender who lacks DMC could be treated involuntarily like any other impaired DMC patient if treatment is in their BI.

Two options can be proposed for a person with an impairment or disturbance of mental functioning who has committed a serious criminal offence:

1. The person can be sentenced to the usual period of imprisonment, but if they were found to lack DMC and need treatment, they could be transferred to hospital for necessary care. If DMC is regained in hospital, the person could continue treatment with consent; if not, transfer to prison for the remainder of their sentence would occur. A sentenced person retaining DMC and who would benefit from treatment in hospital could be offered it, but would need to accept it voluntarily.
2. The court could make an involuntary treatment order without a concurrent sentence, which would deem the person lacking DMC to be subject to an equivalent civil order. The responsible clinician would terminate the order when the necessary conditions for civil patients were no longer met.

Some object that the FL provides no equivalent of a "restriction" order to ensure long-term treatment, usually extending well beyond the period of treatment in hospital. However, discharge from hospital does not mean that a person deemed dangerous would have no more than a referral to a mental health service. Under the first option above, in some jurisdictions, as in England, the sentence might be an "extended sentence" for persons convicted of a serious offence who are deemed to pose a risk beyond the term of a normal sentence. If so, the person would subsequently be under some form of post-discharge supervision in the community, possibly for life. Even if supervision cannot compel treatment, at the very least the person would be regularly monitored and appropriate action could be taken if there is a relapse of illness. Involuntary treatment could be initiated if the conditions are met. This kind of order is non-discriminatory as it applies to all dangerous offenders with DMC, whether or not they have a mental impairment.

A special problem is presented by criminal defendants found "unfit to plead" or "not guilty by reason of insanity" who are subsequently assessed to have capacity and refuse voluntary treatment and who are deemed dangerous. There is not the space to treat this complex question here. Please see Szmukler et al. (2010) for a discussion.

The Burden of New Regulations in General Medical Settings

Since the FL proposal is for generic legislation, it could impose a set of novel, potentially burdensome regulations governing patients lacking DMC on general hospital wards, some who would now require an involuntary treatment order. The challenge is to formulate a law that is practicable so that all with impaired DMC are covered by the same principles. The domains covered in the FL could vary in the range of requirements – supports, advocacy, consultation with a range of others, reviews – and time intervals for their implementation. It should prove possible to find a combination applicable across the whole range of services. An important contextual factor is the accreditation of health and social care institutions and our confidence in their validity.

7. What Do We Mean by "Decision-Making Capability" and "Best Interests"?

DMC and best interests in the FL proposal carry a heavy burden in justifying coercive interventions. The concepts thus need to be clear enough to meet this use. In medicine, one expects investigations to have a high degree of objectivity. Many slip into expecting the same quality in a test of DMC. However, the judgment is of a different kind. A standardized "objective" test of cognitive functioning such as the Mini Mental State has a modest correlation with a person's ability to make a specific decision at a particular time. As we shall see, assessing DMC may involve an "interpretation" of complex phenomena such as beliefs and values in a particular context. Nevertheless, the research evidence on the inter-rater reliability of DMC assessments points to very good reliability, especially when made by clinicians with a similar training (Cairns et al. 2005). Nonetheless, there will always be difficult cases.

Earlier I presented a common definition of DMC, such as appears in the English Mental Capacity Act (MCA) 2005 or in the MacArthur Competence Assessment Tool (Grisso and Appelbaum 1998): The ability to understand and retain information about the nature of the treatment, why it is being proposed, and the consequences of accepting it or not; the patient "appreciates" the relevance of the information to his or her predicament and is able to weigh the consequences of accepting or rejecting the proposed treatment in the light of what is important for that person.

This kind of assessment has been criticized as being too "cognitive," thus failing to take account of the role of values and emotions in decision-making (Tan et al. 2006). While a large proportion of patients, even those with a psychosis, have an impairment of understanding or retention – that is, they are unable to repeat in their own words the information they have just been given – or they are unable to articulate a decision or make a choice (Owen et al. 2013), there are many instances where the assessment is more problematic. In particular, the patient's beliefs and values call for consideration. The problem here is that the assessment of DMC should respect a person's beliefs and values and not be subordinated to the beliefs and values of the assessor. Thus what has been aimed for, explicitly in the thinking behind the MCA 2005 (as in the Code of Practice), is that the test of DMC should be essentially "procedural," tracking the processes used by the patient, regardless of the substantive content. It restricts itself to how the person manipulates the relevant information in the light of the beliefs and values the person holds, which in themselves are not to be overridden by those of the assessor. Such a procedural test is a laudable aim as it prevents clinicians from deeming a person to lack DMC because they make a seemingly unwise decision. If the decision-making process is intact, the patient is entitled to freely decide.

Unfortunately, a procedural view does not take us as far as our intuitions lead us. For example, a person may refuse treatment because of a paranoid idea that the medication offered is intended to deliberately harm him, or a person with anorexia nervosa may accept the risks of dying through self-starvation since she claims that being thin is more important to her than life itself. Their behavior is "rational" if one accepts their guiding beliefs or values. In these cases it appears that judgments about the content of these beliefs or values cannot be avoided. However, psychiatric diagnoses and treatments can be controversial – disagreeing with a medical recommendation is not necessarily evidence of a failure to appreciate normatively significant facts about one's condition; it may be the result of reflecting critically on the expertise offered. So a key question is: When assessing DMC, how might evaluative judgments about a person's beliefs, values, desires, and decisions be understood, and what degree of "objectivity" can be achieved?

At this point one soon confronts the idea of "autonomy." Decisions that are "autonomous," it is said, should be respected. The problem for the non-philosopher (and perhaps for some philosophers) is the range of understandings of "autonomy." Onora O'Neill, whom a group of us working on DMC invited to give a seminar on the subject, has put it as follows:

> Informed consent in medical ethics is commonly viewed as the key to respecting patient autonomy. This claim is endlessly repeated but deeply obscure. There are many distinct conceptions of individual autonomy in circulation, and even more views of the value and importance of these various conceptions. In a survey of views of autonomy, Gerald Dworkin noted that it has been equated with: Liberty (positive or negative) … dignity, integrity, individuality, independence, responsibility and self-knowledge … self assertion … critical reflection … freedom from obligation … absence of external causation … and knowledge of one's own interest. The list could be extended in many ways, and the feasibility and the value of all conceptions of individual autonomy are hotly contested. It seems to me, however, that if informed consent is ethically important, this cannot be because it secures some form of individual autonomy, however conceived. Informed consent procedures protect choices that are timid, conventional, and lacking in individual autonomy (variously conceived) just as much as they protect choices that are self assertive, self knowing, critically reflective, and bursting with individual autonomy (variously conceived).
>
> *(O'Neill 2003)*

There is clearly a relationship between DMC and autonomy in some senses; varying accounts suggest that autonomy may be foundational for capacity or that having capacity is a necessary condition for autonomy (Freyenhagen and O'Shea 2013). However, the question for the clinician in the situation I am describing can be relatively circumscribed and perhaps made slightly simpler – how far does the person's specific decision at a particular time have the property of being "self-determined" or of being "owned" by the person. Buchanan and Brock (1990), pointing to what this might mean, stated that "a competent decision-maker also requires a *set of values* or *conception of what is good* that is at least minimally consistent, stable and affirmed as his or her own." Clearly required then is that an evaluation of an unusual or apparently imprudent treatment decision must go beyond a simple examination of the content of the decision and the immediate explanation offered by the patient. A complex judgment, or interpretation, may be required.

8. Decision-Making Capability and the Role of Interpretation

I was fortunate, a few years ago, to come across Natalie Banner, a young philosopher who had drawn on Donald Davidson's theory of "radical interpretation" (RI) in thinking about DMC (Banner 2010, 2012). In my view, this approach offers a very helpful way of understanding what an assessment of DMC involves (Banner and Szmukler 2014). RI seeks to make sense of people's utterances and intentional actions from a third-person perspective that does not depend on a prior grasp of substantial theory or knowledge (Davidson 1973a, 1994). Davidson's project examines the conditions for interpretation of a radically unfamiliar speaker. It would thus seem to have applicability to the clinical situation where a person expresses seemingly unusual ideas that lie behind an apparently imprudent treatment decision. If such conditions for interpretation exist, they could shed light on normative standards disciplining how we can assess the intelligibility of a patient's decisions.

Davidson generated an idealized method for understanding the utterances of a radically unfamiliar speaker without any prior knowledge of the speaker's language or his mental states. He argues that the interpreter is licensed to make certain assumptions about the speaker's beliefs and language, owing to the fact that there are intrinsic, normatively governed relationships between the meanings of the speaker's utterances, the beliefs he holds, and the actions he performs, on the basis of which the interpreter can frame his attempts to understand the speaker: "[I]nterpretation depends on reading some of the norms of the interpreter into the actions and speech of those he interprets" (Davidson 1994: 123). Without these normative structures, it would be impossible to understand anyone.

Davidson's account of these norms is known as the *Principle of Charity*. It states that "we must assume that a speaker is by and large *consistent* and *correct* in his beliefs." (Davidson 1973b: 238) These conditions of consistency and correctness are termed "coherence" and "correspondence," respectively. A person's beliefs, intentions, and actions hang together broadly as a more or less coherent whole, and they largely reflect what is true. An interpreter is thus guided by these norms as a first step in trying to understand the speaker. The caveat of "by and large" reflects the fact that an interpretation of a behavioral act is imprecise, may be subject to revision, and need not be rigidly bounded by demands for correspondence and coherence. Our mentality is inherently messy: we form beliefs on partial, perhaps conflicting, evidence; we may act against our own avowed interests; and we may make decisions based on emotional rather than rational thought processes. Davidson's theory allows significant scope for errors. What the standards of Charity do imply is that there must necessarily be a broad background of true and coherent beliefs in order for a speaker to be interpretable at all. Indeed, it is only against this background of largely true and coherent beliefs, shared by an interpreter, that incoherence, errors or irrationalities can be recognized.

A significant consequence of Davidson's view is that the mental realm is holistically constituted; that is, elements within that realm are explicated only through the relations they bear to other elements within that system. Rather than focus on the content of a belief for identifying a mental dysfunction, we need to examine the relations it bears to the person's other beliefs, values, and actions. Exploring the context in which such beliefs arise, their history, and their connectedness with other beliefs, values, and behaviors will identify whether they broadly cohere and are thus capable of supporting, rather than undermining, decision-making capacity.

The assessment thus takes substantive content of beliefs and values into account. However, this need not lead to unwarranted paternalism as the judgment is not arbitrary but normatively governed – interpretation according to Davidson is based on the normative, relational structure of a patient's beliefs, values, and decisions. Thus it is clearly nonsensical to generate a context-independent checklist for determining DMC. Taking the broader holistic context into account points towards the kinds of questions a clinician conducting an assessment of DMC ought to bear in mind. For example, one might examine the consistency of the patient's decision-influencing beliefs with his broader worldview and other values reflecting his or her deep commitments, the empirical support offered for such beliefs, whether they are amenable to revision or argument, and the cultural meaningfulness and rationality of the values impinging upon decision-making, to name but a few possible considerations. It is only if we acknowledge the context surrounding each decision and the relational nature of the beliefs and values impacting on decisions that we are in a position to identify where anomalies occur that might indicate impairment of DMC. Whilst a clear-cut prescription for how capacity judgments should work cannot be offered, there are nonetheless strong grounds for employing a wider scope of enquiry than the "procedural" conception of capacity permits. This assessment is most pertinent to the ability to "use or weigh" component of capacity in the Mental Capacity Act 2005; or to "appreciation" and "reasoning" in the account given by the influential MacCAT-T test of capacity.

A consequence of this method of interpretation is the active role played by the interpreter in attributing belief and meaning to the speaker. It might seem this risks leading to unwarranted paternalism. However, it is better to acknowledge the implicit influences on clinical judgment rather than laboring under the illusion they can be simply procedural. The norms guiding interpretation are the general constraints of attributing broad coherence and correspondence in the patient's overall psychology.

Davidson recognized an inherent "indeterminacy" in interpretation. Perhaps something that thus far appears not coherent may not remain so with further probing of the person's beliefs and values. This is certainly a consideration, but in a real-world clinical encounter, where a decision needs to be made whether a person lacks DMC carrying important consequences, the aim is to reach a point in the dialogue where it is reasonable to conclude whether there is a significant enough breach in the relational structure of the patient's beliefs and values. A degree of "objectivity" appropriate for this purpose is the goal. The assessment can be further tested by asking others (for example, those who know the patient well, or a tribunal or court) whether the evidence is sufficiently convincing. Freyenhagen and O'Shea (2013) suggest the possibility of a process of institutional oversight involving among others those with mental disorders. They propose that those previously affected should have a voice in deciding how evaluations should be interpreted.

If the assessment of capacity, especially in difficult cases, involves more than a reductionist procedural approach, there are some important practical implications. First, understanding the principles of the approach outlined, although based on shared norms of interpretation, probably requires training that goes beyond simple interview skills. Second, a DMC assessment may require substantial time. Observing the actions of the person, as well as consulting with others who know them well, may be important. Such procedures do not fit easily with time constraints imposed by emergency departments, for example. Nor do they comport well with trends in clinical practice to devise straightforward algorithms, checklists or "decision-aids" to assist, standardize, and speed-up clinical decision-making.

9. "Substitute Decision-Making," "Best Interests," and the UN Convention on the Rights of Persons with Disabilities

A significant international development in thinking about the rights of persons with disabilities finds expression in the UN Convention on the Rights of Persons with Disabilities (United Nations 2006) (CRPD). At least some forms of mental illness, most clearly those that may lead to involuntary treatment, are taken by the Committee on the Rights of Persons with Disabilities, the authoritative body, to fall under the Convention. They are termed "psychosocial" disabilities. A fundamental objective of the CRPD is the elimination of discrimination against persons with disabilities. Countries that have ratified the CRPD (139 by January 2014) are placed under a variety of obligations to take measures to modify or abolish existing discriminatory laws, regulations, and practices.

Especially in need of remedy is the loss of rights in many countries of disabled persons placed under various forms of guardianship. These may encompass virtually every sphere of persons' lives with decisions being made for them by others. It is clear that in many instances the legal criteria and safeguards governing such guardianship are highly unsatisfactory (Drew et al. 2011). The social model of disability adopted by the CRPD holds that "disability" is not an attribute located within an individual but that it "results from the interaction between persons with impairments and attitudinal and environmental barriers that hinders their full and effective participation in society on an equal basis with others," and that, with support of varying degrees, these significant barriers can be counteracted.

The emphasis is thus placed on "supported" rather than "substituted" decision-making. A formal system is required to ensure that such support is offered so that the "will and preferences" of the person can be realized.

The aspect of the CRPD that concerns us here is the challenge presented to the use of compulsion in mental health practice. Involuntary treatment is clearly a form of substituted decision-making. Is it also discriminatory? Article 4 states there should be "no discrimination of any kind on the basis of disability." Article 12 requires that persons shall "enjoy legal capacity on an equal basis with others in all aspects of life." Legal capacity means not only possessing rights, but also being able to exercise them. Article 14.1 (b) states that the "existence of a disability shall in no case justify a deprivation of liberty" (United Nations 2006).

Some have interpreted the Convention as apparently ruling out "substitute decision-making" entirely (United Nations Committee on the Rights of Persons with Disabilities 2014).[2] The view is that all persons retain legal capacity and that, with varying levels of support, they can express their "will and preferences." Others, such as the UN High Commissioner for Human Rights, have taken a less extreme position on the possibility of involuntary treatment but argue that, if it is to be justified, it must be non-discriminatory, "disability-neutral". Article 14.1(b) is thus taken to mean that a disability must not be a criterion for involuntary treatment, even if it is linked with other criteria, for example, those relating to the risk of harm to self or others. The requirement that a person have a "mental disorder" thus violates Article 14.

The FL proposal, I suggest, is "disability-neutral" (Szmukler et al. 2014). Recall that it is aimed at eliminating discrimination against persons with mental illness. There is no criterion stipulating a "mental disorder"; it applies to everyone. Any person, whether they suffer from a disability or are completely fit, may experience a period of impaired decision-making capability, for example, following a head-injury, infection, or an adverse reaction to a medication. There might be an argument about whether the impaired DMC itself constitutes a "disability" in the CRPD sense, but if it were so, it would rule out any intervention, no matter the circumstances, where a person was rejecting or resisting treatment. This would not be compatible with moral intuitions in most societies about preventing harms to persons where, due to an impairment of some kind, they are not able to do so themselves.

The CRPD emphasis on support is valuable as it forces us to think more deeply about how it might be offered. Advance statements could play a significant role by clarifying a person's preferences for treatment when they are well, anticipating a time in the future when they are unwell and unable to express them. At this stage we do not know how effective these approaches might be in reducing the need for non-consensual interventions, but it could be substantial (Thornicroft et al. 2013). Research in this area should be given high priority.

The CRPD might also prove helpful in offering a new language for considering involuntary treatment. Instead of talking about "decision-making capacity" or "capability" and "best interests," it might perhaps be better to frame our concepts in terms of "will and preferences." Where a person appears to be having a difficulty with a decision that might carry serious consequences, one would ask "What are the person's will and preferences?" and "Is the decision consistent with these?" If, for any reason, it is not possible to ascertain what the person's will and preferences are, or if there is good reason to believe that the currently expressed will and preferences are at variance with the person's enduring or "authentic" will and preferences, then an intervention might be justified. The aim of the intervention where the person's decision is not in accordance with their will and preferences is to give expression to their "authentic" will and preferences. Such a formulation for the justification of involuntary treatment, no matter the condition or the setting, might indeed prove more satisfactory than one based on our current concepts of "decision-making capacity" and "best interests." It could be argued that facilitating a person's will and preferences at a time when they are unable to do so unassisted and when all attempts at support have failed, is not, in effect, "substituted" decision-making at all. Bach and Kerzner (2010) have proposed that this form of intervention be termed "facilitated" decision-making.

Some of the key problems discussed above obviously remain despite such a change in formulation. Ascertaining what are the person's "authentic" will and preferences may still offer the same challenges to interpretation. Sometimes it may not be possible to determine a person's will and preferences at all, or with much confidence, for example, where someone has a severe life-long intellectual disability. Under these circumstances a decision might need to be made on the basis of what would be most consistent with some notion of "human flourishing." There is not the space here to go into this question any further.

10. Conclusions

The conceptualization of "coercive" interventions, their justifications, and their practice have been neglected in mental health care, despite their baleful effects on both patients and staff. Clinical teams when considering decisions to act against the wishes of a patient – for example, whether to make an uninvited home visit, to initiate involuntary treatment, and so on – usually lack a conceptual framework to assist in their deliberations. This contrasts with the rich discussions about what drug or psychological intervention would be most appropriate. Making good decisions about the use of pressures to further a patient's treatment requires such a framework. I have mapped out a conceptual schema of "treatment pressures," ranging through "persuasion," "interpersonal leverage," inducements, threats and compulsion, which form a rough hierarchy. An examination of current justifications for coercion in health care reveals a gross disjunction between those applied in psychiatric practice versus the rest of medicine. The former fail to respect patients' self-determination in the same way as the latter, and reflect deeply embedded discriminatory stereotypes of people with a mental illness. I have proposed a schema for thinking about coercive interventions based on "decision-making capability" and a version of "best interests" that gives predominance to what the patient would have chosen if their DMC had been retained. The proposed regime, termed the "Fusion Law" model, would apply in all instances where there is an impairment of decision-making, whatever its cause or its setting. It is thus non-discriminatory against persons with a mental disorder. A number of problems raised by this approach have been discussed, especially the limits of a purely "procedural" test for DMC and thus the way in which a person's beliefs and values enter into its assessment. I argued that a form of "interpretation" is required and that Donald Davidson's "radical interpretation" offers a helpful approach to the problem. Finally, I discussed the compatibility of the Fusion Model with the landmark UN Convention on the Rights of Persons with Disabilities (2006) that aims at remedying discrimination against persons with disabilities, including forms of mental illness. I argue that the language of the Convention, particularly the use of the terms "will and preferences," may help in clarifying our thinking about non-consensual interventions and their justifications.

Notes

1 I will consider the case of the person who lacks decision-making capacity later.
2 See the recent General Comment from the UN Committee on the Rights of Persons with Disabilities on "Article 12: Equal Recognition Before the Law" (UN Doc. CRPD/C/GC/1, 11 April 2014).

References

Bach, M., and Kerzner, L. 2010. *A New Paradigm for Protecting Autonomy and the Right to Legal Capacity*. Law Commission of Ontario.

Banner, N.F. 2010. "Judging by a Different Standard? Examining the Role of Rationality in Assessments of Mental Capacity." Doctoral thesis, University of Central Lancashire. Available at www.clok.uclan.ac.uk. Accessed April 23, 2015.

——. 2012. "Unreasonable Reasons: Normative Judgements in the Assessment of Mental Capacity." *Journal of Evaluation in Clinical Practice* 18(5): 1038–44.

Banner, N., and Szmukler, G. 2014. "'Radical Intepretation' and the Assessment of Decision-Making Capacity." *Journal of Applied Philosophy* 30: 379–74.

Bonnie, R.J., and Monahan, J. 2005. "From Coercion to Contract: Reframing the Debate on Mandated Community Treatment for People With Mental Disorders." *Law and Human Behavior* 29(4): 485–503.

Buchanan, Allen, and Brock, Dan. 1990. *Deciding for Others: The Ethics of Surrogate Decision Making*. Cambridge: Cambridge: University Press.

Cairns, R., Maddock, C., Buchanan, A., David, A.S., Hayward, P., Richardson, G., Szmukler, G., and Hotopf, M. 2005. "Reliability of Mental Capacity Assessments in Psychiatric in-Patients." *British Journal of Psychiatry* 187: 372–78.

Campbell, T., and Heginbotham, C. 1991. *Mental Illness: Prejudice, Discrimination and the Law*. Vermont: Dartmouth.

Claassen, D. 2007. "Financial Incentives for Antipsychotic Depot Medication: Ethical Issues." *Journal of Medical Ethics* 33(4): 189–93.

——, Fakhoury, W., Ford, R., and Priebe, S. 2007. "Money for Medication – Financial Incentives to Improve Medication Adherence in Assertive Outreach Patients." *Psychiatric Bulletin* 31: 4–7.

Davidson, Donald. 1973a. "Radical Interpretation." *Dialectica* 27(3–4): 313–28.

——. 1973b. "Psychology as Philosophy." Reprinted in *Essays on Actions and Events*, pp. 229–45. Oxford: Oxford University Press, 2001.

——. 1994. "Radical Interpretation Interpreted." *Philosophical Perspectives*: 121–28.

Dawson, J. 2005. *Community Treatment Orders: International Comparisons*. Dunedin, New Zealand: Otago University Press.

——, and Szmukler, G. 2006. "Fusion of Mental Health and Incapacity Legislation." *British Journal of Psychiatry* 188: 504–9.

Drew, N., Funk, M., Tang, S., Lamichhane, J., Chavez, E., Katontoka, S., Pathare, S., Lewis, O., Gostin, L., and Saraceno, B. 2011. "Human Rights Violations of People With Mental and Psychosocial Disabilities: An Unresolved Global Crisis" *Lancet* 378(9803): 1664–75.

Fazel, S., and Grann, M. 2006. "The Population Impact of Severe Mental Illness on Violent Crime." *American Journal of Psychiatry* 163(8): 1397–403.

Freyenhagen, Fabian, and O'Shea, Tom. 2013. "Hidden Substance: Mental Disorder as a Challenge to Normatively Neutral Accounts of Autonomy." *International Journal of Law in Context* 9(01): 53–70.

Grisso, T., and Appelbaum, P.S. 1998. *Assessing Competence to Consent to Treatment: A Guide for Physicians and Other Health Professionals*. New York: Oxford University Press.

HMSO. 1959. "The Mental Health Act 1959." London: Her Majesty's Stationery Office.

——. 1983. "The Mental Health Act 1983." London: Her Majesty's Stationery Office.

Large, M., Smith, G., Swinson, N., Shaw, J., and Nielssen, O. 2008. "Homicide Due to Mental Disorder in England and Wales Over 50 Years." *British Journal of Psychiatry* 193(2): 130–33.

Large, M.M., Ryan, C.J., Singh, S.P., Paton, M.B., and Nielssen, O.B. 2011. "The Predictive Value of Risk Categorization in Schizophrenia." *Harvard Review of Psychiatry* 19(1): 25–33.

Mayer, R. 2007. "What's Wrong With Exploitation." *Journal of Applied Philosophy* 24: 137–50.

O'Neill, O. 2003. "Some Limits of Informed Consent." *Journal of Medical Ethics* 29(1): 4–7.

Owen, G.S., Richardson, G., David, A.S., Szmukler, G., Hayward, P., and Hotopf, M. 2008. "Mental Capacity to Make Decisions on Treatment in People Admitted to Psychiatric Hospitals: Cross Sectional Study." *British Medical Journal* 337: a448.

Owen, Gareth S., Szmukler, George, Richardson, Genevra, David, Anthony S., Raymont, Vanessa, Freyenhagen, Fabian, Martin, Wayne, and Hotopf, Matthew. 2013. "Decision-Making Capacity for Treatment in Psychiatric and Medical in-Patients: Cross-Sectional, Comparative Study." *The British Journal of Psychiatry* 203(6): 461–67.

Rhodes, M. 2000. "The Nature of Coercion." *The Journal of Value Inquiry* 34: 369–81.

Szmukler, G. 1981. "Compulsory Admissions in a London Borough: II. Circumstances Surrounding Admission: Service Implications." *Psychological Medicine* 11(4): 825–38.

——. 2009. "Financial Incentives for Patients in the Treatment of Psychosis." *Journal of Medical Ethics* 35(4): 224–28.

——. 2014. "Fifty Years of Mental Health Legislation: Paternalism, Bound and Unbound." In *Psychiatry: Past, Present, and Prospects*, edited by S. Bloch, S.A. Green, and J. Holmes. Oxford: Oxford University Press.

——, and Appelbaum, P. 2001."Treatment Pressures, Coercion and Compulsion." In *Textbook of Community Psychiatry*, edited by G. Thornicroft, and G. Szmukler, 529–43. Oxford: Oxford University Press.

——, and Appelbaum, P. 2008. "Treatment Pressures, Leverage, Coercion and Compulsion in Mental Health Care." *Journal of Mental Health* 17: 233–44.

——, and Rose, N. 2013. "Risk Assessment in Mental Health Care: Values and Costs." *Behavioral Sciences and the Law* 31(1): 125–40.

——, Bird, A.S., and Button, E.J. 1981. "Compulsory Admissions in a London Borough: I. Social and Clinical Features and a Follow-Up." *Psychological Medicine* 11(3): 617–36.

——, Daw, R., and Dawson, J. 2010. "A Model Law Fusing Incapacity and Mental Health Legislation & Outline of the Model Law." *Journal of Mental Health Law* Special Issue Ed 20: 11–24; 101–28.

——, Daw, R., and Callard, F. 2014. "Mental Health Law and the UN Convention on the Rights of Persons With Disabilities." *International Journal of Law and Psychiatry*: 37(3): 245–52.

Tan, D.J., Hope, P.T, Stewart, D.A., and Fitzpatrick, P.R. 2006. "Competence to Make Treatment Decisions in Anorexia Nervosa: Thinking Processes and Values." *Philosophy Psychiatry and Psychology* 13(4): 267–82.

Taylor, P.J., and Gunn, J. 1999. "Homicides By People With Mental Illness: Myth and Reality." *British Journal of Psychiatry* 174: 9–14.

Thornicroft, G., Farrelly, S., Szmukler, G., Birchwood, M., Waheed, W., Flach, C., Barrett, B., Byford, S., Henderson, C., Sutherby, K., Lester, H., Rose, D., Dunn, G., Leese, M., Marshall, M. 2013. "Clinical Outcomes of Joint Crisis Plans to Reduce Compulsory Treatment for People with Psychosis: A Randomised Controlled Trial." *Lancet* 381: 1634–41.

United Nations. 2006. *Convention on the Rights of Persons With Disabilities*. Available at www.un.org/disabilities/documents/convention/convoptprot-e.pdf. Accessed April 23, 2015.
United Nations Committee on the Rights of Persons with Disabilities. 2014. General Comment on "Article 12: Equal Recognition Before the Law." Available at www.ohchr.org/EN/HRBodies/CRPD/Pages/GC.aspx. Accessed April 6, 2015.
Wertheimer, A. 1987. *Coercion*. Princeton: Princeton University Press.
——. 1993. "A Philosophical Examination of Coercion for Mental Health Issues: Some Basic Distinctions: Analysis and Justification." *Behavioral Sciences and the Law* 11: 239–58.
——. 1996. *Exploitation*. Princeton, NJ: Princeton University Press.
——. 2001. "Exploitation." *Stanford Encyclopedia of Philosophy*. Available at http://plato.stanford.edu/entries/exploitation. Accessed April 23, 2015.

5b

Commentary on Szmukler: Mental Illness, Dangerousness, and Involuntary Civil Commitment

Ken Levy and Alex Cohen

1. Introduction

Dr. George Szmukler has written a very thought-provoking and enlightening chapter. After distinguishing among five different levels of "treatment pressures" – persuasion, interpersonal leverage, inducements/offers, threats, and compulsion (see p. 127) – Dr. Szmukler focuses mostly on the last of these. In both the United Kingdom and the United States, an individual cannot be compelled to receive "involuntary outpatient treatment" (IOT)[1] or be committed to a hospital unless she satisfies three criteria: (a) she is deemed by the authorities to constitute a danger to herself or others or (b) she is dangerous to others (c) because of a mental illness (see p. 130–31).[2] Most of Dr. Szmukler's paper is concerned with (c). He argues, in line with the United Nations Convention on the Rights of Persons with Disabilities (see pp. 141–42), that it is both unnecessary and "unfairly discriminatory"; that the idea that compulsory treatment or commitment requires mental illness rests on the popular myth that there is a significant correlation between mental illness and dangerousness (see p. 132–34).

The solution that Dr. Szmukler proposes is to replace the mental-illness criterion with two tests: one to determine if an individual is suffering from an impairment of "decision-making capability" (DMC) and the other to determine if a given treatment is in the patient's best interests (BI). As compared with current application of the mental-illness criterion, Dr. Szmukler argues, application of DMC and BI would help to minimize the risk of stigma and unfair discrimination and promote greater respect for patients' decisions, preferences, values, and autonomy (see pp. 131, 134, 137-41).

Dr. Szmukler's position regarding the mental-illness criterion advances a debate that has been raging in the literature for the last five decades concerning the tension between individual rights and involuntary commitment for individuals with putative mental illness. We appreciate Dr. Szmukler's clear concern for patients and for their rights, reputations, and general well-being; we agree with his thesis that involuntary treatment is not always the optimal approach; and we are sympathetic to his proposal that we reconsider the conditions triggering involuntary civil commitment. We do, however, take issue with Dr. Szmukler's treatment of the dangerousness criterion. Dr. Szmukler does not really make clear what role it should play. He does suggest that non- or pre-criminal dangerousness "could be covered by the BI requirement" and suggests that if treatment either does not eliminate the danger of violence or is refused by an individual with impaired DMC, then "recourse to the criminal justice system would be necessary" (see p. 135). But this is all a little too quick; recourse to the criminal justice system is often unwarranted if the individual merely poses a danger to herself or others and has not (yet) committed any crime. What, then, should we do in these situations?

We will attempt to answer this question in section 3. (The preceding section, section 2, will explicate the different purposes of criminal punishment and of involuntary civil commitment.) In sections 4 and 5, we will discuss different approaches to the definition of mental illness and offer further reasons in support of Dr. Szmukler's skepticism about the mental-illness requirement. And in section 6, we will offer some final thoughts about the causal epistemology of mental illness. The reader should note that we are writing about involuntary commitment from an American perspective. So there will be some nuanced differences between our approach and that of Dr. Szmukler, who is writing from a more British perspective.

2. Constitutional Limits on Individual Freedom: Criminal Punishment and Involuntary Civil Commitment

Involuntary civil commitment, which we consider to be a necessary evil, is a deprivation of liberty for the purpose of protecting either the patient from self-destructive behavior or society from the patient. Because Western societies greatly value individual liberty, there must be a rigorous test for imposing this deprivation. In order to determine whether a given individual poses a danger to herself or others, at least one qualified expert must apply this test, and both the content and application of this test must be consistent with the individual's constitutional rights—specifically, with the 5th Amendment ("No person shall be … deprived of life, liberty, or property, without due process of law … ") and the 14th Amendment ("[N]or shall any state deprive any person of life, liberty, or property, without due process of law … ").[3]

This last point bears emphasis. Few would argue that arrest following probable cause or imprisonment following a criminal conviction is unconstitutional. Of course, she may argue that a particular arrest or conviction is constitutionally invalid. But arrest and imprisonment in and of themselves are perfectly consistent with the Constitution, despite the premium that the Constitution places on individual liberty. And the reason for this consistency is that constitutional rights are not absolute. There are several reasons. First, as George Washington stated in the cover letter transmitting the Constitution to the Congress: "Individuals entering into society must give up a share of liberty to preserve the rest."[4] In other words, individual liberty must be restricted to make society and social harmony possible. Second, the Constitution permits further restrictions of the right to liberty under certain circumstances. These circumstances include arrest, conviction, curfew, and military draft.

Whether the Constitution permits restrictions of the right to liberty under another circumstance—namely, the determination that a given individual poses a danger to herself or others—is less clear. The patient may have done nothing wrong, certainly nothing that warrants arrest or conviction. Yet involuntary civil commitment involves treating the patient in a manner that superficially resembles incarceration. Just like the criminal offender, the patient is "locked up" against her will. How, then, can we justify treating the patient like an offender? Isn't this an obvious violation of her constitutional due process rights? In a word: no. The reasons justifying involuntarily committing an individual outweigh her constitutional right to liberty. To understand what these reasons are, we first need to understand the reasons why we imprison convicted offenders.

The first reason that we imprison offenders is "consequentialist": to bring about good consequences. The main consequentialist goal of incarceration is to protect society from further crime. Incarceration contributes to this goal in three different ways. First, incarceration incapacitates; it protects society (at least society outside prison)[5] from the person who is incarcerated. Second, specific deterrence and rehabilitation: criminal punishment is designed to discourage the recipients of this punishment from committing further crimes if and when they return to society. Third, general deterrence: criminal punishment is designed to discourage all other similarly situated individuals from committing the same kinds of crime. Both kinds of deterrence, specific and general, presuppose that convicted criminals and most similarly situated individuals are rational (enough) actors who can weigh the risk of punishment for committing (further) crimes against the benefit of avoiding punishment, decide that the latter is more conducive to their well-being, and then act on this decision by choosing to comply with the law rather than violating it.

The second reason that we lock up offenders is "retributivist": to give offenders what they deserve. This second reason intersects with the first (consequentialism) insofar as they both rest on the premise that the convicted offender was responsible for her criminal act. Retributivists assume that responsibility is necessary for (just) punishment because, without it, the person would not *deserve* punishment in the first place. Likewise, consequentialists generally assume that responsibility is necessary for punishment but for a different reason: (a) punishment cannot deter criminal activity unless the people whom the punishment is designed to deter can be motivated by the threat of punishment, and (b) this kind of motivation requires threshold levels of control and rationality, both of which are arguably sufficient for responsibility.

The third reason is "expressivist": to communicate both to offenders and to the rest of society that the kind of behavior for which they are being punished is unacceptable. On this view, punishment is a kind of language that is used to communicate disapproval and impose stigma. One might argue that expressivism reduces to consequentialism because (a) communication is itself a consequence, and (b) it is desired as a means to further consequences (such as deterrence). But at least with regard to (b), the expressivist may maintain that communication is intended not merely as a means to the end of deterrence but also as an end in itself. On this view, it is intrinsically, not just instrumentally, valuable for a community to speak its mind about criminal transgressions.

When it comes to cases of involuntary civil commitment that do not involve a crime being committed, the retributivist and expressivist justifications for criminal punishment simply do not apply. Once again, we involuntarily commit certain individuals for the very consequentialist reason of protecting either patients themselves or others from the patients. This is not specific deterrence because we assume that the patients suffer from serious cognitive, behavioral, and functional deficits and therefore cannot conduct, and then act upon, a rational risk/benefit analysis. Instead of hoping that we can influence them by incentivizing them to act rationally (through the threat of punishment), we need to directly control them. Nor does involuntary civil commitment involve general deterrence. We cannot hope to discourage similarly situated individuals from engaging in self-destructive or other-destructive behavior because similarly situated individuals are equally non-responsible and therefore equally immune to rational incentivization. Put very crudely, patients who are involuntarily committed are not "bad," a term that connotes responsible wrongdoing, but "mad," a term that connotes an inability to think or act rationally. As a result, we cannot appeal to their reason. Instead, we must resort to sheer brute force.

3. Should We Treat Homicide as a Public Health Threat?

Given the presumption of liberty that the Constitution guarantees to every citizen, there are three main reasons why this presumption will sometimes be overridden: arrest, criminal conviction, and involuntary civil commitment. For the remainder of this reply, we will concentrate on involuntary civil commitment. Involuntary civil commitment is authorized if and only if the individual either: (a) carries, or is reasonably expected to carry, a dangerous and infectious disease;[6] (b) is dangerous to herself; or (c) is dangerous to others because she is mentally ill.[7]

Consider (a).[8] Both the federal and state governments have the power to isolate and quarantine individuals whom they reasonably suspect carry a communicable disease.[9] The primary rationale for this power is to prevent the spread of the disease and thereby protect other members of society. The secondary rationale is to treat the individual herself.

Interestingly, while presenting a threat to the public is sufficient justification for involuntary commitment (isolation or quarantine) when the source of the threat is (suspected) infectious disease, presenting a threat to the public is *not* sufficient justification for involuntary commitment when the source of the threat is the person's disposition to homicide. In the latter situation, as we noted in the Introduction, two other conditions must also be satisfied: the person must be mentally ill, and the person's homicidal disposition must be attributable to this mental illness.[10]

Why are these two additional criteria required? Why aren't threats of homicide considered to be, and treated just like, public-health threats? Isn't, for example, a person's statement that he will kill others just as dangerous as a person's carrying of an infectious disease? And if it is just as dangerous, why isn't a disposition to murder sufficient for civil commitment? Why must mental illness and a causal relationship also be satisfied?

There are three main reasons. First, the scale of the threat posed by homicide is far less than the scale of the threat posed by an infectious disease. While the most "successful" serial killers in history have killed hundreds of people, some diseases can easily kill thousands to millions. So as a matter of public policy, if the State wishes to minimize premature deaths, it should make sure to focus much more of its efforts on quarantining dangerous-disease carriers than it does on ferreting out and committing likely murderers. Indeed, as a public-policy priority, homicide prevention should lose out to suicide prevention as well. Despite what the media would lead us to believe, suicides happen to occur much more frequently than homicides.[11]

Second, the chance that a disease will spread if a host remains in the population is much higher than the chance that a given individual will act on her homicidal intentions or threats. If a person carries a highly infectious disease, the chance that she will spread this disease (if left free) is nearly 100 percent. If, however, a person is considered homicidal but not mentally ill, the chance that she will attempt to commit homicide is considered to be much lower—certainly not 100 percent.

Third, while isolation and quarantine are sometimes the only measures that society can implement to stop the spread of certain diseases, methods other than involuntary commitment such as anger management, restraining orders, threats of criminal punishment, and rational dissuasion can be used to "talk down" a would-be killer.

All of this is not meant to suggest that homicidal threats should not be taken seriously or that temporary detainment is not often appropriate to prevent these threats from being executed. It is only to say that the mere threat of homicide is not equivalent in scale, probabilities, or preventability to the dangers presented by communication of an infectious disease and therefore does not necessarily warrant the same kind of preventive response (i.e., involuntary commitment).

4. Defining Mental Illness: Medical vs. Legal Perspectives

The American Psychiatric Association published the Fifth Edition of the *Diagnostic and Statistical Manual of Mental Disorders* (DSM-5) in 2013. The DSM-5 is rather unwieldy. It is approximately 1,000 pages long and lists over 300 kinds of mental disorders. These 300+ mental disorders are placed into 21 separate categories running the gamut of severity—from relatively minor disorders such as adjustment disorders to relatively severe disorders such as those involving dementia, psychosis, and neurodegenerative diseases.

DSM-5 offers one of the two major taxonomies of mental disorders. The other is the International Classification of Diseases (ICD-10), which is published by the World Health Organization. Because the DSM-5 and ICD-10 are so complicated, experts are needed to understand and apply them. As the DSM-5 states, "It requires clinical training to recognize when the combination of predisposing, precipitating, perpetuating, and protective factors has resulted in a psychopathological condition in which physical signs and symptoms exceed normal ranges"[12] (see also Szmukler,

p. 141). Similarly, DSM-5 later states, "Use of DSM-5 to assess for the presence of a mental disorder by nonclinical, nonmedical, or otherwise insufficiently trained individuals is not advised."[13]

The DSM-5 defines *mental disorder* as follows:

> A mental disorder is a syndrome characterized by clinically significant disturbance in an individual's cognition, emotion regulation, or behavior that reflects a dysfunction in the psychological, biological, or developmental processes underlying mental functioning. Mental disorders are usually associated with significant distress in social, occupational, or other important activities. An expectable or culturally approved response to a common stressor or loss, such as the death of a loved one, is not a mental disorder. Socially deviant behavior (e.g., political, religious, or sexual) and conflicts that are primarily between the individual and society are not mental disorders unless the deviance or conflict results from a dysfunction in the individual.[14]

At least two terms in this definition are necessarily vague: *significant* (twice) and *dysfunction* (twice). So are some exceptions to this definition: "[s]ocially deviant behavior (e.g., political, religious, or sexual) and conflicts that are primarily between the individual and society" that are not the results of "a dysfunction in the individual."

Legal definitions of mental illness are quite different from the ones found in DSM-5 or ICD-10. While psychiatrists and psychologists must consider over 300 kinds of mental illnesses spanning the entire thousand-page DSM-5, law tends to focus only on that narrow part of the mental-illness spectrum that correlates with criminal activity or undermines consent. For example, Ohio's criminal code defines mental illness as a "substantial disorder of thought, mood, perception, orientation or memory that grossly impairs judgement, behavior, capacity to recognize reality or ability to meet the ordinary demands of life."[15] Importantly, the vast majority of mental illnesses in the DSM-5 fall short of this legal definition. Few of them either involve substantial impairment of judgment, of behavior, or of other domains of functioning or are associated with violent (or suicidal) behavior. Individuals diagnosed with, for example, a learning disability or an adjustment disorder are not necessarily likely to engage in dangerous behavior.

5. Why is Mental Illness Required for Involuntary Commitment?

Consider two scenarios. In "Suicidal Scenario," Suicidal Sam announces to his co-workers Connie and Clarence that he will hang himself after the close of business. When they laugh uncomfortably, he shows them a rope with a noose, tells them that he is quite serious, and asks them to make sure that he is cremated rather than buried. In "Homicidal Scenario," Homicidal Harry announces to the same co-workers, Connie and Clarence, that he is going to kill his superiors at a meeting the next morning. When they laugh uncomfortably, he shows them the loaded pistol that he legally purchased a week ago and the hole-riddled targets that he shot up at the local firing range. Both Suicidal Scenario and Homicidal Scenario are paradigmatic examples of danger to self and danger to others respectively.

The mere fact that Suicidal Sam threatened to commit suicide is not necessarily sufficient to warrant the conclusion that he suffers from mental illness. The notion that nobody "in her right mind" would prefer to die rather than to live is false. First, some individuals wish to die because they are terminally ill and suffering great physical pain. Their desire to die on their own terms and thereby minimize not only their own but also their family's suffering is arguably quite rational. It is for this reason that the State may not force such individuals to receive life-saving medical treatment.[16] Second, some individuals who have just suffered great trauma—for example, losing a loved one, accidentally injuring or killing another person, or being accused or convicted of a serious crime—might be suicidal. Depending on the circumstances, their wanting to die in order to relieve themselves of great psychic pain (e.g., grief, guilt, or shame) may be rational enough that a diagnosis of mental illness would be inaccurate.[17]

For our purposes, however, assume that Suicidal Sam does not fit into either (rational) category. That is, he is suicidal not because he is terminally ill or because he just suffered great trauma but for a reason that society would consider irrational—that is, not strong enough to warrant a desire to die. (For example, Suicidal Sam is seriously distraught after his girlfriend broke up with him.) Suicidal Sam, then, probably qualifies as mentally ill. The question remains, however, why it matters whether or not Suicidal Sam is mentally ill. The fact that he is irrationally suicidal should be sufficient reason for conviction. Whether his suicidal impulses arise from mental illness or from something else—for example, nihilism or grief—should not matter. Suicide is suicide; it is such a tragic event that if the State has an opportunity to prevent it from occurring through involuntary commitment, it should be authorized to exercise this opportunity—again, whether or not the individual is mentally ill.[18]

Homicidal Harry's situation is more difficult for the State.[19] He has a better chance of remaining free than does Suicidal Sam. Of course, the police may detain Homicidal Harry; ask him questions; and obtain a search warrant to search his person, office, home, and car. But if they cannot find any incriminating evidence—that is, evidence sufficient to warrant probable cause that Homicidal Harry has committed a crime—they cannot arrest him. The best that they can do is give him a stern warning, impose a restraining order on him (protecting his superiors), and then release him. This conclusion, however, assumes two things: (a) that Homicidal Harry's purchase of a weapon, target practice, and stated intent of committing homicide do not, all together, qualify as attempted murder; and (b) that Homicidal Harry is not in one of the few jurisdictions that criminalize communications of intended violence against others even when the intended targets are not the recipients of these communications.[20]

Of course, the State may compel Homicidal Harry to undergo a psychological evaluation. And if the evaluation results in a determination that Homicidal Harry is mentally ill, then—given the danger that he poses to others—he may be involuntarily committed. But if the evaluation does not result in this determination, then—once again—the State's hands are tied; they must release him. And in contrast to Suicidal Sam, whose irrational suicidal intent is generally considered to be presumptive, if not dispositive, evidence of mental illness (e.g., clinical depression), Homicidal Harry's homicidal intent will not necessarily lead to the same conclusion. This is a curious asymmetry that probably stems from the notion that while suicide is generally fundamentally irrational, homicidal behavior is (much) more "natural" and "normal." As it turns out, this assumption may just be correct. There is a weaker correlation between mental illness and homicide than there is between mental illness and suicide.[21] The fact of the matter is that many more or less mentally stable people kill. Examples include domestic violence, bar fights, drug-turf battles, and drunk driving. Still, even if many "normal" people kill, certain kinds of abnormality heighten the probability of killing. The "risk of violence is three-fold among those with psychosis" and the predictors of violence include "acute psychiatric symptoms" (such as mania, depression, delusions, hallucinations, and violent fantasies), Antisocial Personality Disorder, and psychopathy (see Szmukler, pp. 133–34).[22]

One might very well argue that that the State *should* have the power to commit Homicidal Harry *whether or not* he is deemed mentally ill. The reason is that, even if he is not mentally ill, Homicidal Harry is very dangerous. He will likely kill at least one person *and* the person(s) he will kill presumably do(es) not wish to die.

We can think of four reasons why involuntarily committing Homicidal Harry requires him to be not merely dangerous but also mentally ill. First, the weakest reason: It might be thought that some sort of symmetry with the criminal justice system must be maintained. The idea is that if a criminal conviction roughly requires dangerousness (in the form of commission of a crime) and responsibility, then involuntary commitment requires dangerousness and *non*-responsibility. And non-responsibility just is, or is caused by, mental illness. But this hypothesis is problematic. Aside from the fact that not all crimes are necessarily dangerous (e.g., drug possession and perjury), it is not clear why there must be this symmetry with the criminal justice system in the first place. If a person makes clear that she poses a serious threat to others, then it should not matter whether this threatening disposition arises from mental illness or from some other cause. The threat is sufficient reason to commit her, and she should be released from commitment only after authorities determine that the threat has fully passed.

Second, mental illness is thought by some to increase the risk that Homicidal Harry will lose control or engage more readily in aggressive behavior. The problem with this hypothesis is that Homicidal Harry has already clearly exhibited homicidal intentions and (therefore) presents a serious enough risk that he will translate these intentions into action. So whether or not Homicidal Harry is mentally ill, the danger to others is quite real. Still, one might argue that if a person has demonstrated an inclination toward violence that is more ambiguous than Homicidal Harry's, then we may not conclude that this person poses a threat to others unless she suffers from a mental illness (such as schizophrenia or psychosis) that increases the risk that this inclination will be realized. For *this* reason, mental illness is required for involuntary commitment. We believe that this argument is credible but leads to two undesirable consequences: (a) it rules out commitment of individuals who pose a clear and serious threat but are not mentally ill; and (b) by requiring mental illness, we perpetuate the myths that mental illness generally causes dangerousness and that dangerousness is generally caused by mental illness.

Third, it has been argued that if dangerousness alone were required, the State would too often be accused of labeling certain people as dangerous for ulterior reasons—not because they really are dangerous but because they are perceived as political opponents or threats whom the State wishes to silence and intimidate. By requiring mental illness as well, the State avoids this appearance of false pretext and creates the much more salutary impression that its sole reason for committing certain people is their own, and others', welfare.

Fourth, mental illness may be required in addition to dangerousness less from principle than from lack of resources. In a personal communication (dated August 31, 2014) to one of the authors, Ed Richards, Clarence W. Edwards Professor of Law and Director of the Program in Law, Science, and Public Health at LSU Law Center, put it this way:

> After the deinstitutionalization movement, there are relatively few places to lock people up. There are lots of private beds for voluntary commitment (if you have insurance) but not even a lot of private beds for involuntary commitment. They do not want actually dangerous patients, and the state does not want to pay the costs of private facilities. ... Involuntary outpatient treatment has been the answer ... It is much less resource intensive. You do not need a facility.[23]

6. Conclusion: The Causal Epistemology Of Mental Illness

Unlike many complementary domains of medicine (e.g., virology), the causal mechanisms underlying mental illnesses are almost completely unknown. The little we know is that each of them is caused by a complicated interplay of genetic, neurobiological, and environmental factors. There are two reasons why we know so little.

First, there is no known genetic marker, neural signature, behavioral anomaly, or abnormal neuroanatomical structure that occurs in all, or often even most, patients with a specific mental illness. For example, only some individuals with schizophrenia suffer from gross impairments in reality testing. Moreover, symptoms of mental illness wax and wane over time. As a result, an individual diagnosed with schizophrenia may show impaired reality testing at one time, or in one context, but not another. Second, many of the symptoms associated with one particular mental illness are associated with other mental illnesses as well. For example, not only patients with schizophrenia but also patients with bipolar disorder and major depressive disorder suffer from gross impairments in reality testing.

Our etiological ignorance has fueled the development of new diagnostic approaches. Foremost among these is the Research Domain Criteria (RDoC) initiative that was undertaken by the National Institute of Mental Health, the world's largest funding agency for research in mental illness. The RDoC initiative is an attempt to (a) construct a "periodic table" of mental illness demarcating isolated domains of psychopathology; and (b) elucidate the genetic, biological, and environmental mechanisms that cause these domains to malfunction. While still in the initial stages, the RDoC initiative has already produced results. For example, measures of emotion derived from automated acoustic analysis of natural speech are helping to predict episodes of anger and hostility and therefore will likely be useful in predicting individuals' risks of acting out.[24] Given its early successes and ambitious agenda, we are optimistic that RDoC will help us to discover other objective markers of mental illness; the biological processes underlying them; and new measures of, and treatments for, mental illness.

Still, it is important to realize that RDoC and related efforts are only in their infancy. In order for an RDoC approach to be applicable to civil commitment, the very definitions of consent, reality testing, suicidality, homicidality, and related constructs will need to be reduced to their most basic elements before they can be empirically evaluated and objective, reliable, and valid forensic measures of these elements can be developed. But all of this is much easier said than done. Reality testing and dangerousness to self or others are very difficult to deconstruct largely because the neural mechanisms that cause them are quite varied and differ both across individuals and within the same individuals across time. For example, impairments in reality testing can reflect dysfunctions in a range of basic cognitive, emotional, and/or impulse control systems, some or all of which may be present in a given individual at any given time. And even specific control systems are themselves difficult to measure. There is evidence, for example, that an important component of reality testing involves "insight." And while identifiable brain structures are associated with poor insight in schizophrenia,[25] insight itself is multidimensional in nature,[26] and different types of insight reflect different neurobiological mechanisms.[27]

Notes

1 In the United States, the term is *Assisted Outpatient Treatment* (AOT). See www.treatmentadvocacycenter.org/solution/assisted-outpatient-treatment-laws.

2 In some parts of the United States, danger to property, grave disability, and disorganized behavior also qualify.

3 We do not mean to limit the discussion to the United States or constitutional democracies. The UK, for example, is a parliamentary democracy, but it equally respects and protects the same due process rights. So by *constitutional rights*, we should be understood to mean due process rights generally.

4 Letter of the President of the Federal Convention, Dated September 17, 1787, to the "President of Congress, Transmitting the Constitution." See http://avalon.law.yale.edu/18th_century/translet.asp#1.

5 See generally Kevin Bennardo, "Incarceration's Incapacitative Shortcomings," *Santa Clara Law Review* 54.1: 1–18 (2014).

6 See Varholy v. Sweat, 153 Fla. 571, 576 (1943) ("The constitutional guarantees of life, liberty and property, of which a person cannot be deprived without due process of law, do not limit the exercise of the police power of the State to preserve the public health so long as that power is reasonably and fairly exercised and not abused. … Not only must every reasonable presumption be indulged in favor of the validity of legislative action in this important field, but also in favor of the validity of the regulations and actions of the health authorities."); In the Matter of the Application of Mrs. A. Arata for a Writ of Habeas Corpus, 52 Cal.App. 380, 383 (1921) ("That the health authorities possess the power to place under quarantine restrictions persons whom they have reasonable cause to believe are afflicted with infectious or contagious diseases … as a general right, may not be questioned. It is equally true that in the exercise of this unusual power, which infringes upon the right

of liberty of the individual, personal restraint can only be imposed where, under the facts as brought within the knowledge of the health authorities, reasonable ground exists to support the belief that the person is afflicted as claimed."); Edward P. Richards and Katharine C. Rathbun, "Making State Public Health Laws Work for SARS Outbreaks," *Emerging Infectious Diseases* 10.3: 356 (Feb. 2004) ("In the case of quarantine due to disease, a judge would determine whether the state has shown that the detained person deserves quarantine. The judge must defer to public health authorities on their choice of public health strategies.") (footnote omitted).

7 See Kansas v. Hendricks, 521 U.S. 346, 347, 363, 372 (1997); Heller v. Doe, 509 U.S. 312, 314–15 (1993). In cases of civil commitment, it is necessary to demonstrate both a temporal and causal link between the mental illness and the dangerous behavior. If a person exhibits dangerous behavior but this danger is not related to her mental illness, then she does not qualify for commitment. For example, an individual diagnosed with schizophrenia—defined in part by gross impairments in judgment, reality testing, and functioning—may present as homicidal for reasons that do not pertain to her manifest diagnosis. Conversely, a soldier that has returned from combat and meets criteria for Post-Traumatic Stress Disorder—a disorder not typically associated with the level or type of impairment characteristic of legally defined mental illness—*would* be appropriate for commitment if she were displaying grossly disorganized and aggressive behavior secondary to flashbacks.

8 The Centers for Disease Control and Prevention website states: "Isolation is used to separate ill persons who have a communicable disease from those who are healthy. Isolation restricts the movement of ill persons to help stop the spread of certain diseases. For example, hospitals use isolation for patients with infectious tuberculosis. Quarantine is used to separate and restrict the movement of well persons who may have been exposed to a communicable disease to see if they become ill. These people may have been exposed to a disease and do not know it, or they may have the disease but do not show symptoms. Quarantine can also help limit the spread of communicable disease." See www.cdc.gov/quarantine/aboutlawsregulationsquarantineisolation.html.

9 See ibid. ("The federal government derives its authority for isolation and quarantine from the Commerce Clause of the U.S. Constitution. Under section 361 of the Public Health Service Act (42 U.S. Code § 264), the U.S. Secretary of Health and Human Services is authorized to take measures to prevent the entry and spread of communicable diseases from foreign countries into the United States and between states. The authority for carrying out these functions on a daily basis has been delegated to the Centers for Disease Control and Prevention (CDC). … States have police power functions to protect the health, safety, and welfare of persons within their borders. To control the spread of disease within their borders, states have laws to enforce the use of isolation and quarantine. These laws can vary from state to state and can be specific or broad. In some states, local health authorities implement state law. In most states, breaking a quarantine order is a criminal misdemeanor. … Centers for Disease Control and Prevention are charged with enforcement of federal laws authorizing isolation and quarantine."). *But see* Edward P. Richards, "The Jurisprudence of Prevention: The Right of Societal Self-Defense Against Dangerous Individuals," *Hastings Constitutional Law Quarterly* 16.3: 329, 337 n.38 (1989) (attributing the States' constitutional power to quarantine not to "any power which the States assume to regulate commerce or to interfere with the regulations of Congress, but because police laws … must of necessity have full and free operation, according to the exigency which requires their interference.") (citing Thurlow v. Massachusetts (The License Cases), 46 U.S. (5 How.) 504, 632 (1847)).

10 Just being mentally ill is also not sufficient for involuntary commitment. There are two reasons. First, if it were sufficient, then—given that over a quarter of the adult population suffer from a diagnosable mental illness in a given year (see www.nimh.nih.gov/health/publications/the-numbers-count-mental-disorders-in-america/index.shtml)—the constitutional presumption of liberty would be rendered meaningless. Second, there is no point. The vast majority of

mentally ill individuals are not threats to themselves or others. So the economic and non-economic costs of involuntarily committing them would far outweigh the benefits, if any.

11 The U.S. Center for Disease Control (CDC) reports that the overall suicide rate is twice the overall homicide rate and twice to three times the homicide rate for adults over 25 years old. See www.cdc.gov/mmwr/preview/mmwrhtml/mm6128a8.htm. One explanation for this disparity might be that homicide is more difficult than suicide. While suicide involves killing a willing participant, homicide does not.

12 American Psychiatric Association, *Diagnostic and Statistical Manual of Mental Disorders*, 5th ed, Washington DC: American Psychiatric Association, 2013, p. 19.

13 Ibid., p. 25.

14 Ibid., p. 20.

15 Ohio's Revised Code (ORC) § 5122.01(A).

16 See Ken Levy, "Gonzales v. Oregon and Physician-Assisted Suicide: Ethical and Policy Issues," *Tulsa Law Review* 42.3 (2007): 699, 701.

17 See American Psychiatric Association, *DSM*-5, xlii (improving upon the DSM-IV by "differentiating bereavement and major depressive disorders").

18 It is possible that the mental-illness requirement for civil commitment to prevent suicide is meant to distinguish between individuals who only seem suicidal and individuals who really are suicidal. This possibility rests on the assumption that mental illness dramatically raises the risk that an unhappy person will follow through on her (stated) intention to commit suicide, an assumption that is supported by the fact that suicide is highly comorbid with mental illness. See www.afsp.org/understanding-suicide/key-research-findings ("[S]tudies have consistently found that the overwhelming majority of people who die by suicide—90% or more—had a mental disorder at the time of their deaths. Still, suicidal behavior is usually difficult to predict unless imminent risk factors are present."); http://ajp.psychiatryonline.org/article.aspx?articleid=170454 ("In young men, completed suicide is linked to specific mental disorders, namely, major depression, borderline personality disorder, and substance abuse. Comorbidity involving any of these disorders is frequently associated with completed suicide."); www.ncbi.nlm.nih.gov/pubmed/8678167?ordinalpos=1&itool=EntrezSystem2.PEntrez.Pubmed.Pubmed_ResultsPanel.Pubmed_DiscoveryPanel.Pubmed_Discovery_RA& linkpos=1&log$=relatedarticles& logdbfrom=pubmed ("[R]isk for suicide increases with age in individuals with major affective illness.").

19 For a more extended discussion of the same issue, see Ken Levy, "Dangerous Psychopaths: Criminally Responsible But *Not* Morally Responsible, Subject to Criminal Punishment And to Preventive Detention," *San Diego Law Review* 48.4 (2011): 1299, 1382–92.

20 See ibid. at 1384 n.187.

21 See supra note 16. When we control for socio-economic status, gender, substance abuse, and other variables, we find that the contribution that mental illness makes to violent crimes is much smaller than the contribution that it makes to suicide. While a significant number of incarcerated individuals in the United States have mental illnesses, there is not necessarily a causal link. In many cases, their crimes are caused more by deinstitutionalization than mental illness per se. See http://depts.washington.edu/mhreport/facts_violence.php.

22 See also http://www.forensicpsychiatry.ca/risk/assessment.htm.

23 Cf. www.bazelon.org/Where-We-Stand/Self-Determination/Forced-Treatment/Outpatient-and-Civil-Commitment.aspx. ("The Bazelon Center opposes outpatient commitment. There is no evidence that it improves public safety. … When people are dangerous due to mental illnesses, they should be hospitalized. … Outpatient commitment is not a quick-fix that can overcome the inadequacies of under-resourced and under-performing mental health systems.")

24 See www.ncbi.nlm.nih.gov/pubmed/23444120.

25 See www.ncbi.nlm.nih.gov/pubmed/22664168.

26 See www.ncbi.nlm.nih.gov/pubmed/23407202.

27 See www.ncbi.nlm.nih.gov/pubmed/17671876.

Bibliography

American Foundation for Suicide Prevention. 2015. "Key Research Findings." Available at: www.afsp.org/understanding-suicide/key-research-findings. Accessed April 27, 2015.

American Psychiatric Association. 2013. *Diagnostic and Statistical Manual of Mental Disorders. 5th ed.* Washington DC: American Psychiatric Association.

Bennardo, Kevin. 2014. "Incarceration's Incapacitative Shortcomings." *Santa Clara Law Review* 54.1: 1–18.

Centers for Disease Control and Prevention. 2009. "Morbidity and Mortality Weekly Report (MMWR): QuickStats: Suicide and Homicide Rates, by Age Group – United States." Available at: www.cdc.gov/mmwr/preview/mmwrhtml/mm6128a8.htm. Accessed April 27, 2015.

Centers for Disease Control and Prevention. 2015. "Legal Authorities for Isolation and Quarantine." Available at: www.cdc.gov/quarantine/aboutlawsregulationsquarantineisolation.html. Accessed April 27, 2015.

Comparelli, A. 2013. "Relationships Between Psychopathological Variables and Insight in Psychosis Risk Syndrome and First-Episode and Multiepisode Schizophrenia." *Journal of Nervous and Mental Disease* 201.3 (March): 229–33. Available at: www.ncbi.nlm.nih.gov/pubmed/23407202. Accessed April 27, 2015.

Conwell, Y., Duberstein, P. R., Cox, C., Herrmann, J. H., Forbes, N. T,. Caine, E. D. 1996. "Relationships of Age and Axis I Diagnoses in Victims of Completed Suicide: A Psychological Autopsy Study." *American Journal of Psychiatry* 153.8 (Aug.): 1001–8. Available at: www.ncbi.nlm.nih.gov/pubmed/8678167?ordinalpos=1&itool=EntrezSystem2.PEntrez.Pubmed.Pubmed_ResultsPanel.Pubmed_DiscoveryPanel.Pubmed_Discovery_RA&linkpos=1&log$=relatedarticles&logdbfrom=pubmed. Accessed April 27, 2015.

Heller v. Doe, 509 U.S. 312 (1993).

Hucker, Stephen J. 2011. "Psychiatric Aspects of Risk Assessment." *Forensic Psychiatry*. Available at: www.forensicpsychiatry.ca/risk/assessment.htm. Accessed April 27, 2015.

"In the Matter of the Application of Mrs. A. Arata for a Writ of Habeas Corpus," 52 Cal.App. 380 (1921).

Judge David C. Bazelon Center for Mental Health Law. 2014. "Outpatient and Civil Commitment." Online at www.bazelon.org/Where-We-Stand/Self-Determination/Forced-Treatment/Outpatient-and-Civil-Commitment.aspx.

Kansas v. Hendricks, 521 U.S. 346 (1997).

Lesage, A.D., Boyer, R., Grunberg, F., Vanier, C., Morissette, R., Ménard-Buteau, C., Loyer, M. 1994. "Suicide and Mental Disorders: A Case-Control Study of Young Men." *The American Journal of Psychiatry* 151.7 (July): 1063–68. Available at: http://ajp.psy chiatryonline.org/article.aspx?articleid=170454. Accessed April 27, 2015.

"Letter of the President of the Federal Convention, Dated September 17, 1787, to the President of Congress, Transmitting the Constitution." Reprinted from *Documentary History of the Constitution, Vol. II.* (1894) pp. 1, 2. The Avalon Project: Documents in Law, History, and Diplomacy. Available at: http://avalon.law.yale.edu/18th_century/translet.asp#1. Accessed April 27, 2015.

Levy, Ken. 2011. "Dangerous Psychopaths: Criminally Responsible But *Not* Morally Responsible, Subject to Criminal Punishment *And* to Preventive Detention." *San Diego Law Review* 48.4: 1299–395.

——. 2007. "Gonzales v. Oregon and Physician-Assisted Suicide: Ethical and Policy Issues." *Tulsa Law Review* 42.3: 699–729.

Lima, C.F., Castro, S. L., Scott, S. K. 2013. "When Voices Get Emotional: A Corpus of Nonverbal Vocalizations for Research on Emotion Processing." *Behavior Research Methods* 45.4 (Dec.): 1234–45. Available at: www.ncbi.nlm.nih.gov/pubmed/23444120. Accessed April 27, 2015.

National Institute of Mental Health. 2015. "Transforming the Understanding and Treatment of Mental Illnesses: Statistics." Available at: www.nimh.nih.gov/health/publications/the-numbers-count-mental-disorders-in-america/index.shtml. Accessed April 27, 2015.

Ohio's Revised Code (ORC) § 5122.01(A).
Raij, T.T., Riekki, T. J., Hari, R. 2012. "Association of Poor Insight in Schizophrenia with Structure and Function of Cortical Midline Structures and Frontopolar Cortex." *Schizophrenia Research* 139.1–3 (Aug.): 27–32. Available at: www.ncbi.nlm.nih.gov/pubmed/22664168. Accessed April 27, 2015.
Richards, Edward P. 1989. "The Jurisprudence of Prevention: The Right of Societal Self-Defense Against Dangerous Individuals." *Hastings Constitutional Law Quarterly* 16.3: 329–92.
Richards, Edward P. and Rathbun, Katharine C. 2004. "Making State Public Health Laws Work for SARS Outbreaks." *Emerging Infectious Diseases* 10.3 (Feb.): 356–57.
Shad, M.U. 2007. "Neurobiological Underpinnings of Insight Deficits in Schizophrenia." *International Review of Psychiatry* 19.4 (Aug.): 437–46. Available at: www.ncbi.nlm.nih.gov/pubmed/17671876. Accessed April 27, 2015.
Thurlow v. Massachusetts (The License Cases), 46 U.S. (5 How.) 504, 632 (1847).
Treatment Advocacy Center. 2015. "Assisted Outpatient Treatment Laws." Eliminating Barriers to the Treatment of Mental Illness. Available at: www.treatmentadvocacycenter.org/solution/assisted-outpatient-treatment-laws. Accessed April 27, 2015.
University of Washington School of Social Work. 2015. "Facts about Mental Illnesses." Mental Health Reporting. Available at: http://depts.washington.edu/mhreport/#. Accessed April 27, 2015.
Varholy v. Sweat, 153 Fla. 571 (1943).

6a
Scrupulous Treatment

Jesse S. Summers and Walter Sinnott-Armstrong

1. Introduction

Imagine an extremely cautious driver. She comes to a complete stop at every stop sign, yields to every pedestrian waiting to cross the street, and never exceeds the speed limit at all. It would be strange, even dangerous, to suggest that she should be *less* cautious, should pay *less* attention to the law. She does not need to take driving lessons to learn how to drive more like other people. To take a non-legal case, what if someone gave almost all of his income to strangers who are worse off, putting himself below the poverty line, passing up most of the goods his peers take for granted? Should we try to talk him into caring less or giving less to the needy? Few of us drive this carefully or give this much to the needy, but is there a problem with them or with us? It seems backwards to advise them to become more like us. If anything, they should advise us to be *more* concerned with safety and *more* generous.

Our question here is when, if ever, people need psychiatric treatment for being "too" concerned about morality. There are surely drawbacks to being moral in an immoral world. It is often personally costly, even distressing, to do what is morally required. Can those costs justify treatment? If these people honestly believe that they are morally required to act as they do, isn't it intrusive and presumptuous of us to try to change their moral beliefs?

This issue is not fiction. In fact, there are people who are much more concerned with morality (or with religious obligations) than most of us. Some of these people are diagnosed as having *scrupulosity*, and they are sometimes treated for this mental disorder. Our central question here is whether this treatment is justified. It seems dangerous to allow our opinions about how moral a person ought to be to guide treatment, especially for those who are more moral than we are. Even if we can justify some treatment, what kind of treatment can we justify? Is it permissible to encourage or even force a person, as part of their treatment, to do what they see as immoral?

Before we answer these questions, we'll begin by explaining in more detail the clinical condition of scrupulosity and why it is thought to be a candidate for treatment.

2. Scrupulosity[1]

Scrupulosity is a form of Obsessive-Compulsive Disorder (OCD) (Nelson, Abramowitz, Whiteside, & Deacon, 2006; Tek & Ulug, 2001) with moral or religious obsessions or compulsions and otherwise the same cluster of features as other forms of OCD.[2] Although scrupulosity is not a common form of OCD (Miller & Hedges, 2008), it is perhaps the earliest identified form. The first clear cases in Judaism are in the 11th century and in Catholicism in the 16th century (Greenberg, Witztum, & Pisante, 1987; Greenberg & Huppert, 2010; cf. Mora, 1969), and the earliest reference of all is in Plutarch (Plutarch, 1951: 373, 5–6, 9; cf. www.ocdhistory.net/biblio.html).

OCD in general is an anxiety disorder in which a person has persistent, intrusive, and unjustified anxiety-evoking thoughts, or "obsessions," that she resists or reduces by repeatedly performing some behavior, or "compulsion." For example, a patient might regularly have thoughts of a break-in at her house, which evoke a great deal of anxiety. Checking the lock temporarily reassures her and soothes the anxiety, but only briefly: her underlying anxiety about the house's security—or perhaps a more general anxiety—returns after, or even persists through, the checking. The thought's repetition and the return of the anxiety lead to more compulsive behavior and more elaborate compulsions in a desperate attempt to soothe the anxiety.

In this description, what begins the obsessive–compulsive cycle is an intrusive thought that the house is susceptible to a break-in.[3] Such thoughts are intrusive to the extent that one views them as unwelcome and perhaps inconsistent with many of one's other beliefs. Intrusive thoughts, so understood, may be present in as much as 90 percent of the population (Rachman & de Silva, 1978; Salkovskis & Harrison, 1984; cf. Rassin & Muris, 2007). For most of the population, we react to such intrusive thoughts by checking the evidence, shifting our attention to something else, trying to analyze why the thought occurred, or discussing the thought with other people (Wells & Davies, 1994). In contrast, those with OCD are more likely to react in two other ways: they worry about the thought or they punish themselves in some way for having the thought (Moore & Abramowitz, 2007; Wells & Davies, 1994). Perhaps the person's reaction is stronger because the thoughts seem to the person more serious, more worrisome, and therefore harder to ignore or dismiss.[4]

Such obsessive thoughts lead to anxiety and then to compulsions. At first, the lock-checker checks the locks as a way to reduce the anxiety and the obsessions. Later, however, the lock-checker might perform the compulsive lock checking as a way of staving off anxiety before any anxiety is felt (Salkovskis, 1999). When she walks near the front door, she checks its lock repeatedly, though not in response to any felt anxiety about a break-in. Or, instead of checking the lock, she may strenuously avoid vulnerable parts of the house, or seek excessive reassurance from locksmiths or security companies that the house is secure from break-in. Or, perhaps to make an increasingly routine compulsion feel more reassuring, her compulsions may develop into rituals: she develops a particular way of checking the lock that she finds more reassuring, checking it a certain number of times while holding a certain neutralizing thought in mind, or never touching the doorknob with the left hand, or always leading with the right foot when stepping into the house. Instead of responding to a specific anxiety, the compulsions and rituals can take on a life of their own.

This general description of OCD also applies to its specific forms, including scrupulosity. Scrupulosity is informally characterized as "seeing sin [or immorality] where there is none" or "focus[ing] on minor details of the person's religion, to the exclusion of more important areas" (Nelson et al., 2006: 1072). However, the condition is more complicated and more closely connected to OCD than this characterization would suggest.

Consider first this religious presentation of scrupulosity in Mary:

> 31-year-old wife and mother of three, … an Orthodox Jew and the daughter of an Orthodox rabbi. She worked in the home, raising her children. Mary's main OCD symptoms included recurrent, persistent doubts that she had not completed religious prayers and other rituals properly. Thus, she engaged in such behaviors repeatedly until satisfied that they had been performed correctly. For example, before eating, she felt compelled to recite (to herself) the ritual blessing 18 times (18 is a significant number in Judaism). If she experienced any stray thoughts, or if there were any distractions during the ritual, she would stop and start over from the beginning. When she was unable to finish rituals, she kept a mental note and completed them after the rest of her family had gone to bed. Frequently, Mary spent several hours each night repeating prayers and other religious rituals that she was unable to complete during the day.
>
> *(Abramowitz, 2008)*

Mary's unwanted, anxiety-inducing intrusive thoughts were about whether she had completed religious rituals correctly. Such religious presentations are the most commonly observed kind of scrupulosity. Scrupulous compulsions are often religious in nature, such as excessive praying, disproportionate attention to religious minutiae, and repeated reassurance-seeking from religious authorities (Abramowitz, 2008, Nelson et al., 2006).[5]

Scrupulosity can also take a secular form. Here is an example:

> At a restaurant where Bridget worked as a waitress she had a recurring fear of accidentally poisoning her customers. Accordingly, she checked the containers of cleaning solvents stored in the kitchen cabinets to ensure she did not inadvertently powder the food she served with a lethal garnishing of chemicals. Despite the fact that her position never involved contact with the solvents, making her involvement in such a fatal faux pas a virtual impossibility, she was tormented by the idea and correspondingly checked the containers at almost every order.
>
> *(Garcia, 2008)*

Bridget's anxieties concern harming others, which is not a distinctively religious concern. Bridget did develop a number of religious rituals, such as making the sign of the cross to stave off harm to loved ones and even strangers. However, her basic motivation in this case—avoiding harm to others—is not distinctively religious but is shared by purely secular people.

Whether secular or religious, both Mary and Bridget have intrusive, anxiety-inducing obsessive thoughts that they respond to with compulsions. Scrupulosity also shares other features with other forms of OCD. For example, the scrupulous share obsessions and beliefs about their excessive responsibility, particularly for controlling intrusive thoughts. Scrupulosity also shares with other forms of OCD contamination fears and disgust sensitivity (especially towards sex and death), which a fuller discussion would consider (Olatunji, Tolin, Huppert, & Lohr, 2005; Fergus, 2014).

In addition to those common features, scrupulosity also has certain characteristic features, especially (a) moral perfectionism, (b) chronic doubt and intolerance of uncertainty (Nelson et al., 2006; Frost & Steketee, 2002; Olatunji, Abramowitz, Williams, Connolly, & Lohr, 2007), and (c) moral thought–action fusion. These traits are not necessary or sufficient, so these traits alone would not diagnose scrupulosity: Minimally, a diagnosis should also assess whether the patient has other OCD traits. Further, these traits alone need not distinguish scrupulosity from non-pathological religious and moral views that also value something similar to each of these conditions (Summers & Sinnott-Armstrong, 2015). Nevertheless, these traits are typical or characteristic of scrupulosity.

Perfectionism involves extremely high moral or religious standards for oneself and, correspondingly, a heightened sensitivity to anything that falls short of such standards. Perfectionism—though understudied—seems to promote and maintain various psychopathologies (Shafran & Mansell, 2001; Egan, Wade, & Shafran, 2011). This is not surprising: having high standards and being sensitive to whether they are achieved can make one ever-vigilant and anxious about possible failures. In many religious cases like Mary's, the person is so sensitive to any defect in near-perfectly said prayers that they repeat them over and over. Or, in Bridget's secular case, her perfectionist standards regarding harm to others led her to go far beyond any normal standards to ensure she didn't poison customers.

The second characteristic feature of scrupulosity is chronic doubt and intolerance of uncertainty about the moral or religious status of one's acts and oneself. If one is antecedently anxious about one's religious or moral life, then one is on the lookout for slight or even imaginary failures, whose importance may become magnified. Many anxious repetitions of the same action may be necessary to alleviate these uncomfortable doubts or fears, to feel confident that an action had been performed adequately.

Perhaps the most striking and surprising characteristic of scrupulosity is moral thought–action fusion. Thought–action fusion is a broad and not yet well-understood problem with some general connections to OCD (Berle & Starcevic, 2005; Shafran, Thordarson, & Rachman, 1996). There are two forms: likelihood thought–action fusion and moral thought-action fusion. Someone with *likelihood* thought–action fusion believes that her thoughts, merely by occurring, make some outcome related to the content of the thought more likely to occur. The scrupulous patient might believe that her thoughts will have such effects, but this is not distinctively characteristic of scrupulosity (Nelson et al., 2006; Rassin & Koster, 2003; cf. Tolin, Abramowitz, Kozak, & Foa, 2001; Berman, Abramowitz, Pardue, & Wheaton, 2010).

In *moral* thought–action fusion, which is more characteristic of scrupulosity, the scrupulous patient sees having thoughts about immoral actions, even if they are uncontrollable and intrusive thoughts, as just (or almost) as bad as having an immoral intention, making an immoral attempt, or even actually performing an immoral action (Abramowitz et al., 2002). The perceived wrongness of having the thought lies simply in entertaining its content, however unwillingly. Consider an example.

> Bob was changing his daughter's diaper when the thought, idea, or image (he wasn't quite sure which) flashed through his mind—"touch her private parts." The first time it happened, he shuddered, tried to dismiss the idea, and hurriedly completed diapering her. All day he tried not to think about it. The next time he changed her diaper, however, the idea came back, but this time in the form of a graphic picture of Bob engaging in the dreaded behavior. This time he felt nausea, became dizzy, and called his wife to finish, saying that he thought he was ill and would pass out. The idea began to torment Bob. He found himself not wanting to be alone with his daughter, lest he "give in" to this impulse. He refused to bathe her or change her diaper. … He talked to his rabbi who tried to reassure him that he was not a child molester and should dismiss the thoughts. When Bob could not do this, the rabbi referred him to a psychiatrist. … He and his therapist also explored how "incestuous" feelings are commonplace. Still Bob was not comforted.
>
> *(Ciarrocchi, 1995: 7–8)*[6]

Although the thought (or idea or image) was disturbing, Bob was reliably and repeatedly informed that there was nothing wrong about the thought's merely having occurred, particularly because he found the thought repulsive. Further, although Bob worried about "giving in" to the idea—which sounds like the expression of likelihood thought–action fusion—it also seems that he had no desire to do so or history of doing so. All he had were thoughts about his doing so. Still, Bob imbued those thoughts with moral significance, worrying that he was doing wrong merely in having them (cf. Rassin & Koster, 2003).

All together, the scrupulous person sets high moral standards for her actions as well as her thoughts and then experiences uncertainty and doubt about whether she meets those standards adequately (Abramowitz et al., 2002; Ciarrocchi, 1995). Of course, these three characteristic features are not independent. Judging thoughts to be equivalent to actions can be seen as one kind of extreme standard that constitutes perfectionism. Perfectionism can produce chronic doubt because it is more difficult to meet perfectionist standards. And uncertainty about which moral standards are correct can lead one to adopt extreme standards in order to make sure that one did not overlook any immorality. These interconnections show how the characteristic features of scrupulosity fuel one another and produce an interconnected and coherent syndrome.

3. Justifications for Treatment

If scrupulosity is a form of OCD, and if psychiatrists are justified in treating OCD, then why aren't they also justified in treating scrupulosity for the very same reasons? There are two major problems with this simple deduction. First, the features of OCD that justify treating other forms of OCD might not be present in scrupulosity. Second, the methods of treating scrupulosity might have costs that do not arise when treating other forms of OCD. We'll consider the first of these problems in this section and the second problem in the next section.

The first argument for treating scrupulosity therapeutically is that scrupulosity, like other forms of OCD, is a mental disorder. This argument is too simple. For one thing, just as with physical illnesses, some mental illnesses lead to only minor problems that are not worth the effort to treat. For example, a claustrophobe who lives on an open farm far from civilization might be happy and only rarely feel anxiety from his mental illness, so treating him might not be worth the effort of his traveling to see a therapist. Similarly, some people with OCD might be able to control their anxiety at little cost, for example by checking their locks or washing their hands more than necessary but not enough to cause significant distress. Furthermore, whether a condition is even labeled a mental illness may depend on one's social environment. It has not been that long since homosexuality was classified as a mental illness by the DSM, and some scholars have argued that schizophrenia is culturally valued in some circumstances (Krippner, 2002). These examples are debatable, but they remind us to be cautious in assuming that our existing categories of mental illness alone are enough to show that a condition should be treated. Even if mental illness usually should be treated, we need to ask what it is about each mental disorder that warrants treatment.

The most natural answer for most mental illnesses, including OCD, is distress. Addicts suffer the distress that comes from increasing dependence. Paranoid schizophrenics suffer the distress of a world that seems to conspire against them. Likewise, OCD creates the distress of easily triggered, stubbornly maintained, or regularly and deeply felt anxiety. When mental illness leads to such distress, this second argument asserts, treatment seems justified at least in part as a way to alleviate that distress. We should consider the probability of the treatment succeeding, the benefits of successful treatment, and the costs of treatment (successful or unsuccessful). Nonetheless, allowing for such cost–benefit calculations, this second argument for treatment is relatively straightforward.

Alleviating distress won't always justify treatment. Even when benefits probably outweigh costs, we still need to consider the patient's autonomy. Typically a distressed patient wants to alleviate that distress by changing something about herself, such as her addiction, her schizophrenia, or her anxiety disorder. Some scrupulous patients share this desire for relief, and the justification for their treatment is then that they are in distress, they request treatment, and treatment will probably bring more benefits than costs. It is easy to justify treatment in those cases.

However, this justification is inadequate for those in distress who do not initiate treatment, or who even refuse it. Their recalcitrance forces the therapist (as well as caregivers, loved ones, and others) to balance a desire to alleviate the patient's distress with respect for the patient's (perhaps limited) autonomy. The patient might not recognize her own distress, might prefer the distress to the costs of treatment, or might even prefer her current condition to the condition that therapy aims to bring about. The patient's distress alone is not enough to justify treatment in those cases. These are the cases that will interest us here.

One can sometimes justify psychiatric treatment over indifference, over refusal to grant permission, or even over objection. For example, the risk of death or severe harm for an extreme anorexic or a patient with a delusion that he can fly sometimes trumps the patient's refusal of treatment. Those are cases in which one is a risk to oneself or others. Even when death or permanent harm is not at stake, one can sometimes justify treatment over objection because it is clear enough that the person will later be grateful that the treatment was administered.

These cases are quite complicated. The first complication is that psychiatric treatment is often much less efficacious when the patient objects, so we need to determine the treatment's likelihood of success not in general but specifically with a recalcitrant patient. Another complication is that we need to determine how to get a patient to submit to treatment over objection: Sometimes repeated attempts at persuasion and family pressure are justified, but involuntary commitment by legal authorities is not. A third complication arises because the patient might object to treatment by certain people. A paranoid patient might have special objections to being treated by the therapist who is best able to help. Similarly, a patient with scrupulosity might want treatment only if it is sanctioned or administered by a religious leader (Huppert & Siev, 2010; Huppert, Siev, & Kushner, 2007). However, we will ignore these complications for now and only ask the general questions of whether, when, and why some kind of psychiatric treatment over objection is justified, assuming it is likely to succeed. We will also assume in each case that the patient has consented to therapy up until now, or that nothing more than an initial interview has taken place; therefore, we are asking whether the therapist is justified in *beginning* or *continuing* treatment *of this particular condition.*

Finally, we will focus on only one special case of psychiatric treatment over objection. There are many reasons that a patient may object to treatment. What interests us is that people with scrupulosity might refuse psychiatric treatment for specifically moral or religious reasons. Patients might think, for example, that psychiatric treatment will make them morally worse, even if it succeeds in making them less distressed. Our question is whether some such treatment can be justified when these patients object for moral reasons in particular.

What justifies such treatment in cases of scrupulosity usually cannot be the prevention of death or permanent physical disability, as in cases of anorexia or flying delusions. Scrupulosity almost never threatens such harms. Bridget might lose her job, Bob's home life might deteriorate, and Mary's health might worsen from her sleep deprivation, but none are likely to die or seriously injure themselves or others from scrupulosity.

Surprisingly, such treatment also cannot be justified merely by the distress and anxiety felt by people with scrupulosity. Morality and religion often require personal sacrifice and make people anxious about living up to moral and religious standards. It is distressing for an honest person to break a promise, to keep a promise that they wish they could break, or even to see someone else break a promise. It is also difficult for a caring person to be polite or helpful to a jerk. Good people also often feel some anxiety about whether they are doing the right thing. These bad feelings don't show that such people need therapy, but only that they are willing to endorse and adhere to certain moral norms at some personal cost. Likewise, patients with scrupulosity might be distressed about many aspects of their lives—that they are pleasing to god, have harmed someone inadvertently, have sinned by thinking about doing something wrong—but that distress by itself is not enough to justify therapy.

Of course, people with scrupulosity might feel greater distress and anxiety than most others. Even this greater degree of distress, however, would not be a general justification for their treatment. It is always problematic to make an assessment that a person is in enough distress to justify treatment over objection (Wakefield, 1992). If a person with scrupulosity thinks that her distress is warranted by her own moral standards, then it is particularly problematic to claim that she is wrong (either because her standards are wrong or because she interprets them wrongly). The job of psychiatrists is presumably not to judge the moral views of their patients. Yet that judgment seems needed in order to justify psychiatric treatment over moral objection on the basis of great distress. So this justification is problematic at best.

Another possible justification for treatment over moral objection is a prediction of future gratitude. Although currently people with scrupulosity are distressed by the slightest possibility of sin, this distress and assessment are due to their mental illness. After successful treatment, they would have less anxiety, distress, and chronic doubt; they would see their former anxiety levels as unjustified because they would then have less stringent moral standards; and they would understand that treatment was in their best interests, so they would be grateful that they had had the treatment.

This justification is problematic for people with scrupulosity. It assumes that the patient is better off after successful therapy because they are no longer as distressed by what was previously distressing. But what *should* a person find distressing? Before treatment, people with scrupulosity might recognize that they will be happier after treatment, but they might see this happiness as the result of lower moral standards, and they might be willing to sacrifice their happiness for the sake of moral goodness. Unless a therapist can show that the patient's moral standards are incorrect and the therapist's moral standards are correct, it is hard to see how the therapist could justify treatment over moral objection. Without such a showing, treatment seems too close to indoctrination into our lax moral culture or to an imposition of the therapist's own moral standards. Even if the patient could be convinced of the therapist's standards, the therapist ventures onto shaky ground when she must rely so explicitly on her own assessment of how moral a person should be.

Yet another justification, which avoids this problem, cites the moral standards of a relevant community. A therapist who applies the standards of the patient's own moral or religious community need not rely on the therapist's own standards, since the therapist need not be a member of that community or endorse its standards. Still, how and how well this justification works depends on the relation between the community's moral standards and the patient's own moral standards.

Consider first a patient who is trying to meet the standards of her own community. Her standards—those she would argue for and defend—she sees as morally or religiously ordinary standards. For example, Mary prays 18 times after each meal and doubts that she has completed the prayers properly, even though she has no evidence of any major error or distraction. If Mary believes that this is what her community requires, and she is wrong about what her community requires, then the therapist (perhaps with help from community leaders) can point out this error in Mary's interpretation of her community's standards without endorsing those community standards and, hence, without imposing the therapist's own standards. Of course, merely being wrong about what is religiously required is not itself grounds for treatment over moral objection.[7] Even if the patient feels great distress, and the therapist can relieve that distress without imposing the therapist's own moral standards but only by applying the community standards that the patient wants to follow, the patient retains more than enough autonomy to make her own decisions about whether to object to treatment. Therapy over moral objection would not be justified in this case.

Likewise, there is no justification for treatment over moral objection for patients who are trying to exceed their community's standards or to endorse and meet a higher standard. Imagine Mary knows that her community requires only one prayer without major error, but she personally sees that standard as too lax. She thinks that her community should endorse a more stringent requirement of 18 prayers after each meal with no error or distraction at all. She believes that she and other members of her community are really required to meet this more stringent standard. In this situation, the therapist cannot simply appeal to the community standard, because Mary knows and rejects that standard. The therapist could not justify treatment over objection without assuming that the community is right and Mary is wrong about the proper standards. Treatment then seems too close to indoctrination, as discussed above, regardless of whether Mary feels distress.

How, then, could a therapist justify treatment over objection for patients whose actions reflect abnormally stringent moral or religious standards? We'll suggest three justifications, each of which cites an internal incoherence in the patient's beliefs or standards. Because the incoherence is internal to the patient's own views, the therapist's own standards are not imposed on the patient. In each case, that incoherence is best explained as the patient's attempt to soothe her own anxiety, and each kind of case can involve great distress. Together, this incoherence motivated by anxiety that causes great distress will provide justifications for treatment over moral objection.

The first possible justification appeals to internal incoherence that arises from the patient's inability to coherently defend her actions or her standards. Imagine that Mary is asked to defend her praying 18 times after each meal. She might cite a standard that she knows is abnormal. But then how could she defend her abnormal standard? Is there some biblical or rabbinic source for saying 18 prayers? Is it required for everyone? Does someone sin by praying only once after each meal? Is everyone else, including her friends and family as well as religious exemplars and leaders in her community, a sinner many times over? Questions like these will often reveal that Mary's own views are incoherent because they are arbitrarily chosen.

How did Mary end up with such arbitrary and incoherent standards? The answer seems to be that she chose those standards to soothe her anxiety rather than in any way that would justify those standards. The description of her case is not detailed enough to know for sure, but here's a suggestion of how Mary arrived at her rituals as a response to her anxiety. Mary had "persistent doubts" that led her to engage in prayers "repeatedly until satisfied that they had been performed correctly" (Abramowitz, 2008). She had doubts about whether she had said a prayer adequately (cf. Bonchek & Greenberg, 2009). She repeated parts of it to reassure herself; then, she repeated all of it. As repeating the entire prayer started to feel ordinary, she felt a need to repeat the entire prayer again. Finally, she decided to try 18 repetitions, since 18 is a number important in her religion, and 18 repetitions did soothe her anxieties.[8] In this story, Mary *feels compelled* to exceed her standard (which requires only one prayer said adequately) because she *doubts* that she has fulfilled that standard, and she feels *anxious* if she does not repeat her prayers.[9]

Notice that this doubt might not only make her exceed her own standards; it might even make her adopt the higher standards, believing that they are in fact required. If she comes to think that she is in fact required to pray 18 times without any error after each meal, those higher standards are part of her understanding as to why she feels so much anxiety and doubt after saying the prayer only once. This rationalization can explain and thus make her anxiety and doubt easier to deal with. However, she settles on these higher standards only in order to explain or cope with her anxiety, not because she has engaged in a theological investigation. In general, then, Mary's abnormal standards and the actions that reflect those standards end up being incoherent because they are motivated primarily by her need to relieve her doubts and anxieties.

This first form of incoherence—when one acts on or endorses standards without justification[10] but only from the motivation to soothe one's anxieties—leads to a justification for treatment over moral objection because the patient cannot coherently defend her own standards, and the underlying explanation for this incoherence is something amenable to psychiatric treatment. To justify treatment in such cases, the therapist does not need to rely on the therapist's own standards but can instead cite the patient's own desire for coherence plus the source of that incoherence in the desire to avoid anxiety as justification for changing the patient's views so as to become more coherent. What get treated are not the patient's moral views or standards themselves but instead the anxiety that is the source of those standards. Of course, treatment will not be justified unless the patient suffers significant distress, but the point here is that therapists can justify relieving that distress over moral objections when those objections are arbitrary and motivated to soothe anxiety.

A second type of incoherence arises from a conflation of ideals with requirements. For an illustration, consider Ezekiel, who cleans all of his orifices for about 20 minutes before praying (Greenberg et al., 1987). He and those in his community agree that one should not begin prayer when very dirty, when one smells of feces, or when one has not showered in a long time. That is a minimal requirement, a standard below which it would not be permissible to pray. In contrast, the ideal level of cleanliness is to be free from every microscopic speck of dirt and feces (and bacteria?). This ideal is practically unobtainable, though one can approach it to varying degrees. Even for people above the minimal requirement, it might be better to come closer to the ideal. However, if one thinks that the ideal is required, then one will never feel permitted to pray, because that standard cannot be met. Even if it could be met, one could never know whether one has met it on a particular occasion. Then, for example, Ezekiel could never be sure that he is entirely clean, so he could not begin prayer without anxiety and doubt.

If a patient's extreme behavior or standard result from a failure to distinguish ideals from requirements, and if that failure is again the result of an underlying desire to soothe the patient's anxiety, and if this condition causes great enough distress, then treatment can be justified despite moral objection without imposing the therapist's own standards. The therapist relies on the patient's standards and helps the patient to see that the patient has confused her ideals with minimal requirements. The therapist relies only on a conceptual distinction, so the therapist's own standards are unimportant in resolving this confusion. This justification does not question the patient's views about what is morally or religiously ideal. It simply reminds the patient that what is ideal need not be required. Hence, treatment over moral objection may be justified in many such cases without presumptuously imposing outside standards.

A third kind of internal incoherence results from perseveration or fixation. OCD patients, including those with scrupulosity, often focus exclusively on a small number of (often unimportant) issues at the expense of many other (more important) issues. Those with scrupulosity focus primarily on the features that relieve their anxiety in the short term, not on features that further their professed goal to be more moral or religious. As a result, people with scrupulosity are more moral or religious in select areas, but their actions are morally or religiously distorted (Summers & Sinnott-Armstrong, 2015). They might be far more observant about making sure no word of a prayer is said incorrectly, but that extra time can lead to problems in other areas, for example in devoting enough time to one's family (Greenberg et al., 1987). They may diligently pull over to the side of the road to cross themselves whenever they hear an ambulance, but they may not think about the danger and inconvenience of those around them as they quickly change lanes (Garcia, 2008). In cases like this, a therapist can justify treatment by appealing to standards that the patient herself endorses but which she has forgotten because she is so fixated on only one part of her overall view.

Consider again Bridget, who "checked the containers at almost every order"—but why? She might say that she wanted to reduce the chances of poisoning her customers, but "her involvement in such a fatal faux pas [was] a virtual impossibility" (Garcia, 2008). If she really wanted to protect the interests of her customers, then she would be more concerned about getting them their meals quickly. Indeed, her regularly checking the levels of solvents that she wouldn't otherwise come near could have made it *more* likely that she would poison the customers. The fact that she continuously checked the containers despite such costs to those customers whose welfare was her professed goal shows that her real motivation to check the containers so often was to reduce her anxiety, not to protect her customers. Because her ritual did not really serve her own goals, the therapist can justify treatment by citing her own goals.

The three types of incoherence cited here—arbitrariness, conflation, and fixation—are important in establishing that the therapist is not imposing the therapist's own goals. But a justification for treatment over moral objection also requires that the patient suffers significant distress and that the underlying explanation of the patient's incoherence is that she is trying to reduce her own anxiety.

This goal of reducing anxiety distinguishes scrupulosity from extreme religious devotion (Taylor, 2002). A devout Catholic might regularly pray the rosary to imitate his favorite saints or to carry out the penance prescribed by a priest during confession. In contrast, a scrupulous Catholic might pray the rosary as a way of preventing bad thoughts or events that would increase anxiety (Abramowitz, 2002; Greenberg, 1984; Tek & Ulug, 2001; Traig, 2004).

This motivation is also what scrupulosity most fundamentally has in common with other forms of OCD. Those with scrupulosity usually focus on those things that also provoke anxiety in other forms of OCD, like sex or death. The scrupulous focus on the religious or moral expression of these common anxiogenic areas.

People with scrupulosity also often suffer from certain cognitive or emotional distortions that are also characteristic of OCD (O'Connor & Robillard, 1995). For example, those with OCD, including the scrupulous, treat themselves as excessively responsible—perhaps feeling responsible for the outcome of events over which they have little control, such as the death of a loved one who lives far away, or for the subsequent "impurity" of someone with whom they interacted. The scrupulous, attracted to a religious expression of this concern, might focus on their own prayers. They might feel strong anxiety if prevented from prayer, might feel a need to say prayers for things about which they are not responsible, and might believe their failure to say such prayers would be especially serious.

Similarly, we should expect the scrupulous to look for reassurance that their actions were morally faultless. This helps to assuage their anxieties and doubts. They might seek reassurance from an authority, as when a patient repeatedly sought his rabbi's reassurance that he had not sinned by swallowing his saliva on Yom Kippur, a day when fasting is required (Abramowitz et al., 2002). Or, they might look for reassurance from secular sources, as did a scrupulous patient who worried that his former date, with whom he had not had sexual intercourse, had become pregnant and subsequently might have had an abortion. He went to great lengths to reassure himself: calling doctors in the area, checking whether she had missed any work (Abramowitz, 2008).

Because the scrupulous are focused on relieving their own anxiety rather than on doing what is moral, a therapist can justify treating most such cases of scrupulosity without imposing her own moral standards on the patient. The therapist can justify treatment by citing the patient's own moral or religious standards or at least the standards that the patient would hold if her view were not distorted by her desire to relieve her anxiety and doubt. The patient is not a moral exemplar but is driven by her emotional distortions. Of course, this justification might not be one that the patient is ready to accept at the beginning of treatment, and we have not resolved the question of what kind of treatment this would justify, but this justification of treatment over moral objection does avoid simply appealing to the therapist's own moral or religious standards.

We have argued that treatment of scrupulosity over moral objection can be justified in various cases by citing incoherence, a source in anxiety, and significant distress. As we said, different justifications might apply in different cases of scrupulosity. Moreover, separate justifications might need to work together. When a patient has an abnormally high moral standard, that by itself is not enough to justify treatment over moral objection. In contrast, when that higher standard is both incoherent and also an attempt to soothe anxiety, and this leads to distress for the patient, then there is a justification for treatment over moral objection. But what if only one of these conditions is met? Someone with incoherent moral or religious standards but whose standards are not motivated by a desire to relieve anxiety seems to need education rather than psychiatric treatment. Similarly, someone whose moral or religious standards are motivated by a desire to relieve anxiety may benefit from psychiatric treatment, but such treatment cannot be compelled if those standards are not incoherent or otherwise defective, or if they lead to no distress, even if they are abnormally stringent. Thus, three conditions—incoherence, the motivation to relieve anxiety, and significant distress—all seem necessary in order to justify treatment over moral objection. The justification is sufficient only jointly.

This triple requirement responds, then, to the puzzle at the outset: Why should we treat someone with high moral standards? Shouldn't we instead praise them? Our answer is that we *do* and *should* praise them in some cases: When their high standards are coherent and they are motivated by recognizably moral motives instead of just the need to soothe their own anxiety, then we should not treat them (unless they want treatment). Take, for example, someone who gives away almost everything she has (Salwen & Salwen, 2010). She makes the case for why this is morally good, maybe even why it is morally required. Most of us will not act as she does, so her actions are statistically abnormal. Perhaps there is even something defective about her actions. She may focus too much on material donations to charity over other moral requirements. Her gifts might cause problems for her family and friends. Nevertheless, her actions are aimed at helping others and not just to soothe her own anxiety, so she is not blinded by her anxiety to other areas that she should and does also care about. If this person's standards are wrong, then we should address this with reasoned debate and discussion, pointing out competing moral requirements or unanticipated consequences of her actions. If the person were offered therapy that she refused for moral reasons, then there is no justification in trying to treat her over such objection. Thus, we are justified in treating some people who have abnormal, extremely high moral standards when the underlying motivation—to soothe anxiety—is what explains those standards and when they suffer significant distress, but we are not justified in treating someone *just because* she has higher moral standards.

4. Types of Treatment

This justification for treatment in general still leaves open the question of which specific kind of treatment is justifiable. As with treatments for physical illnesses, some forms of treatment might raise special problems, even if they are effective. In particular, the short-term costs of one form of treatment are that the therapist asks the patient to do something she judges potentially immoral. In the long term, successful therapy might make the patient less sensitive to morality. Such costs are potentially significant.

One effective means of treating various forms of OCD (alone or in combination) is Exposure and Response Prevention. This treatment requires exposing OCD patients to something that, given their OCD, will provoke their anxiety, then having them follow instructions not to perform actions designed to soothe the anxiety their prior actions raised. For a lock-checking form of OCD, the therapist might instruct the patient to leave the door unlocked for a while, and not to perform any rituals, including mental rituals, that would soothe anxiety about the unchecked lock. By experiencing and noticing that her action brings about anxiety, but not then doing anything to ease that anxiety, the patient avoids reinforcing the anxiety with her compulsions, and she may recognize that her anxiety will diminish naturally over time (Abramowitz, Deacon, & Whiteside, 2012; Abramowitz, 1996).

For patients with scrupulosity, the exposure is to an act that the patient sees as at least potentially immoral. This kind of exposure seems problematic. Should a therapist instruct a patient to do something that the patient judges to be potentially immoral, particularly when given the additional instruction not to do anything to compensate for the supposed moral transgression?

The short-term costs seem less problematic if we remember the justification for treatment, which justification is also shared with the patient. The patient's extreme view of moral or religious obligations reflects her attempt to soothe her own anxiety, not simply her strong desire to be moral. In addition, the patient's moral view is incoherent in ways discussed above (arbitrary, conflated, fixated). Unless the therapist is also a religious authority, she might need to consult a relevant religious authority to show this in particular cases.[11] Given this justification for treatment, the therapist does have some flexibility to ask the patient to act in a way that the patient prefers not to act for moral or religious reasons, but which is not immoral by the overall standards of the patient. If the patient remains concerned about the immorality of the action the therapist requests, the therapist can remind the patient of the larger goals and techniques of this form of therapy, which are important to make clear to the patient. This reminder should not itself be a form of reassurance, but the patient should be made to understand that the goal of treatment is not to make the patient act immorally. The short-term costs of such treatment therefore seem minimal, given the above justifications for treatment.

Potential long-term risks are another matter. Treatment—exposure therapy or any other form of treatment for scrupulosity—might make a person less sensitive to real moral or religious obligations. Even if the patient's moral views are abnormal, there is no way to target only those disproportionate moral positions. If Bridget comes to be less anxious about harming others, this will keep her from checking unnecessarily for poisons, but she might also become less attentive to harms that a moral exemplar might continue to worry about. These dangers arise because such patients' moral and religious practices are motivated (at least in part) to soothe some underlying anxiety. If therapy is successful in reducing that anxiety, then their motivation to be moral or religious may also decrease, and perhaps not just in the misguided or disproportionate cases.

Luckily, this danger is probably not terribly serious because most people are not moral or religious primarily as a way of soothing anxiety. Philosophers have long debated what exactly motivates people to be moral, but there is good reason to think anxiety is not the only or the primary motivation. Similarly, there are motivations other than the desire to soothe anxiety (such as concern for others and love of god) that lead people to be religious. Most people are capable of being moral and religious with normal levels of anxiety. This suggests that successful therapy need not eliminate an adequate motivation to be moral and religious.

Nevertheless, for some patients who are motivated largely by their anxiety, there is some theoretical threat that the long-term effects of reducing anxiety might be to reduce their moral or religious motivation more broadly. We are unaware of any research showing this to be a real danger, so we suggest this only as a theoretical possibility. It is nevertheless instructive to consider how to address even this theoretical danger.

One way to diminish this theoretical danger is to supplement therapy with steps to help the patient calibrate her moral responses to the moral and religious responses that she or those in her community consider normal and justified. (Remember, in many cases the scrupulous exceed even their own moral standards.) In the case of morality, the person's regular interactions with ordinary people over time should be adequate for this purpose, and the patient may learn over time how to discuss what is morally required without doing so simply to reassure her own anxiety. If the therapist can continue discussions of how best to negotiate morally fraught situations without thereby simply reassuring the patient, then this role might be appropriate for the therapist. It would require the therapist to take substantive moral stands, and the therapist should exercise caution here. In the religious case, a religious community could serve a similar role. Indeed, there are sometimes even support groups for people with scrupulosity within religious communities, such as the Roman Catholic Scrupulous Anonymous (Ciarrocchi, 1995). Steps like these can reduce the theoretical dangers of treating scrupulosity.

5. Conclusion

Initial appearances might incline some to think of the scrupulous as exceedingly moral or religious, but we have argued that scrupulosity is, instead, a form of mental illness, specifically OCD. Even so, there remains a question of whether this particular form of OCD warrants therapeutic treatment. We argued that such therapy cannot be justified simply by pointing out that scrupulosity is a mental illness, that it causes distress, that the patients will be grateful after therapy, or that patients with scrupulosity go beyond what their communities require. Nonetheless, therapy for scrupulosity can be justified, sometimes even over moral objection. Therapists need not invoke their own moral or religious judgments or claim that scrupulosity patients are too moral or religious. The reason is that patients with scrupulosity are not simply more moral or religious than other people, but, as a result of underlying anxiety that they try to soothe, they are disproportionately and inflexibly concerned with certain areas of morality and religion at the expense of others that they themselves often recognize as important, so their views become internally incoherent. Thus, one may justify their treatment based on the significant discrepancy between the moral or religious standards to which they themselves are ostensibly committed and their behavior manifesting their obsessions and compulsions, which manifest that underlying anxiety, and which create distress. Finally, we considered a potential short-term cost of exposure therapy, that the person is asked to do something she sees as immoral, and one possible long-term cost of any form of treatment, that she may in fact become less moral. We argued that neither cost is a terribly serious danger. We thus conclude that, contrary to initial appearances, treatment of the scrupulous even over moral objection is morally justified in most cases. There still might be some cases of scrupulosity where treatment is not justified, but they will be exceptional.

Notes

1 This section borrows from the authors' previously published work (Summers & Sinnott-Armstrong, 2015; Summers & Sinnott-Armstrong, forthcoming-a; Summers & Sinnott-Armstrong, forthcoming-b).

2 DSM-IV-TR considers scrupulosity within Obsessive-Compulsive Personality Disorder (OCPD), in which—among other things—such extreme morality or religiosity is not subjectively resisted (DSM-IV-TR 301.4). OCPD is generally ego-syntonic, that is, the patient finds no particular distress from the condition, whereas OCD is generally ego-dystonic; and distress might affect the need for treatment. DSM-5 is more concerned with the degree of insight the patient has into her own condition. Regardless, the research on scrupulosity shows little interest in these diagnostic categories (Summers & Sinnott-Armstrong, forthcoming-a).

3 OCD can be described in several ways, some more cognitive than others. The cognitive theory of OCD and its variants presented here seem to be the most common theory among psychologists who work on scrupulosity (cf. Salkovskis, 1999; Abramowitz, Huppert, Cohen, Tolin, & Cahill, 2002). Possibly problematic is the order of causal explanation: for example, do thoughts of future harms cause anxiety or does the feeling of anxiety lead some people to notice and fixate on thoughts of future harm as a way to justify why she feels anxiety? There also might be feedback or mutual support. We will write as if the thoughts cause the anxiety, though we later consider some complications that arise if the anxiety causes the thoughts.

4 For simplicity, we won't consider whether someone with OCD could have beliefs that are in fact true but different from widespread false beliefs. For example, the lock-checker could have a better understanding of the true burglary rate in the area than most of her neighbors do, and then it would be unclear whether she worries too much or her neighbors worry too little (Taylor & Brown, 1988; Taylor & Brown, 1994).

5 Why are religious presentations more common than secular presentations? Perhaps because the religious are more prone to develop OCD, because those with OCD tend to be attracted to religion, or because so many people are religious and then use their religion to rationalize their anxieties and compulsions—or perhaps all three. It is also possible that there is much more secular scrupulosity than we have noticed, because we expect scrupulosity to be religious, so we overlook secular cases. This is a topic for future research.

6 Notice that Bob's motivations and moral standards seem secular, even though he went to a rabbi for guidance.

7 What about being wrong about what morality requires? Does that error justify therapy? The answer is complicated. It may be grounds for *detainment* if someone is wrong about moral issues in ways that endanger others, for example, someone who believes that killing innocent people is morally good (at least if the person does or is likely to act on that belief). And someone's being radically wrong about important moral issues certainly *suggests* some

underlying psychological problem. It's hard to imagine someone who endorses murdering innocents but has no underlying psychopathology. However, this intersection of morality, rationality, and psychology is far more than we can discuss here. Therefore, we will focus primarily on religious examples, since a failure to be religious is not itself indicative of psychopathology.

8 Would it have continued to soothe her anxiety if she hadn't sought therapy?

9 A subtle question that we have to gloss over here is what should count as a belief. When a person "feels compelled" to repeat a prayer 18 times, does she *believe* that she should or must repeat it 18 times? Does a compulsive hand-washer *believe* that his hands are still dirty, or does he just *feel compelled* to continue washing them despite knowing how clean they are? We raise these questions to suggest a distinction between what one believes one should do and what one is motivated to do (Grayson, 2014).

10 To be clear, Mary probably could give *some* justification as to why she should pray 18 times after a meal, but that justification is best explained as a rationalization of the desire to alleviate anxiety, that is, if the person weren't trying to alleviate anxiety, she would likely not even herself find her justification persuasive. Certainly, those in her community will find it to be a weak justification. As a short-hand, then, we will say that there is no justification, but that should be understood as meaning that the justification is weak and primarily a rationalization of an underlying desire.

11 Consulting respected authorities is a common part of treatment for scrupulosity (Huppert & Siev, 2010). However, a therapist must be careful not to let the consultations with a religious authority serve as reassurance to the patient. That would defeat the response-prevention aspect of the treatment. The therapist should also be aware that asking the patient to replace the prayer repetitions with more religiously acceptable activities would similarly risk turning those replacements into their own anxiolytic compulsions.

References

Abramowitz, J. S. (1996). "Variants of exposure and response prevention in the treatment of obsessive-compulsive disorder: A meta-analysis." *Behavior Therapy, 27(4)*, 583–600.

Abramowitz, J. S. (2002). "Treatment of scrupulous obsessions and compulsions using exposure and response prevention: A case report." *Cognitive and Behavioral Practice, 8(1)*, 79–85.

——(2008). "Scrupulosity." In *Clinical handbook of obsessive compulsive disorder and related conditions* (pp. 156–72). Baltimore: Johns Hopkins University Press.

Abramowitz, J. S., Deacon, B. J., & Whiteside, S. P. H. (2012). *Exposure therapy for anxiety: Principles and practice*. Guilford Press.

Abramowitz, J. S., Huppert, J. D., Cohen, A. B., Tolin, D. F., & Cahill, S. P. (2002). "Religious obsessions and compulsions in a non-clinical sample: the Penn Inventory of Scrupulosity (PIOS)." *Behaviour Research and Therapy, 40(7)*, 825–38.

Berle, D., & Starcevic, V. (2005). "Thought–action fusion: Review of the literature and future directions." *Clinical Psychology Review, 25(3)*, 263–84.

Berman, N. C., Abramowitz, J. S., Pardue, C. M., & Wheaton, M. G. (2010). "The relationship between religion and thought–action fusion: Use of an in vivo paradigm." *Behaviour Research and Therapy, 48(7)*, 670–74.

Bonchek, A., & Greenberg, D. (2009). "Compulsive prayer and its management." *Journal of Clinical Psychology, 65(4)*, 396–405.

Ciarrocchi, J. W. (1995). *The doubting disease: Help for scrupulosity and religious compulsions*. Mahwah, NJ: Paulist Pr.

Egan, S. J., Wade, T. D., & Shafran, R. (2011). "Perfectionism as a transdiagnostic process: A clinical review." *Clinical Psychology Review, 31(2)*, 203–12.

Fergus, T. A. (2014). "Mental contamination and scrupulosity: Evidence of unique associations among Catholics and Protestants." *Journal of Obsessive-Compulsive and Related Disorders, 3(3)*, 236–42.

Frost, R. O., & Steketee, G. (2002). *Cognitive approaches to obsessions and compulsions: Theory, assessment, and treatment.* New York: Pergamon Press.

Garcia, H. A. (2008). "Targeting Catholic rituals as symptoms of obsessive compulsive disorder: A cognitive-behavioral and psychodynamic, assimilative integrationist approach." *Pragmatic Case Studies in Psychotherapy, 4(2)*, 63–74.

Grayson, J. (2014). *Freedom from obsessive compulsive disorder (Updated Edition).* New York: Penguin.

Greenberg, D. (1984). "Are religious compulsions religious or compulsive: A phenomenological study." *American Journal of Psychotherapy, 38(4)*, 524.

Greenberg, D., & Huppert, J. (2010). "Scrupulosity: A unique subtype of obsessive-compulsive disorder." *Current Psychiatry Reports, 12(4)*, 282–89.

Greenberg, D., Witztum, E., & Pisante, J. (1987). "Scrupulosity: Religious attitudes and clinical presentations." *British Journal of Medical Psychology, 60(1)*, 29–37.

Huppert, J. D., & Siev, J. (2010). "Treating scrupulosity in religious individuals using cognitive-behavioral therapy." *Cognitive and Behavioral Practice, 17(4)*, 382–92.

Huppert, J. D., Siev, J., & Kushner, E. S. (2007). "When religion and obsessive–compulsive disorder collide: Treating scrupulosity in ultra-orthodox Jews." *Journal of Clinical Psychology, 63(10)*, 925–41.

Krippner, S. C. (2002). "Conflicting perspectives on shamans and shamanism: Points and counterpoints." *The American Psychologist, 57(11)*, 962–78.

Miller, C. H., & Hedges, D. W. (2008). "Scrupulosity disorder: An overview and introductory analysis." *Journal of Anxiety Disorders, 22(6)*, 1042–58.

Moore, E. L., & Abramowitz, J. S. (2007). "The cognitive mediation of thought-control strategies." *Behaviour Research and Therapy, 45(8)*, 1949–55.

Mora, G. (1969). "The scrupulosity syndrome." *International Psychiatry Clinics, 5(4)*, 163.

Nelson, E. A., Abramowitz, J. S., Whiteside, S. P., & Deacon, B. J. (2006). "Scrupulosity in patients with obsessive-compulsive disorder: Relationship to clinical and cognitive phenomena." *Journal of Anxiety Disorders, 20(8)*, 1071–86.

O'Connor, K., & Robillard, S. (1995). "Inference processes in obsessive-compulsive disorder: Some clinical observations." *Behaviour Research and Therapy, 33(8)*, 887–96.

Olatunji, B. O., Tolin, D. F., Huppert, J. D., & Lohr, J. M. (2005). "The relation between fearfulness, disgust sensitivity and religious obsessions in a non-clinical sample." *Personality and Individual Differences, 38(4)*, 891–902.

Olatunji, B. O., Abramowitz, J. S., Williams, N. L., Connolly, K. M., & Lohr, J. M. (2007). "Scrupulosity and obsessive-compulsive symptoms: Confirmatory factor analysis and validity of the Penn Inventory of Scrupulosity." *Journal of Anxiety Disorders, 21(6)*, 771–87.

Plutarch. (1951). *Plutarch: Selected lives and essays* (L. R. Loomis, Trans.). Roslyn, NY: Walter J. Black.

Rachman, S., & de Silva, P. (1978). "Abnormal and normal obsessions." *Behaviour Research and Therapy, 16(4)*, 233–48.

Rassin, E., & Koster, E. (2003). "The correlation between thought-action fusion and religiosity in a normal sample." *Behaviour Research and Therapy, 41(3)*, 361–68.

Rassin, E., & Muris, P. (2007). "Abnormal and normal obsessions: A reconsideration." *Behaviour Research and Therapy, 45(5)*, 1065–70.

Salkovskis, P. M. (1999). "Understanding and treating obsessive-compulsive disorder." *Behavior Research and Therapy, 37(supplement)*, s29-s52.

Salkovskis, P. M., & Harrison, J. (1984). "Abnormal and normal obsessions—A replication." *Behaviour Research and Therapy, 22(5)*, 549–52.

Salwen, K., & Salwen, H. (2010). *The power of half: One family's decision to stop taking and start giving back.* Houghton Mifflin Harcourt.

Shafran, R., & Mansell, W. (2001). "Perfectionism and psychopathology: A review of research and treatment." *Clinical Psychology Review, 21(6)*, 879–906.

Shafran, R., Thordarson, D. S., & Rachman, S. (1996). "Thought-action fusion in obsessive compulsive disorder." *Journal of Anxiety Disorders, 10(5)*, 379–91.

Summers, J. S., & Sinnott-Armstrong, W. (forthcoming-a). "Scrupulous characters and mental illness." In I. Fileva (Ed.), *Character: Perspectives from philosophy and psychology*. Oxford: Oxford University Press.

——(forthcoming-b). "Scrupulous agents." *Philosophical Psychology*.

——(2015). "Scrupulous judgments." In M. Timmons (Ed.), *Oxford studies in normative ethics*. Oxford: Oxford University Press.

Taylor, C. Z. (2002). "Religious addiction: Obsession with spirituality." *Pastoral Psychology, 50 (4)*, 291–315.

Taylor, S. E., & Brown, J. D. (1988). "Illusion and well-being: A social psychological perspective on mental health." *Psychological Bulletin, 103(2)*, 193–210.

——(1994). "Positive illusions and well-being revisited: Separating fact from fiction." *Psychological Bulletin, 116(1)*, 21–27.

Tek, C., & Ulug, B. (2001). "Religiosity and religious obsessions in obsessive-compulsive disorder." *Psychiatry Research 104(2)*, 99–108.

Tolin, D. F., Abramowitz, J. S., Kozak, M. J., & Foa, E. B. (2001). "Fixity of belief, perceptual aberration, and magical ideation in obsessive–compulsive disorder." *Journal of Anxiety Disorders, 15(6)*, 501–10.

Traig, J. (2004). *Devil in the details: Scenes from an obsessive girlhood*. New York: Little, Brown.

Wakefield, J. C. (1992). "Disorder as harmful dysfunction: A conceptual critique of DSM-IIIR's definition of mental disorder." *Psychological Review, 99(2)*, 232–47.

Wells, A., & Davies, M. I. (1994). "The Thought Control Questionnaire: A measure of individual differences in the control of unwanted thoughts." *Behaviour Research and Therapy, 32 (8)*, 871–78.

6b

Commentary on Summers and Sinnott-Armstrong: Scrupulosity and the Shady Morality of Psychiatry

Hanna Pickard

Can you be too moral? Certainly, you can be too *moralistic* – a prude, a prig, a rigid stickler to rules, moral and otherwise. Equally, you can be too prone to perfectionism, irrational doubts, and anxiety, lacking the ability to cope well with these traits in various aspects of life – again, moral and otherwise. But is it possible either to have so much *care or concern for morality* or to have *moral standards* that are so high that you have a problem that may need psychiatric treatment? In their rich and nuanced paper, Jesse Summers and Walter Sinnott-Armstrong argue that, when a person has a condition called *scrupulosity*, it is appropriate to treat patients who exhibit too much moral care or concern, or whose moral standards are too high, even over their objections when certain conditions are met. This commentary aims to raise some questions about their characterisation of scrupulosity as a disorder involving, among other things, *too much care or concern for morality* or *too high moral standards*, and their arguments for the appropriateness of treatment over patients' objections. But, in so doing, it also considers some of the broader connections between morality and psychiatry, bringing the monsters that lurk in the shadows of psychiatry to light.

Scrupulosity is not a self-standing disorder according to the DSM-5. Rather, it seems to combine one of the traits characteristic of Obsessive-Compulsive Personality Disorder (OCPD) with some of the symptomatology of Obsessive-Compulsive Disorder (OCD). The personality trait in question is excessive conscientiousness, "scrupulosity", and inflexibility about matters of morality, which is out of keeping with a person's religious or wider moral community. The symptomatology in question is persistent and intrusive thoughts – particularly thoughts about real or possible failures to meet the demands of morality – which cause anxiety and distress and lead to compulsive and repetitive patterns of behaviour that aim, but ultimately fail, to cope with the underlying thoughts and emotions.

To give a flavour of the condition, Summers and Sinnott-Armstrong describe an Orthodox Jewish woman who feels compelled to recite a ritual blessing 18 times before eating; a religious man who obsessively cleans his orifices for at least 20 minutes before praying; and a waitress who checks that the containers of cleaning solvents are sealed before serving every order to make sure she does not poison her customers. Certainly such behaviour and correspondingly its underlying motivation appear unusual. But do these people really have too much care or concern for morality or moral standards that are just too high?

Consider a non-religious and non-moral but otherwise comparable pathological example: a person who checks the lock on the door 22 times when leaving the house to make sure it is secure. Would we say this person cares or is concerned too much about household security or has overly high security standards? I don't wish to deny that, speaking loosely, we might put the problem this way. But on consideration, this characterisation does not seem apt, because it suggests that the behaviour in question *promotes household security*. We would certainly expect a person who cares about household security or has high security standards to ensure the door is locked before leaving. But, if indeed it is locked the first time they check, nothing security-wise is gained by a further 21 checks. Rather, when linked to a diagnosis of OCPD or OCD, this behaviour seems better characterised as a way of *coping with anxieties about household security*, which the person feels compelled to perform even though the repeated behaviour does nothing to decrease the likelihood of a break-in. This is not a person who *cares or is concerned too much* about household security or whose *standards* are too high, but a person who is *anxious* about household security and has developed an obsessive–compulsive coping strategy.

Let us return now to the religious and moral examples more characteristic of scrupulosity. Do these people have too much care or concern for morality or have moral standards that are too high? Again, this characterisation does not seem apt, because moral ends are not in fact served by such highly rigid, repetitive, and fixated behaviour. Of course, all things being equal, Orthodox Jews believe that they should recite a ritual blessing before eating; many religious people believe that they should not pray in a dirty, squalid state; and morally decent people believe that we should all take precautions to ensure we don't kill other people, which will involve responding appropriately to possible risks. But, just as household security is not promoted by checking the lock 22 times, morality would not seem to be promoted by saying the ritual blessing 18 times, cleaning orifices for at least 20 minutes before praying, or checking that the containers of cleaning solvents are sealed before serving every order. If the ritual blessing has been recited, the body normally cleaned, and there is no evidence of possible risk of poisoning, then 17 further blessings, extra time spent cleaning, and incessant checks on the containers are neither morally required nor morally desirable. Rather, as Summers and Sinnott-Armstrong indeed emphasise, these patterns of behaviour instead seem to be *aimed at coping with anxieties about morality*, which scrupulous people feel compelled to act on even though the behaviour arguably does nothing to increase the likelihood that moral ends are in fact promoted.

Indeed, morality may, in certain contexts, demand precisely that people *not* behave in such ways. This will be so whenever the behaviour – perhaps due to its rigidity, repetitiveness, and fixation – *interferes* with genuine moral demands and so bears a *moral cost*. This may happen, for example, if the compulsion to recite the blessing 18 times before dinner impedes attending to one's child at dinner; or if obsessive washing pre-prayer results in less time or focus on praying itself; or if incessantly checking the cleaning solvents means that food gets cold and goes to waste. In general (and among other things), acting morally requires the flexibility to adjust principles to particular contexts and circumstances; the capacity to balance multiple considerations as opposed to fixating on one thing in particular; and the ability to manage any unhelpful desires and emotions so that these interfere minimally with doing the right thing. The scrupulous people described by Summers and Sinnott-Armstrong do not seem to evidence such qualities. Rather, their OCPD or OCD seems to *compromise* their capacity for morality, not make them *more* moral.[1]

Scrupulosity, then, is not well characterised as a disorder involving, among other things, *too much care or concern for morality* or *too high moral standards* insofar as that suggests that scrupulous behaviour *promotes* morality. The scrupulous people described by Summers and Sinnott-Armstrong are not more moral than their religious or wider community. Like others in their community, we can suppose, they want to do things right. The difference between them and others seems to be that, even when there is no reason whatsoever to doubt that they have done things right, they are extremely anxious about this, and have developed obsessive–compulsive ways of coping that repeat behaviour in a rigidly specified way, but that do not in fact serve moral ends.[2] So, as Summers and Sinnott-Armstrong describe, their problem is that, like others with OCPD and OCD, they are prone to rigidity, perfectionism, irrational doubts, and anxiety, and lack the ability to cope well with these.[3] But – and this is the crux – this does not make them more moral than ordinary, even if the focus, in these cases, of the rigidity, perfectionism, irrational doubts, and anxiety, is on behaviour pertaining to religious and common morality.

Why does this matter? The answer is that it matters because there is only a distinctive puzzle and need to justify treatment for scrupulosity if it really does involve an extra dose of morality, as we might put it. Rigidity, perfectionism, irrational doubts, anxiety, and poor coping skills are all problems that psychiatrists commonly treat. On the whole, we do not consider these traits good to have. Equally, they often and understandably cause clinically significant distress and impairment – a core marker of psychiatric disorder and one of the cornerstones for the justification of treatment. Morality, in contrast, is generally considered to be good to have. It comes as a surprise to hear it characterised as part of the cause of clinically significant distress and impairment. Of course, sometimes doing the right thing is hard and causes discomfort – for example, when it requires forsaking selfish pleasures for the sake of others. But how could doing the right thing cause clinically significant distress and impairment? And, if it did, would we really want psychiatrists to interfere in such cases, to help people do the right thing *less* and stop caring so much about morality or having such high moral standards?

If it is correct that scrupulosity is not rightly characterised as involving *too much care or concern for morality* or *too high moral standards*, then the puzzle and need for a special justification for treating scrupulosity, over and above the treatment considerations relevant to OCPD and OCD, collapses. However, treatment for scrupulosity may nonetheless require psychiatrists to challenge and try to change beliefs and behaviour that patients themselves view as morally important – for instance, by helping them to understand their obsessions and compulsions as unhelpful ways of coping with anxiety and distress, as opposed to morally required or desirable. And, even if this would not *in fact* make patients *less* moral – notwithstanding their own view of the matter – it is yet something that, at least instinctively, it may seem wrong for psychiatrists to do.

Summers and Sinnott-Armstrong state: "The job of psychiatrists is presumably not to judge the moral views of their patients" (p. 168). It is at this point that the monsters lurking in the shadows of psychiatry need to come to light. History reveals psychiatry to have been the perpetrator of terrible human rights abuses – a willing, coercive tool of tyrants and evil states, and an impressively systemic instrument for social control that has been used to violate and harm individuals whose beliefs or lifestyles do not conform to the norm.[4] Psychiatry is a branch of medicine. Its aim is to alleviate suffering and to help and care for people, not harm them. Summers and Sinnott-Armstrong are absolutely right that the job of psychiatrists is not to be *morally judgemental* any more than it is to serve tyranny, oppression, and conformity. Yet, morality and psychiatry are intertwined, in the very nature of psychiatric disorder, diagnosis, and treatment. We cannot address this fact and protect people against the risk psychiatry poses unless we bring this monster out of the shadows and face up to it in broad daylight.

Many of the personality disorders – including Obsessive-Compulsive Personality Disorder, to which scrupulosity is connected – are diagnosed via personality traits that link to immoral actions or display a lack of moral qualities. Lack of empathy, lack of remorse, cruelty and callousness, a willingness to exploit others and violate their rights, a history of criminal activity and violent behaviour, impulsivity, recklessness, extreme and inappropriate anger, a tendency towards unjustified suspicion and distrust, obedience to rules at the expense of the good of others, and a desire for interpersonal control – these are some of the traits by which some personality disorders are diagnosed. Hence, in order to make a diagnosis, psychiatrists must attribute traits to people that are not morally neutral, but which invite moral condemnation. In order to treat people for these traits, psychiatrists will in effect be offering a form of moral improvement – treatment ipso facto makes people *morally better*. Of course, psychiatrists do not typically view the process of diagnosis and treatment in these terms, especially outside of forensic contexts. These personality traits typically cause terrible distress to those who have them and create chaos and impairment in their lives because of their impact on the possibility of stable and caring relationships with others, a sense of belonging to a community, employment and educational opportunities, and more. So the aim of helping and caring for people, and alleviating suffering, can be achieved by diagnosing and treating these traits, without any need to explicitly focus on their moral status. Yet, morality lurks in the shadows of this process, no doubt inviting psychiatrists to step out of the role of doctor and carer, and into the role of judge and oppressor.[5]

Hence psychiatrists may need to attribute and address morally relevant traits to people in order to do their job, even though the aim of their job is not to judge people morally. In principle, this is true whether the traits are morally negative or positive. Either way, psychiatrists need to act for the good of the people they treat, and be alive not only to individual differences and people's right to choose how to live, but also to the diversity of ways of living that are conducive to wellbeing. On the whole, and as a rule of thumb, psychiatric treatment is in practice seen as justified when the following conditions obtain: a psychiatric diagnosis can be made or the person in question has problems that fit within the domain of psychiatry well enough; they suffer from sufficient distress and impairment to warrant psychiatric intervention; a form of treatment is available that there is evidence or reason to think will help them; and, crucially, they want to be helped.

There is no question that many cases of scrupulosity will meet these conditions, with the form of treatment in question likely being an individually tailored variety of intervention for Obsessive-Compulsive Disorder or Obsessive-Compulsive Personality Disorder. But Summers and Sinnott-Armstrong want to argue that treatment for scrupulosity may be justified even when people do not want to be helped. They state explicitly that they are interested in cases where treatment might be justified in particular "over objection" and "over moral objection" (p. 168). The cases they have in mind appear to involve a person refusing treatment out of a conviction that it would result in them becoming *less* moral. I am unsure how common it is to find scrupulous people refusing treatment on precisely these grounds when they are genuinely distressed and struggling to function due to their scrupulosity. When this is the case, psychiatrists who press treatment will indeed be (implicitly or explicitly) challenging and hoping to change beliefs and behaviour that patients view as morally important. But, however common such refusal is, it is extremely important to draw a very sharp distinction between two different kinds of action that psychiatrists can take when patients do not want to be treated, and that require correspondingly different forms of justification. The distinction is between the action of *offering* treatment over a patient's objection – and, perhaps, even more, endeavouring to persuade the patient to accept it – and the action of *forcing or otherwise coercing* a patient to undergo treatment.

In ordinary cases of scrupulosity, I can see no justification for a psychiatrist to force or otherwise coerce an unwilling patient to undergo treatment. There are two standard ethical and legal forms of justification for involuntary treatment. The first is when the patient lacks decision-making capacity to consent to treatment that is judged to be in their best interests. Given the standard criteria for assessing decision-making capacity, it seems unlikely that most scrupulous patients fail to have it in relation to a decision as to whether or not to undergo treatment for scrupulosity. The second is when there is a sufficient risk of serious harm to self or others if treatment is not forced to warrant the violation of patient autonomy that involuntary treatment constitutes. Again, it seems extremely unlikely that the average scrupulous patient poses such a risk to self or others. Of course, there may be particular cases where one or other of these two standard concerns arises, and a justification for involuntary treatment is therefore available in that particular case. But Summers and Sinnott-Armstrong do not discuss cases where scrupulous patients lack decision-making capacity or pose a sufficient risk of serious harm to self or others, and I cannot see how, in absence of such concerns, involuntary treatment for scrupulosity could ever be justified.[6]

Perhaps, then, Summers and Sinnott-Armstrong mean to focus not on whether a psychiatrist would be justified in forcing or coercing treatment for scrupulosity over objection, but rather on whether a psychiatrist would be justified simply in offering treatment – or trying to persuade a patient to be treated – over objection.

Well, why wouldn't they be justified in offering treatment? There are indeed circumstances where, even if a person has come to a psychiatrist for help and wants treatment, it should not be offered. For instance, if the person's distress and impairment, that core marker of psychiatric disorder and cornerstone for the justification of treatment, is not sufficient to warrant psychiatric intervention, or if no treatment exists of which there is evidence or reason to think it will help. But this is not the kind of issue Summers and Sinnott-Armstrong consider. Rather, they seem to be concerned, as suggested above, with the impropriety of a psychiatrist judging a patient's moral views or "imposing [their] own moral standards on the patient" (p. 172) merely in virtue of offering treatment for scrupulosity. I think we can here see how psychiatry's monsters are lurking in the shadows – the concern seems to be that psychiatry should not be an instrument of oppression and conformity, "imposing" its own so-called "moral standards" on patients. Above, I claimed that moral ends are not served by 17 further blessings, extra time spent cleaning, and incessant checks on the containers. But people disagree about morality. So, one might wonder, how do I know my claims are right? And, if there is a possibility that I am wrong and scrupulous patients are right, how could a psychiatrist be justified in imposing this view on patients?

Both concerns – how to respond to moral disagreement, and how to protect against the risk of psychiatry being an instrument of oppression and conformity – are well taken. But imposing a moral view on patients is not what *offering* treatment – as opposed to forcing or otherwise coercing treatment – for scrupulosity amounts to. If a person suffers distress and impairment due to rigidity, perfectionism, irrational doubts, anxiety, and poor coping skills – with respect to any matters, moral or otherwise – it is surely justifiable for psychiatrists to offer help and try to persuade the person to accept it. Psychiatrists do this all the time – with all forms of obsessions, compulsions, and irrational thinking processes. Indeed, arguably, offering treatment and aiming to persuade a person to accept it (while always acknowledging that the choice is theirs) can be a sign of respect for that person – a way of engaging with them as a rational and participant member of our shared social and moral community, developing a genuine relationship with them, and expressing care and concern. What would not be justified is to force or in some way coerce treatment – to violate a person's autonomy and right to choose – because they suffer distress and impairment due to some combination of rigidity, perfectionism, irrational doubts, anxiety, and poor coping skills in relation to any domain, moral or otherwise.

Summers and Sinnott-Armstrong argue in detail that treatment over objection – whether this is to be understood as forced treatment or the offer of treatment – is only justified when the person meets three conditions: they are in significant distress, their beliefs are internally incoherent and they cannot adequately justify them, and this incoherence is driven by anxiety or underlying emotional needs. Alongside impairment, significant distress is, as mentioned above, part of the rule-of-thumb justification for diagnosis and treatment, and rightly emphasised by Summers and Sinnott-Armstrong. Equally, their account of how and why scrupulosity can develop as a way of coping with anxiety or underlying emotional needs is insightful, and can be nicely linked to clinical practice. The conceptualisation of many of the behaviours that are diagnostic of or contributory to psychiatric disorders as unhelpful ways of coping with underlying emotions is both prevalent within psychiatric contexts and may straightforwardly contribute to the rationale for offering treatment. However, I am not convinced of the relevance of finding a person's beliefs to be internally incoherent, and the person themselves being unable to justify their beliefs, to the justification of treatment. This seems to place a demand on people with scrupulosity that few of us without it ever meet. Do most of us really have internally coherent beliefs, especially as pertaining to religious or moral domains? And could most of us, even if our beliefs are coherent, justify them adequately to others, especially others who do not already hold a similar set of beliefs? Honest reflection on our own shortcomings, together with the findings of social and cognitive psychology, suggest that we typically possess, alas, a mish-mash of poorly integrated beliefs, which we may have limited access to, which stem from different origins, and which we have acquired via diverse processes.[7] It's not easy to sort through them, and, even if we manage to achieve this, we may yet lack the articulacy and argumentative skills to justify ourselves adequately to others. Unquestionably, the consistency and justification of our (religious, moral, and other) beliefs is an ideal to which we may aspire. But if there is really a question as to whether (forced or merely offered) psychiatric treatment can be justified, I do not think it can be answered by pointing to the fact that a person fails to live up to this ideal.

So, does scrupulosity involve caring or being concerned about morality too much or having moral standards that are too high? No, it is a condition where people suffer from rigidity, perfectionism, irrational doubts, anxiety, and poor coping skills, particularly with respect to matters that pertain to religious and common morality. Is it scrupulous to treat scrupulosity? Absolutely, if the person suffers sufficient distress and impairment to warrant psychiatric intervention, and if they want treatment. If they don't, psychiatrists should yet go ahead and offer it, and explore with the person why it is at least possible, on the one hand, that they are mistaken if they genuinely believe their behaviour is morally required or desirable, and on the other, that their rigidity, perfectionism, irrational doubts, anxiety, and poor coping skills are getting in the way of a better life. But, presuming the person retains decision-making capacity and the risk of harm to self or others is not severe, there is no justification for forcing or coercing treatment over objection. This cannot be emphasised enough, because it's absolutely essential to controlling the monsters lurking in the shadows of psychiatry. When capacity is present and risk is not high, psychiatrists ought to talk to people openly about their assessment of their problems, and try to engage them in treatment if their best judgement – meaning their judgement when they have done all they can to be sensitive to the other person's (moral and other) perspective, and alive to their own biases and preconceptions – really is that the person would benefit from treatment despite their misgivings about having it. But when capacity is present and risk is not high, psychiatry cannot be granted the power forcefully or coercively to interfere in people's lives. Let's relegate the monsters to history.[8]

Notes

1 In this respect, scrupulous patients appear more like the informal characterisation of scrupulosity that Summers and Sinnott-Armstrong quote but reject as "seeing sin [or immorality] where there is none" or "focusing on minor details of the person's religion, to the exclusion of more important areas" (p. 163). Summers and Sinnott-Armstrong rightly emphasise the over-simplicity of this characterisation, due to its failure to understand scrupulosity in connection with OCPD or OCD. But this characterisation nonetheless emphasises the way scrupulosity *interferes with* morality, rather than seeing it, as Summers and Sinnott-Armstrong do, as *servicing* morality.

2 It is a good question why scrupulous people are especially anxious and prone to irrational doubts *about morality in particular*. A psychodynamic explanation might posit unconscious, immoral impulses, which could be traced both to general features of our species and individual developmental trajectories, as the source. Scrupulosity could then be understood as a defence against these impulses. But such an account is not part of the standard conception of scrupulosity.

3 Note that pathological perfectionism – the sort that warrants clinical attention – with respect to any domain does not in fact make patients "perfect" or enable them to meet their expectations or achieve their goals – unlike our intuitive understanding of non-pathological perfectionism. Non-pathological perfectionists typically have high standards and push themselves very hard, but often meet (at least some of) their expectations and goals. Patients who struggle with pathological perfectionism typically have expectations and goals that they fail even to try to meet – or give up trying to meet very quickly – due to their intolerance of lapses, mistakes, and failures, and low self-esteem and self-efficacy. When I first started working clinically, I was often struck by the oddity of patients who describe themselves as perfectionists, yet were highly dysfunctional and very far from "perfect". They often failed to meet ordinary expectations or achieve even the most ordinary goals. As I have come to understand it, such patients seem to feel that they are bound to fail no matter what, and in response opt to fail by not even trying, rather than to fail by trying but not succeeding. Pathological perfectionists are therefore typically far less "perfect" than non-pathological non-perfectionists.

4 Standard examples include the diagnosis of runaway slaves as suffering from drapetomania; homosexuals as suffering from a form of perversion and sexual deviance; and political dissidents as suffering from psychopathology and madness.

5 For further discussion of issues of morality within psychiatry and in relation to personality disorders in particular, see Pearce and Pickard (2009) and Pickard (2011, 2013).

6 It is also important to mention, as Summers and Sinnott-Armstrong equally note, that forced treatment for scrupulosity is very unlikely to be effective, since treatment outcomes typically depend on patient motivation and engagement.

7 The literature on this topic is copious, but for two excellent books written for a general audience, see Khurzban (2012) and Wilson (2004).

8 Thanks to Jesse Summers and Walter Sinnott-Armstrong for very generous and helpful comments on an earlier version of this commentary.

References

Khurzban, R. (2012) *Why Everyone (Else) is a Hypocrite: Evolution and the Modular Mind*. Princeton, NJ: Princeton University Press.

Pearce, S. and Pickard, H. (2009) "The moral content of psychiatric treatment". *British Journal of Psychiatry* 195: 281–82.

Pickard, H. (2011) "Mental illness is indeed a myth". In L. Bortolotti and M. Broome, (Eds.) *Psychiatry as Cognitive Science: Philosophical Perspectives*. Oxford: Oxford University Press, 83–101.

——(2013) "Responsibility without blame: Philosophical reflections on clinical practice". In K. W. M. Fulford et al. (Eds.) *Oxford Handbook of Philosophy and Psychiatry*. Oxford: Oxford University Press, 1134–52.

Summers, J. and Sinnott-Armstrong, W. (this volume) "Scrupulous treatment."

Wilson, T. O. (2004) *Strangers to Ourselves: Discovering the Adaptive Unconscious*. Cambridge, MA: Harvard University Press.

7a

The Place of Ability to Value in the Evaluation of Decision-Making Capacity

Scott Y. H. Kim

1. Introduction

Patients' authority to make their own medical decisions is ordinarily presumed, but when there are concerns about potential decisional impairment, the modern practice is to assess whether they retain a sufficient amount and type of abilities relevant to decision-making. This function-oriented framework—in contrast to an appeal to a diagnosis or a label ("unsound mind")—for determining patients' decision-making capacity (DMC) reflects the high priority we now place on patient self-determination. Although this move toward a functional assessment of DMC is ethically necessary, it also makes capacity assessment much more difficult. Indeed, psychiatric consultants in the United States find that capacity evaluations are some of the more challenging consultations to perform (Seyfried et al. 2013).

One reason why capacity evaluations are so challenging is that the criteria for capacity are very broad and much is left to the judgment of the evaluator (Kim 2010). Although a considerable amount of judgment will always be necessary in DMC evaluations, there is still a need to better explicate the structure and elements of some of the standards or abilities that make up DMC. Two issues make this need evident. First, the criteria for DMC found in statutes of various jurisdictions often vary (Kim 2010: 26–28). For example, England and Wales adopted a comprehensive law addressing DMC (Mental Capacity Act 2005) recently. Despite the shared culture, medical knowledge, and historical legal roots, the criteria used in the MCA are, at least on the surface, different from the dominant model taught in the United States. MCA's criteria are the abilities to understand, to retain information, to use or weigh information, and to communicate a decision; the criteria from a model widely taught in the United States (Grisso and Appelbaum 1998; Berg, Appelbaum and Grisso 1996) are the abilities to understand, to appreciate, to reason, and to communicate a choice. Naturally, the question becomes: Are the abilities to appreciate and reason the same as the ability to use or weigh information, as some seem to assume (David et al. 2010)? It is not clear.

Second, there has been a small but persistent literature reflecting concerns that the dominant models of DMC fail to capture something essential. These criticisms tend to focus on concerns that the dominant models are too "cognitive"(Charland 1999; Vollmann 2006; Elliott 1997) and fail to take into account issues of "authenticity," "identity"(Tan et al. 2006a), and "valuing" (Elliott 1997). Others frame it as a problem of "value-laden" criteria of capacity (Holroyd 2012).

Thus, although it is broadly agreed (Grisso and Appelbaum 1998) that the abilities necessary for DMC include the abilities to understand (i.e., intellectually absorb) the relevant information and to communicate a choice, how to evaluate DMC processes that occur in between the two need more discussion (Kim 2013). In this chapter, my goal is not to reconcile MCA with the US model, nor to review the various arguments for a more inclusive model of DMC that accounts for concerns about emotions, valuing, identity, authenticity, and so on. Instead, my goal will be to provide an overarching structure to the space between understanding (intellectual comprehension) and communicating a choice by showing how the themes of authenticity, emotions, motivation, and values could fit into a model of DMC. I propose an integrated framework, rather than the more familiar list-based one—that is, a framework that explains how the various components fit together in a process rather than simply a legal checklist. The goal is to provide an overall framework and to show, at least in outline, what such a model must look like, even if some of the details will require much more work elsewhere to delineate.

2. A Simple Model for DMC

Figure 7a.1 shows the proposed conceptual model. Although the model proposes a sequence or a process, it is not intended to be a psychological model per se; its main purpose is conceptual, with only the minimal process assumptions to make the conceptual model coherent. The process begins with the disclosure of the needed information for the patient's decision-making. The disclosure elements are well described legally and ethically, and will not be discussed here (Kim 2010).

Ability to Understand

The first ability is the ability to *understand*—that is, the ability to intellectually comprehend information. This is perhaps the most intuitive of the criteria for DMC since, unless information is absorbed and comprehended by the patient, no informed decision is possible. Unfortunately, writings on capacity—indeed even statutes on capacity—often use the same terms in different ways. For example, I am using the term "understand" in a technical, narrow sense roughly equivalent to "intellectually comprehend" rather than in the more broad everyday sense that tends to include a person's application of what has been comprehended to one's own situation (Kim 2010). The dominant model in the United States (the four abilities model of Grisso and Appelbaum (1998)) uses it narrowly. Thus, in this model, a person can understand that the doctors are recommending a treatment for her medical condition (demonstrated by the patient's

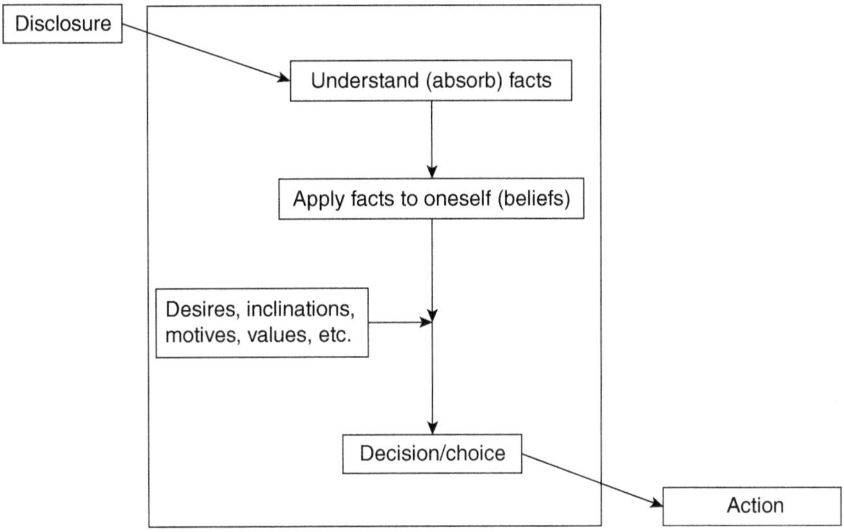

Figure 7a.1 Abilities Necessary for Decision-Making Capacity. (The ability to reason is not located in a specific place in the model; instead, it is assumed to underlie processes in various places in the model. See discussion in text.)

ability to discuss in her own words the rationale and character of the treatment) but does not believe she has the condition or that the treatment is an actual medical treatment (say, because she believes the "doctors" are actually CIA agents out to harm her).

Ability to Appreciate

Assuming that the disclosed information has been adequately understood, there are two further components necessary for the patient to arrive at a decision or a choice. One necessary ability is the application to one's own situation the facts that have been absorbed (i.e., facts that have been intellectually comprehended in the first step). This is what has been known as the *appreciation* ability. This requires the formation of beliefs since to apply the facts to one's own situation means to believe that the facts are relevant to oneself and one's situation. For example, if the medical team has disclosed that the risk of a proposed treatment is a low probability of a stroke, then the patient either does or does not believe that this is true of *her*.

Ability to Value

But the mere application of the facts (e.g., regarding a proposed treatment) to oneself is not sufficient to arrive at a choice regarding that treatment. A person may be able to absorb the information that the doctors believe she needs a treatment to prevent a great medical harm. She may even believe that such a harm would in fact occur to her without the treatment. But that does not automatically translate into a decision to accept the treatment. This is because there has to be a propelling force or motive which, in combination with the application of the relevant facts, leads to a choice or decision. For the moment, I will use the mechanical metaphor of force and propulsion to refer to concepts such as motive, desire, inclination, and even value. (This will need some more distinctions to make the model workable, but that comes later.) This is the component that can involve emotions although not always, since we do not always have to act out of emotion. We can have cool, calculating motives, after all. In fact, I will try to avoid the use of the term "emotion" if possible because it tends to evoke the false dichotomy of "cognitive" vs "emotional" elements of our psyche, which is not a useful dichotomy given the obviously complex cognitive judgments or construals that our emotions reflect. We can talk about motives or desires that may or may not have a strong emotional component, but the important aspect is the motivational component. This component is the ability to value.

Ability to Reason

Although the model I propose has a component called the "ability to reason," it is not possible to give a succinct definition or description of it. At least in the United States, the most pertinent thing to say about this standard is that it is a procedural standard that reminds us not to judge people's choices as "irrational" simply because their choice is apparently self-defeating or is not something (we or) most people would want. Beyond these two elements of content neutrality and procedural focus, there is little firm guidance on what the reasoning ability is. As Berg, Appelbaum and Grisso (1996) have noted, no US court has used the reasoning standard as the sole criterion to find someone incapable. This suggests that it is usually or perhaps even always accompanied by deficits in domains that are marked in boxes in Figure 7a.1. Any impairment of reasoning severe enough to be a factor will likely manifest itself as an impairment in understanding, appreciation, or valuing. Also, as I have discussed elsewhere, the measurement of reasoning is not straightforward, and is best conceived of as an opportunity to probe the patient's statements (Kim 2010). In the UK, the idea of a "reasoning" ability has had a different understanding from the one I have drawn for the US situation. Some have interpreted the ability to "weigh" in the MCA criterion of "use or weigh" to mean "being able to *reason* with information in accord with her life choices, preferences, and values" (David et al. 2010, italics added). As will become clear below (see Section 5), this makes the "weigh" criterion more like the ability to value, while equating this with at least a part of the reasoning criterion. This may account for the peculiar result in a recent study in the UK that shows that a sizable number of patients are found to lack DMC solely based on what is perceived to be (by UK evaluators) lack of reasoning ability (Owen et al. 2013a, 2013b; Kim 2013). This is a good reminder that in the literature on DMC, one cannot assume that even the most familiar words are used uniformly.

Thus, I have not created a separate box for the ability to reason in Figure 7a.1. But this should not be taken to mean that it is not an important ability (or, more likely, set of abilities), only that to delineate the issues involved would take us too far afield from the central issue of this chapter—namely, the ability to value. I refer the reader to other places where this complexity is discussed in more detail (Kim 2010: 24–26). For the purposes of this chapter, the reader can assume that the ability to reason is best conceived as a set of process-related abilities that may play a role in understanding, appreciation, and valuing, or in the integration of those abilities into a final decision.

3. Impaired Ability to Value versus "Pathological Value"

Given that we have a sketch of an integrated model of DMC in front of us, we can now flesh out a bit what it means to have intact or impaired "valuing ability." The reader should not, however, infer that any degree of impairment in the ability to value is sufficient for finding someone incapable. Such a judgment of incapacity will depend on the risk–benefit context, the degree of impairment in valuing ability as well as in any other impaired ability, the prospect (or lack) of recovery from the underlying pathology, and so on. It is important to keep separate the distinction between finding someone's valuing ability impaired and categorically finding someone lacking DMC.

Perhaps the first issue to deal with head on is the common objection that it is not the business of the capacity evaluator to judge another person's values. Some state this as the issue of whether DMC assessment can be value-neutral (Holroyd 2012), and others have discussed it as the problem of pathological values (Tan et al. 2006a). This is an understandable concern since, in a modern liberal society such as ours, the idea of restricting another's exercise of choice based on someone else's judgment of that person's values is quite disturbing (especially when that someone else has the implicit or explicit backing of the state). The capacity evaluator really does need to be quite careful and clear that she does not judge an impaired patient incompetent merely based on a disagreement about the patient's values. But this cautionary note should not prevent us from the seeing the following rather mundane point: *As long as the ability to value is an ability that can go wrong in certain types of neuropsychiatric pathology, the idea of assessing a person's ability to value is no more (or less) disturbing than the idea of assessing a person's capacity to make a decision.* What we must assess is the *ability* to value, not the value itself. Thus, I think the term "pathological values" is unfortunate (Tan et al. 2006b; Vollmann 2006). It suggests that we are passing judgment on the worthiness of the values that the person holds, when in fact we should be directing our attention to the underlying *ability* to value.

How does one evaluate a person's ability to value? We can make some limited progress by way of analogy with the ability to apply facts to oneself. The contours of this "appreciation" (Grisso and Appelbaum 1998) ability are a bit better worked out, and an analogy, although not perfect, can get us started. Recall that appreciation is essentially an ability to form adequate beliefs. Note again that the very idea of judging someone else's beliefs as part of assessing his DMC (and thereby determining whether he retains decisional authority) feels rather abhorrent to our liberal sensibilities. Indeed, it is reported (Grisso and Appelbaum 1998) that in some jurisdictions this appreciation standard is not used. But if we reflect on the fact that there is really nothing offensive about the fact that a person's ability to apply facts to oneself can be derailed by certain types of brain malfunction, such a law is, I think, well meaning but ultimately mistaken. One would have to believe that a distinction between evaluating someone's beliefs and evaluating that person's ability to form adequate beliefs does not exist.

Figure 7a.2 provides a flow diagram for the capacity evaluator in assessing this ability to apply relevant medical facts to one's own situation. It specifically shows how to avoid a paternalistic judgment by restricting what types of beliefs are to be taken as manifestations of an impaired ability to appreciate. The diagram makes clear that a mere disagreement with the recommended treatment is insufficient to declare someone as being unable to apply facts to themselves. The key is to determine the *basis* for the lack of belief, which must be shown to be both sufficiently irrational *and* based on a cognitive or psychiatric pathological process. The classic case is the delusional patient who can absorb that the doctors are recommending treatment X for condition C but does not believe she has C or does not believe the doctor's opinion because, in fact, she believes the doctor is a hostile alien from another planet. This belief is not only substantially irrational, it is likely a manifestation of an underlying psychotic process, for example, delirium, dementia, or a psychotic disorder.

The assessment of the ability to value or form motives can be analyzed in a similar way. For instance, suppose that the treatment team is recommending an intervention that has a high likelihood of significant benefit and low likelihood of harm but that the patient is refusing the treatment. Suppose that the person is able to intellectually absorb the information (by phrasing in his own words the facts given to him), and even is able to state (and believe) accurately what the potential medical benefits and risks are, as applied to him. Yet he still refuses the recommendation.

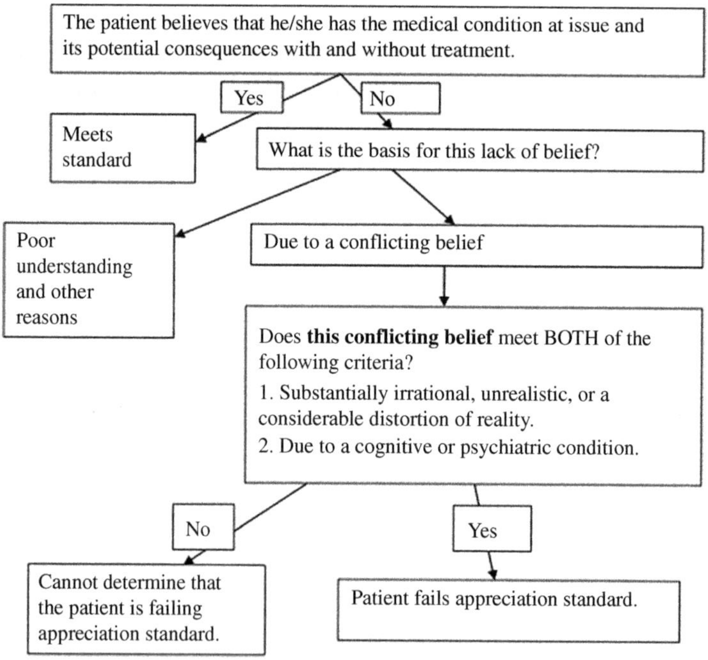

Figure 7a.2 Flow Diagram for Assessment of Ability to Apply Facts to Oneself (Ability to Appreciate). From S. Kim, *Evaluation of Capacity to Consent to Treatment and Research*, Oxford University Press, 2010. Used with permission.

Suppose further assessment showed that the reason for the patient's refusal is a new "value," of very recent origin, coinciding with the initiation of, say, high-dose systemic corticosteroids for treatment of obstructive lung disease. The patient believes that without treatment he will likely suffer the medical harm predicted by the doctors yet feels sure ("I have faith … ") that the "Universal Force of All Reality" will reverse that harm in due course. Suppose further that he is known never to have been religious or even spiritual. Indeed, his wife says "this is definitely not like him at all."

Perhaps some will say that this is not really an example of lack of valuing ability but rather a case of impaired appreciation (failure to form adequate beliefs regarding how the facts apply to oneself). The "belief" that he will be harmed is not really genuine, since he feels he will recover. Perhaps cases like this can be handled as cases of impaired appreciation ability. It may even be true that if we dig and probe enough, many or most cases of impaired ability to value could also exhibit some belief that is a manifestation of the ability to appreciate. Perhaps this is why in most clinical situations a special appeal to impaired ability to value is not needed (Grisso and Appelbaum 2006). But this is an empirical issue, and I am just speculating.

Suppose that, instead of a new spiritual belief, the patient is suffering from a severe depression. He agrees that without the treatment he would suffer medical harm. But he feels so tired and worn out, and wonders if it is worth it to get the treatment. We need not speculate or suppose that he doesn't "really" believe the medical recommendation. He actually doesn't care if he lives or dies. He recognizes he might die without treatment. He no longer values his life. This case illustrates someone who understands the medical facts and seems to be able to apply them to himself. What is wrong is that, under the grip of his depression, he is failing to value his own life. Let's assume also that his attitude about his life is temporally tied to his discontinuing his medications three months ago with increasing severity of his depression since then.

Drawing on an analogy with the ability to appreciate, we can articulate at least two conditions that need to be present for a determination of "impaired ability to value."

One necessary condition is some type of pathology, psychiatric or cognitive, or malfunctioning of brain processes that can reasonably be determined to be the source of the impaired ability to value. This is the same condition as condition 2 in Figure 7a.2 for assessing the ability to form adequate beliefs regarding how the facts apply to oneself. I find it odd that some writers think that it is desirable to construct or have a DMC assessment that does not have to appeal to a "conceptually prior idea of mental disorder" (Tan et al. 2006b; Vollmann 2006). Indeed, if there is no suspicion whatsoever of a mental or brain disorder, it will be very difficult to escape the problem of judging the values of a person rather than evaluating that person's ability to value. As discussed below, an assumption about the "reality" of mental disorders (broadly construed, ranging from psychiatric to cognitive disorders) is necessary for any theory of DMC. If one believes that a person can become decisionally incompetent, then one must also be a realist about psycho-cognitive pathology.

What is the corresponding analogy for condition 1 in Figure 7a.2, if we are to apply a similar scheme to the ability to value? Here the analogy cannot be fully sustained since a motive or a desire is not something that can straightforwardly have truth content and be judged as "substantially irrational, unrealistic, or a considerable distortion of reality." One's belief that God exists can be true or false; one's commitment to God is not false or true in the same way. How then can one evaluate values or desires without falling into unjustified paternalism? The obvious candidate is some form of authenticity—broadly speaking, one's desire could be seen as arising out of an impaired ability to value if that desire is due to a pathology and is patently inconsistent with the set of values and history that roughly constitute the person's identity (Elliott 1997; Tan et al. 2006b). The underlying spiritual value that trumps the value of medical benefits for the patient refusing a recommended therapy is inauthentic in the sense that, were the person not suffering the psychopathology, he would not have such a value or desire. A severely depressed patient's failure to value his life when it is so closely tied to his depression is best seen as not part of his identity but as an enemy within. If the value is out of line with the person's prior set of values *and* arises out of a psychopathologic or cognitive dysfunction, then it seems reasonable to say that the person's ability to value is impaired. Thus, the judgment here is not that the person fails to conform to the values dictated by society but rather that, due to a pathology, she is being prevented from being herself, as it were.

I want to be clear that the notion of authenticity espoused here must not be a strong one. It would be a mistake to tie DMC to a high standard of authenticity in the sense that a person's decision must be part of some tight set of identity-conferring "projects, relationships, and life plans" (Kim 2010). The burden of proof is on those to show that a value is inauthentic, and not the other way round, and we should be very careful in requiring too high a level of consistency. The *presumption* about a person's motive and desire is authenticity, even if the "new" desire seems out of character. The questioning of that presumption should arise only when there are compelling reasons, such as obvious psychopathology, leading to self-destructive choices.

4. Some Underlying Assumptions of the Model

First, the model espouses value-neutrality, but only of a certain kind. The ideal of value-neutrality drives the modern conceptions of DMC. This is why the reasoning standard is discussed primarily negatively: The content of the choice is not what is being evaluated but rather the process. The reason why some states have rejected the appreciation standard is the fear that allowing an evaluation of a person's beliefs encroaches too much upon that person's right to self-determination, to live "according to one's own beliefs." This reasoning goes even further when it comes to values and commitments that people hold. There is a presumption that values are person-relative, and people (especially not the state, nor its instrument in the form of capacity evaluators) should not "impose" their values on others.

Of course, it is unrealistic to have a completely value-neutral conception of DMC. Value-neutrality of DMC assessments are delimited by two issues. First, to the extent that we incorporate welfare considerations in setting capacity thresholds (Kim 2010: 34–36), some type of value comes into play. This is unavoidable. We must make assumptions about some objective (or at least inter-subjectively reasonable) notion of welfare, if only to agree that some degree of instrumental welfare is necessary for anyone to exercise meaningful self-determination. Elliott, for example, argues that the very notion of informed consent assumes certain empirical facts, such as that each individual will exhibit and exercise some minimal degree of self-interested behavior (Elliott 1997).

Second, the model assumes that we are not "neutral" about psychopathology. It assumes that cognitive and psychopathology are not mere socially constructed conventions, either as political tools of oppression or as alternative lifestyles. For those who believe that schizophrenia is just another way of living, as normal as not having schizophrenia, this model will not be convincing. Of course, the state of science is such that we cannot pinpoint the underlying pathology that is responsible for most psychiatric illnesses. And of course there are political, historical, and economic incentives that shape some, or in some cases significant, aspects of our diagnostic scheme. But if a skeptic rejects the proposed DMC model because he does not "believe in" psychiatric illness, the problem is much bigger than a dispute over DMC, a problem that needs to be addressed elsewhere.

5. Applying the Model: Easy and Difficult Cases

So far, for simplicity, I have not distinguished between the variety of "motive forces" that people are subject to, and have treated the terms "values," "motives," "desires," "impulses," "inclinations," and so on, interchangeably. However, since it is possible, for example, to have a desire or an impulse that a person sincerely wishes he did not have—indeed, intensely disvalues—we need to make some important distinctions.

Valuing as endorsing or identifying with (or as "accountability" (Elliott 1997)) can be conceptualized as involving several factors. First, there is the motive or impulse or a desire—the motive force, as it were. Second, there is the endorsing or identifying with a motive (or resisting it). I do not mean to suggest a simplistic model of endorsement. The idea of an internal rational evaluator who coolly anoints one desire and dismisses others is not very realistic. Life is much more complicated. But the distinction between a desire one endorses or identifies with, and acts on on that basis, is different from acting on that desire despite another desire not to do so. Just because one acts from a desire does not imply that the motive that drove the action is something that the agent fully endorses or identifies with. The main point here is that intuitively we generally accept the distinction between endorsing a desire and not (Frankfurt 1971).

Third, since ambivalent motivations are all too common (suppose one wants A, which is incompatible with B, which one also wants), there is also an element of comparing, contrasting, weighing, or choosing between different motives or values. It is natural to think of these tasks as "reasoning" or even "weighing." All of these components could theoretically "go wrong" and could reasonably be seen as necessary for the ability to value. For example, Owen and colleagues, in a careful phenomenological analysis, have recently described how some severely depressed persons seem unable to compare or even consider different "possible futures" (Owen et al. 2013a, 2013b). Once we recognize that the ability to value can have these different components—perhaps for simplicity's sake we could call them the impetus, the endorsement, and the weighing functions—the evaluation of that ability can get quite complicated. I suspect that much work will be needed to spell out the role of these elements in the assessment of the ability to value.

In the remainder of this section, I will briefly describe several hypothetical cases and explore how the model sketched above might apply. The point is not to provide a definitive analysis of each scenario—in fact, much of what I say will be speculative and impressionistic—but to briefly demonstrate the points of usefulness that the model might have and to show how some of the distinctions in the DMC model might come into play.

1. *Delusional belief as the basis for impaired valuing.* As in the case of our patient above who is delirious from steroids and has a psychotic belief leading to his refusal of treatment, what starts the ball rolling is the psychotic belief, which disorders the ordinary values that one holds. If one did not have that psychotic belief, then he wouldn't disvalue the harm from refusing the treatments. Such cases are probably best handled by an appeal to the appreciation standard. It is likely that these probably comprise many cases of "impaired valuing." If it were possible to eliminate the pathological belief, then the impaired valuing would disappear as well. Thus, if anti-psychotics reduce or eliminate the new "spiritual belief" that is part of a steroid induced delirium, then presumably the person's previous state of valuing would be restored.

   It is unlikely that all cases of impaired valuing are derivative of a psychotic belief. In fact, even when there is a psychotic belief associated with an impaired ability to value, it is possible that the belief is derivative of the distorted value, rather than the reverse.
2. *Depressive disorder directly distorts, creates, or eliminates a drive, desire, or inclination* the person would otherwise have, as in a severely depressed person with no desire to live, or with a desire to die. Here, the pathology is located in the mechanism of desire or impulse itself. Thus, this is the paradigmatic case of an impaired ability to value. And it is common but can have different manifestations.

2a. *Severely depressed patient who is at imminent danger to self* or others. In most jurisdictions, such a case does not even require a determination of incapacity to provide urgent, involuntary intervention of hospitalization. However, once the immediate danger is over, the question of providing ongoing treatment will generally require an assessment of DMC. And then the question of impaired ability to value will play a greater role in the evaluation. To the extent that the lack of desire to live (or wish to die) is due to one's depression and is "inauthentic" (would not have that desire if not depressed), the ability to value is impaired.

2b. *Severely depressed person with new onset cancer, but able to weigh options.* Suppose a patient has been diagnosed with cancer. It requires a long and arduous course of chemotherapy and surgery, with a moderate chance of prolonged survival; let's assume almost everyone with such a cancer chooses treatment. Our patient, however, has been battling severe, chronic depression all of his adult life. He has had 15 courses (each with 12 sessions) of ECT. He has tried virtually every combination of antidepressants, mood stabilizers, and antipsychotics. Fortunately, with the help of his doctors, he has been able to manage working most of his life, and his children are now grown. With each course of ECT, the length of remission has decreased, while the cognitive side effects have remained or increased. The likelihood of future bouts is very high. He feels that this cancer is actually a gift from God (he has always been a religious man) to end his suffering, and refuses cancer treatment.

This patient is severely depressed, but has insight into the situation, and it would be difficult to say that his depression is *impairing* his desire to live. A better interpretation would be that his willingness to accept death could be a considered, endorsed judgment consistent with who he is. By "who he is," we need not mean that the pathology of depression is constitutive of his identity—rather, what is endorsed is his assessment of his life, including his life lived with depression.

2c. *Severely depressed person refusing depression treatment.* Now imagine that our patient from 2b does not have cancer. Instead, he is suffering from another severe episode of depression. The doctors propose another course of ECT to bring him out of this episode. The patient refuses. He knows he is suffering from depression, and even acknowledges that his wishes may be colored by his mood. But he feels that he has fought his illness long enough. If he dies, that is okay with him. He insists he is not seeking death, just that he doesn't think the benefits of ECT would outweigh the burdens. He is not eating much, and not drinking enough water. Although it would depend on other details, this person may very well have sufficient DMC. He is influenced by his depression but he seems able to take stock of his overall situation. He may be in danger of making a poor decision but it would be difficult to say that this person's ability to value is so impaired that his DMC is lacking. The main issue here for me as a psychiatrist would not be a question of DMC but whether the patient is making a considered choice and how to therapeutically discuss his treatment options so that his choice is not unduly influenced by the depression itself.

2d. *Severely depressed person without insight.* Imagine the same patient from 2c but who only repeats that he wishes to die and says, "I don't care about what ECT does. I'm just tired. Don't bother me." He does not engage any more than this, and does not eat or drink. For such a patient, a DMC assessment is necessary. It is possible that the person's motivational mechanism is so impaired by his depression that his ability to value is too dysfunctional for competent decision-making. There is no evidence that he is weighing his options, or any evidence that he can evaluate his own state of depression. He is simply in the grip of it, and cannot step outside it. An excellent phenomenological analysis of such behavior can be found in a recent study by Owen et al. (2013a, 2013b).

3. *Overwhelming emotion makes it difficult to compare and act on values*—for example, a fear of needles that leads to refusal of needed treatment. This seems an inability to weigh or compare options due to a fear that disrupts its normal function. One is bowled over by a fear. Such cases can be very difficult to evaluate because the person's cognition may seem to be intact (i.e., understands and discusses the situation with accuracy). Much will depend on whether the person is operating

entirely "within" the emotion, unable to take an evaluative stance at all about it. For instance, would the person be open to treatment or intervention to reduce that fear?

4. *A person with anorexia nervosa.* The case of the anorexia nervosa patient can become quite complicated. At one level, she is like the person who is in the grip of a fear or depression—there is a desire that has pathologic origins and can control the filter through which one experiences and interacts with her world. There is also a strong false-belief component as well: the misconception that one is fat when in fact one might be dangerously thin and underweight. Thus, such a belief might lead one to analyze the person's DMC mostly via the appreciation ability. One complicating factor is that a person with anorexia may have mostly intact cognitive functions and indeed even exhibit, at times, insight into her illness. She could even verbalize that she knows that she has an illness and that without treatment she could die. This could be genuine insight, with a retained ability to take an evaluative stance toward one's pathologic perceptions and consequent behaviors. But then again, given the relentlessly pervasive impact of anorexia nervosa on one's view of reality, perhaps these statements are still driven by anorexia to satisfy her doctors in order to avoid certain types of treatment. Thus, when a patient with anorexia says she knows she could die, that she has an illness, but that she does not care (Tan et al. 2006b), this apparent "insight behavior" itself could be a manifestation of her condition. The assessment of the ability to value in such situations will be, to say the least, quite challenging.
5. *Psychopathology consists of a pathological drive which one does not (at least in some sense) want.* He may try to resist acting on the impulse but yet succumbs to it. "Succumbing" to pathological impulse seems different from an "endorsement" or "identifying with" the desire. A person who is trying to fight an addiction would fit into this category. As a matter of practice, we tend not to find this person incompetent to make a medical decision, even if he makes predictably unwise and self-defeating decisions. A person who shows weakness of will actually is able to take an important evaluative stance toward his unwanted desire and even resist it to some degree. We may wish to not hold him entirely responsible for his actions, but that is different from saying that he lacks capacity due to that weakness. However, when the failure to resist becomes so overwhelming that the person is not able to care for one's basic needs, a reassessment of the situation will be needed.
6. *The object of one's desire seems irrational.* For example, in body integrity identity disorder (BIID), a person desires the amputation of a healthy limb: "My limbs do not feel like they belong to me, and should not be there" (Blom et al. 2012). The patient feels that the limb is not his, not part of him, and alien, causing distress. The pathology here is the feeling of alienation toward one's own limb. If we accept that such a feeling does exist, then the desire to get rid of that feeling is not irrational. What is disturbing is the means of reducing this feeling. But if the removal of the limb—for the sake of argument—does lead to better overall functioning and satisfaction (Blom et al. 2012), then the apparently higher value one places on one's overall function and sense of well-being over the

burdens and costs of becoming an amputee does not indicate an impaired ability to value. The case of BIID is intriguing because, while the source of the desire for amputation (the feeling of alienation toward one's own body part) is clearly pathological, the overall valuing ability appears to be intact.

The case of BIID is useful in comparison with the situation in anorexia nervosa. The anorexic patient feels that her body is overweight when in fact she is very thin. Given that perception of self, it makes sense to want to restrict one's intake. Thus, why not treat her the way we just suggested for BIID? Mainly because whereas for persons with BIID the surgical solution does seem to lead to psychological relief and higher functioning (Blom et al. 2012), a person with anorexia nervosa desires to restrict intake no matter how thin she becomes—indeed, as she becomes thinner, the desire for restriction does not abate and can even become greater. The fear of becoming fat does not abate with loss of weight, and the perception of one's body is out of touch with reality (American Psychiatric Association 2013). This suggests that there is an inherent distortion in the evaluative capacity that has no connection to reality. The person with overwhelming fear of needles is also distinguishable from the person with anorexia. If it is possible to accomplish the medical procedure by avoiding the use of needles, then presumably the patient should allow the procedure.

7. *A patient with TBI whose pattern of decisions show impaired ability* to weigh and implement decisions. Such a patient can discuss the medical facts with apparent understanding and even voice choices that reflect application of facts to self and a desire to make a good decision. Yet, the overall pattern of decision-making is very poor—they cannot carry out the tasks. This person can talk about it but can't carry out the task of weighing options, stringing together steps to achieve an aim, and so on. Here, the ability to weigh and act on one's values is impaired but only manifests itself over the longer run than what one can detect in an interview. Thus, in some situations, the assessment of DMC will require more than just direct interviews about a specific decision but an overall longitudinal evaluation.

No doubt there are other relevant cases that touch on the ability to value and its various components. The above cases, however, help us to see that an impaired ability to value is a clearly recognizable phenomenon. How one evaluates and determines its impact on the overall assessment of DMC will be very fact sensitive, however.

6. Conclusion

To the extent that the ability to value (and the various components that make up that ability) is (1) essential to decision-making and (2) can be impaired due to pathology, it is not a controversial claim that DMC evaluation must include an assessment of that ability. Although as a matter of empirical fact that some or a substantial portion of persons with impaired ability to value could also be described as having an impairment in appreciation, it seems clear that the two abilities are distinct. My hope is that the framework provided in this chapter—that shows how the abilities to comprehend the relevant facts, to apply those facts to oneself, to integrate those facts with one's values and desires, to reason, and to evidence a choice—will be useful for future discussions on how to reconcile and flesh out the various "criteria for capacity" that are now operative in various jurisdictions.

Acknowledgments

This chapter contains the opinions of the author and does not represent the views or policies of the National Institutes of Health, Department of Health and Human Services, or the US government. The author acknowledges helpful comments from David Wendler, David DeGrazia, and Gareth Owen on earlier drafts of this chapter. Figure 7a.2 is published with the permission of Oxford University Press.

References

American Psychiatric Association. *Diagnostic and Statistical Manual of Mental Disorders: DSM-5.* 5th ed. Arlington, VA: American Psychiatric Association, 2013.

Berg, Jessica Wilen, Paul S. Appelbaum, and Thomas Grisso. "Constructing Competence: Formulating Standards of Legal Competence to Make Medical Decisions." *Rutgers Law Review* 48 (1996): 345–96.

Blom, R. M., R. C. Hennekam, and D. Denys. "Body Integrity Identity Disorder." *PLoS One* 7, no. 4 (2012): e34702.

Charland, L. C. "Appreciation and Emotion: Theoretical Reflections on the Macarthur Treatment Competence Study." Kennedy Institute of Ethics Journal *Inst* 8 (1999): 359–76.

David, Anthony S, Matthew Hotopf, Paul Moran, Gareth Owen, George Szmukler, and Genevra Richardson. "Mentally Disordered or Lacking Capacity? Lessons for Management of Serious Deliberate Self Harm." *BMJ* 341 (2010): 587–89.

Elliott, C. "Caring About Risks: Are Severely Depressed Patients Competent to Consent to Research?" *Archives of General Psychiatry* 54, no. 2 (1997): 113–16.

Frankfurt, H. "Freedom of the Will and the Concept of a Person." *Journal of Philosophy* 68 (1971): 829–39.

Grisso, T., and P. S. Appelbaum. *Assessing Competence to Consent to Treatment: A Guide for Physicians and Other Health Professionals.* London: Oxford University Press, 1998.

——. "Appreciating Anorexia: Decisional Capacity and the Role of Values." *Philosophy, Psychiatry, Psychology* 13, no. 4 (2006): 293–97.

Holroyd, J. "Clarifying Capacity: Values and Reasons." Chap. 7 in *Autonomy and Mental Disorder*, edited by Lubomira Radoilska. New York: Oxford University Press, 2012.

Kim, Scott Y. H. *Evaluation of Capacity to Consent to Treatment and Research.* New York: Oxford University Press, 2010.

——. "Varieties of Decisional Incapacity: Theory and Practice." *The British Journal of Psychiatry* 203, no. 6 (December 1, 2013): 403–5.

Mental Capacity Act 2005. Online at www.legislation.gov.uk/ukpga/2005/9/contents. Last accessed April 28, 2015.

Owen, Gareth S., Fabian Freyenhagen, Matthew Hotopf, and Wayne Martin. "Temporal Inabilities and Decision-Making Capacity in Depression." [In English]. *Phenomenology and the Cognitive Sciences* (June, 2013a): 1–20.

Owen, Gareth S., George Szmukler, Genevra Richardson, Anthony S. David, Vanessa Raymont, Fabian Freyenhagen, Wayne Martin, and Matthew Hotopf. "Decision-Making Capacity for Treatment in Psychiatric and Medical In-Patients: Cross-Sectional, Comparative Study." *The British Journal of Psychiatry* 203, no. 6 (December, 2013b): 461–67.

Seyfried, Lisa, Kerry A. Ryan, and Scott Y. H. Kim. "Assessment of Decision-Making Capacity: Views and Experiences of Consultation Psychiatrists." *Psychosomatics* 54 (2013): 115–23.

Tan, Jacinta O. A., Anne Stewart, R. Fitzpatrick, and T. Hope. "Competence to Make Treatment Decisions in Anorexia Nervosa: Thinking Processes and Values." *Philosophy, Psychiatry, & Psychology* 13, no. 4 (2006a): 267–82.

——. "Studying Penguins to Understand Birds." *Philosophy, Psychiatry, & Psychology* 13, no. 4 (2006b): 299–301.

Vollmann, J. "'But I Don't Feel It': Value and Emotions in the Assessment of Competence in Patients with Anorexia Nervosa." *Philosophy, Psychiatry, & Psychology* 13, no. 4 (2006): 289–91.

7b

Commentary on Kim: Decision-Making Capacity and Value

Jennifer Hawkins

1. Introduction

In his contribution to this volume, Scott Kim claims that our current criteria for assessing decision-making capacity (DMC) are incomplete. The problem is not what the existing criteria tell us to look for, but rather there are key aspects of decision-making that current criteria simply do not assess at all. Moreover, Kim claims the problem is, at root, *evaluative*, meaning that in certain cases the problem with an individual's decision-making stems from her evaluative outlook. For this reason, Kim thinks we need to formulate a new, additional criterion to use in capacity assessment. We should add assessment of what he calls "the ability to value" (p. 189) and he goes on to offer an interesting sketch of how such assessments might work in practice.

I am deeply sympathetic to Kim's general project. I agree both that current criteria are incomplete and that many of the problematic cases are evaluative. No doubt some theorists still need convincing on these points, but I can't hope to do that here. For the purposes of this essay, I shall simply assume that there are some such cases. What I find interesting are questions about how to appropriately craft guidelines for something so controversial. How can we assess a person's evaluative outlook (or aspects of it) as part of capacity assessment? More importantly, how can we hope to do so in a way that respects the key values that have shaped contemporary medical ethics?

Unfortunately, the problem is usually articulated in a very unhelpful way as the problem of maintaining "value neutrality" in capacity assessment. Kim himself introduces the problem this way. He rightly recognizes that many people's first reaction to his proposal will be to raise an objection along these lines. As he states it, the worry is that those who assess capacity are not supposed to be in the business of "judging a person's values." Kim is confident, however, that he has an answer to this worry. He emphasizes that on his proposal we are not directly assessing a person's outlook or the particular choices that flow from it. Rather we are assessing something more basic, namely her *ability* to value. However, I do not think this answer succeeds. Let me be clear: I *do* think an answer is possible. But Kim has not done enough to show us how this is possible. My aim is to present my own alternative understanding of the ethical constraints, and then demonstrate how, consistent with these constraints, we can sometimes ethically assess an individual's evaluative outlook as part of assessing capacity.

It remains to be seen, of course, whether Kim (or others) will want to accept my particular way of framing the issues. As I hope to show, my formulation does have a number of virtues. In addition to making it clearer what we can and cannot do in terms of assessing values, my account is able to save Kim's theory from several possible objections.

2. Evaluative Outlooks

Throughout this essay, I refer to a person's "evaluative outlook." I wish to be clear that the phrase is mine and not Kim's. However, I see no reason why he would object to it. Nothing significant turns on our different terminological choices. "Evaluative outlook" is simply the phrase I use to simplify discussion of a side of our psychology that is complex.

The complexity I refer to is simply this. At any given time an individual has numerous mental attitudes of various sorts all of which could count as evaluative or quasi-evaluative. Moreover, there can sometimes be internal conflicts between attitudes that have to be resolved in some way. For our purposes it does not matter how conflicts are resolved or how the different elements of a person's evaluative psychology come together, but simply that they do. When all the various types and kinds of evaluative input are taken account of and all contradictions and conflicts resolved, what we have is what I refer to as a person's *overall sense of what matters*. An important aspect of having a sense of what matters is one's sense of *relative* value, a sense of what things matter more than others. Most of us do not have a completely worked-out sense of what matters. Nonetheless, to be able to make practical decisions at all a person must have at least a partial, internally coherent vision of what matters, a sense of what matters *in this context here and now*. I use the phrase "evaluative outlook" to refer to these kinds of partially worked-out visions, a person's sense of what matters in a particular decision-making context. Though internally consistent with itself, a particular evaluative outlook may or may not be consistent with past decisions a person has made or with other aspects of her overall sense of what matters. And most importantly, it may or may not be stable. I assume that insofar as we are interested in how evaluative psychology contributes to decision-making, it is evaluative outlooks that concern us.

3. Evaluative Outlooks and Judgments of Personal Good

Before we can tell whether it is possible to assess evaluative outlooks as part of DMC assessment, we need to be clear what the ethical requirements in this area really are. Talk of "value neutrality" and of "not judging values" is unhelpful for various reasons. The reference to "value" is too vague. And the rationale—the reason *why* we are not supposed to judge values is left obscure.

We need a better framework for thinking about what patients are doing when they make decisions, and how evaluative thinking plays into this. Rather than talk vaguely about value, I propose to talk about what is *good for a person*, and about the relationship between evaluative outlooks on the one hand, and judgments of personal good on the other. I assume that in the context of medical decision-making the aim of decision-making is to promote the individual patient's overall good. I take it that this is the patient's aim, but also that it is the proper aim of those who assist patients in making decisions. To avoid certain common misunderstandings of my views, I need first to say a bit about what I mean by personal good, why I think personal good is the proper aim of medical decision-making, and the sense in which judgments about personal good can be wrong.

I use the phrases "personal good" and "prudential good" to talk about the special kind of value that is at stake when we say that something is good *for* a particular person. I also assume that the more general, guiding notion that makes sense of talk about "good for" is the notion of a good life. Other things—choices, events, relationships, achievements, and so on—are good because they contribute to a good life. And some are better than others in virtue of making a life even better. This is the kind of value that self-interest seeks to realize, but it is also the kind of value beneficent individuals seek to realize for others. It is also the kind of value that is diminished when an individual is harmed, and increased when she is benefited.

Of course, we all have very different conceptions of what a good life for us would look like. But it is still safe to say that other things being equal we want good lives, in the sense that we want lives good for us in a way that we can recognize as good. Moreover, we use our own particular vision of a good life as a background constraint on our more immediate decision-making, in the sense that decisions must, minimally, be consistent with the requirements of such a life.

Though medical decisions are not typically focused directly on questions about personal good, it is still true that good medical decisions must be consistent with the individual's pursuit of a good life. It can, however, be easy to lose sight of this, particularly given that medicine has a number of internal ends that shape medical thinking and in terms of which particular choices are routinely evaluated as good or bad. Physicians may seek to prolong a patient's life, they may seek to alleviate a patient's suffering, or they may seek to improve a patient's ability to function despite chronic ill-health. Most of the time the pursuit of these ends is consistent with what the patient wants. But it is possible for these medical ends to conflict with pursuit of the overall good, and when that happens medical ends may have to be revised or abandoned, since the more important end is the patient's overall good.

As I think of it, facts about personal good are highly individually relative. There are many explanations of why this so. People vary dramatically in what they value, but also in terms of their temperaments and in terms of the circumstances and opportunities they find themselves facing. I do not need to defend a detailed account of personal good here. I simply hope to sketch a few broad outlines. I conceive of prudential goodness as depending on a kind of "fit" between a person and the conditions of her life. A high degree of fit disposes a person to evaluate her own life positively, to find value in it. Although fit is what grounds positive attitudes, it is the attitudes themselves that really matter. Since fit is a degree notion, various ways of living might contribute to fit, and more than one path through life might be "good." The notion of "fit" is helpful, for it can give us a way of understanding the goodness of choices. If a person is trying to choose between two options, and if it is true that she would find significantly more value in her life if she chose A over B (because A has a much higher degree of fit), then on my view A is a better choice for her. Some cases will still seem puzzling, for example, cases in which a person is choosing death. After all, any alternative will have more positive value than death because death has no experienced value of any kind. But we don't want to say that death is always a bad choice. The alternatives to death may also have a lot of negative value. In such cases there is presumably a fact of the matter about whether there is some possible future for the individual such that in the living of it she would find more value than disvalue. What we should say is this: If there is such a future (one with a significant balance of positive over negative value), then in choosing death a person makes a mistake. But when no such future is available, death is the better choice.

My account of personal good is relative, but it still leaves room for the notion of prudential mistake. The view on offer is both relative and *objective*, in the sense that I think there are answers to questions about personal good. Our beliefs about the answers could be correct or incorrect. There is something—fit and the attitudes it produces—we are aiming at when we try to make prudentially wise decisions. Mistakes are possible because the consequences of our decisions are frequently not fully realized or experienced until some time later. Thus we often think we are choosing well, only to later discover we were wrong. The important point is that it is not merely third parties who can be mistaken about what would be good for a particular individual A. Individuals can be mistaken about their own good.

4. Ethical Constraints

Against this backdrop we can now say something more concrete and helpful about the role of values in medical decision-making and about what it is that capacity assessors are supposed to avoid.

There are three important constraints. Two of these are *epistemic* constraints—that is, they are constraints on the kinds of inferences we can safely make, given the tenuous nature of our knowledge of certain facts. These two serve as reminders to be *epistemically humble* given the complexity of what we are dealing with. The third is also a constraint on inference, but it derives more directly from facts about our existing moral framework.

The first constraint has to do with what we can conclude simply on the basis of *what* an individual chooses. The answer is: nothing. We must keep in mind that facts about personal good are incredibly diverse. Many quite surprising ends—ends one might be tempted to think could never be in someone's interest—have nevertheless turned out in some cases to be good for people. Given how diverse human good is, and how limited our knowledge of the variety of its forms, we can never conclude that an individual is making a prudentially poor choice simply on the basis of *what* she chooses. The constraint on capacity assessment derives from this more general one. Historically, not only were people tempted to infer that bizarre ends were a sign of prudential mistake, but they also tended to infer that such a mistake must indicate a lack of decision-making capacity. So the constraint on capacity assessors is this: *We cannot infer anything about decision-making capacity simply on the basis of what someone chooses.*

The second constraint is a more general epistemic constraint. It tells us that even if we look more closely at the relationship of "fit" between an individual and her choice—which is, admittedly, the better way to think about decisions of personal good—we cannot make judgments about a person's good with any great certainty. So many factors are relevant to such decisions and human good is so complex that we need to be incredibly humble about our ability to make such judgments. This gives rise to a general constraint that applies to all physicians (and indeed all people) in all contexts, namely that we must always be epistemically humble about judgments of personal good, that is, always open to the possibility that even our most thoughtful, well-intentioned judgments could be wrong. The more specific constraint for capacity assessment is: *An assessor's judgment about whether an individual is making a prudential mistake either should not figure at all in assessments of capacity, or, if it does, it must be given very little weight. Given the possibilities for error, we can never decide that someone lacks capacity simply on the basis of the fact that we think she is making a mistake.*

The third constraint overlaps with this one to some extent, for it is also a reminder not to infer lack of capacity from (supposed) prudential mistake. But it has a different rationale. In our society we have decided that competent adults have the right to make their own decisions. Though not typically formulated this way, we should think of this as *the right to make prudential mistakes.*

It is important to frame the rationale for this right properly. As most people know, a dramatic shift occurred in medicine in the late twentieth century with the result that we came to accept that patients should have the final say about their own healthcare. This was motivated in part by a growing recognition of just how complex individual good is, and the recognition that physicians are often poorly placed to make decisions consistent with a patient's overall personal good. But there is more to the story. For although it is difficult for physicians to make such decisions, patients find it difficult as well and they make mistakes too. Nonetheless, in our culture most people *want* to make such decisions for themselves, even though they might make a mistake. As a society we have come to accept something like the following reasoning: Since these are decisions about an individual's life and since the consequences of such decisions (typically) fall (primarily) on her, if she is willing to assume that responsibility, then we ought to let her make the decision.

If prudential mistakes are protected—if even competent adults make, and have the right to make, prudential mistakes—then it follows that even if we could know when people are making mistakes, we would not be able to infer that a person lacks DMC simply because she is making a mistake. For capacity assessors this means that *even if a mistake is occurring, we must base a decision about decision-making capacity on something else.*

5. An Alternative Proposal for Assessing the Role of Evaluative Outlooks

The three constraints outlined above offer a clear account of what we must avoid. They also, I think, point to a way forward.

Consider again the story about how we came to accept a right to make prudential mistakes. As a society we concluded that most people should be allowed to make their own decisions, even if they make mistakes. The significant fact is that we did not start with an independently grasped understanding of decisional capacity and then apply it to real people, letting the facts about who would be allowed to make personal decisions turn out to be whatever they might be. Nor do I think we should have approached capacity that way. Instead, from the beginning, a practical, pragmatic constraint has been imposed on theorizing about DMC, namely any theory of DMC must have the implication that most ordinary adults are competent. Since ordinary people make a fair number of prudential mistakes, one way of thinking about decisional capacity is as follows. Psychological features that make a person *much more prone to prudential mistakes than even ordinary people are* may undermine decisional capacity.

This in turn suggests a way of thinking about the role of evaluative outlooks. People sometimes find themselves in what, for lack of a better word, I shall call "psychological conditions." I am using what I hope is a neutral word because I want to remain open on the questions of whether conditions in my sense are illness, or disorders. What makes something a psychological condition is that it is more durable than a mere mood, and causes alterations in a person's evaluative outlook. Although conditions in my sense alter evaluative outlooks, not all conditions will be bad or of concern to those assessing capacity, since the alterations caused by some conditions will be minor. In other cases, though the alterations may be more significant, it may still be true that they do not have an overly negative impact on a person's prudential decision-making. *My suggestion is that we try to identify those conditions that alter people's evaluative outlook in such a way that they are more prone to prudential mistakes than even ordinary people are.* We could then formulate my proposal by saying that a necessary (though not sufficient) requirement of finding someone to be lacking DMC on evaluative grounds is that she have such a condition, one known to generally affect prudential decision making in this way. Many mental disorders, such as depression, would count as conditions in my sense. Depression is known to cause people to see the world through a dominantly negative lens, and in virtue of this they often abandon many aspects of their own good. But something like extreme grief might also count as a condition in this sense, since grief also casts a strongly negative light that can undermine a person's ability to make good choices.

The proposal is not yet complete, however. Although the presence of such a condition should be thought of as necessary, it is not sufficient. If we allowed it to be sufficient then we would have to say, for example, that a depressed person is incapable of making a prudentially wise choice (except perhaps by accident). We would have to discount *all* of the decisions of such individuals. But that would be too strong.

I propose instead that we use the presence of such a condition as the primary factor, but then add that in order for a person to be found lacking DMC with respect to a particular decision, we must also have some good reason for suspecting that she is making a prudential mistake. In other words, we must have some reason for thinking that the person is making a decision that does not fit her, or fit her nearly as well as other options open to her. Alternatively, in the case of someone who is choosing death, we would have to have some good reason to suppose that the individual is passing up a real possibility for a dominantly positive existence (positive in a sense that she *herself* will experience it as positive if she chooses it). In a case where we already know that a person is in a condition that typically causes people to be poorer than usual prudential decision-makers, what we need is something else to suggest that this is actually happening in the particular case at hand. And although we cannot ever know with certainty that someone is making a prudential mistake, we can sometimes have good reasons for suspecting this. My proposal is that such reasons, which could *never* in themselves lead us to judge someone to be lacking DMC, may in certain cases tip the balance in favor of such a decision.

This proposal does not violate any of the ethical constraints sketched in the last section. There is no attempt to infer anything simply on the basis of *what* the individual is choosing. Nor is there any attempt to infer lack of decision-making capacity simply on the basis of prudential mistake. The proposal is consistent with acknowledgement of how difficult and uncertain judgments about personal good must always be. Capacity assessors need not claim knowledge of what is good for a person. Moreover, it is designed to recognize and honor the fact that most ordinary adults have the *right* to make prudential mistakes. The majority of the work is done by direct appeal to conditions. And conditions are to be identified, and shown to be relevant to capacity assessment, prior to and thus independently of our assessment of any particular individual. They are to be picked out as alterations in evaluative outlook that are known to lead a great many people to make decisions that do not fit them.

6. A Friendly Amendment to Kim's Proposal?

At the outset I claimed that Kim does not do enough to convince us that it really is possible ethically to assess evaluative outlooks as part of capacity assessment. He emphasizes that he wants to assess "the ability to value" as opposed to judging the worthiness of particular values. However, by itself this answer is inadequate. To begin with, the phrase "ability to value" suggests a contrast between those who have some evaluative outlook or other, and those who entirely lack one. But for the most part, the cases that interest us are not cases in which a person lacks any sense that things matter. Rather the problem is that her sense of what matters is off-base, flawed, mistaken, or bad. Kim's actual proposal suggests that he hopes to avoid saying such things by focusing on the origin of certain attitudes in illness. But we still need an explanation of why illness *matters*. The story here will, I think, have to say that certain illnesses distort our values in ways that make them off-base, flawed, mistaken, or simply bad. If, as I think, such claims are unavoidable, we need more of an explanation than Kim provides for why it is really okay to say that a person's evaluative outlook is flawed.

I have tried to give such an explanation. Given that the proper end of medical decision-making is the individual's own overall good, there is a straightforward sense in which evaluative outlooks can be problematic. They can lead people to make prudential mistakes. Moreover, I have also taken care to show that the mere fact that a person makes an evaluative mistake is not a sufficient reason for thinking she lacks DMC, since many ordinary people make prudential mistakes. Having once explained the sense in which an evaluative outlook can be criticized, I have also shown that as assessors of capacity we must be careful not to infer lack of capacity simply from (apparent) prudential mistake. To understand the link between flawed evaluative outlooks and DMC, we have to recognize that there are some *psychological conditions* that radically alter a person's evaluative outlook in predictable ways and *that are known to make a person a much worse prudential judge than normal.*

In many ways Kim's proposed account is much like the one I have sketched. It has two parts, that is, two necessary conditions that together would be sufficient for finding someone to lack DMC on the basis of evaluative considerations. The first necessary requirement is that the person must have a recognized form of "pathology, psychiatric or cognitive, or malfunctioning of brain processes that can reasonably be determined to be the source of the impaired ability to value" (p. 195). The second necessary requirement is an authenticity requirement. Namely, the choice the individual is making, or the desire she is expressing, must be "patently inconsistent with the set of values and history that roughly constitute the person's identity" (p. 196).

Kim's focus on brain disorders is on the right track in one sense. For it suggests that he is thinking about broad alterations to a person's psychology, alterations of some duration. But it is still left unclear why precisely brain disorders are the focus. What precisely is the link between brain disorders and poor judgment (as opposed to just unusual judgment that is not necessarily poor)? As a result, his requirement seems to face several difficulties. First, I must say that I do not accept that all mental disorders are brain disorders, even though I am a realist about mental disorder. But let us set that aside. Even if mental disorders are brain disorders, it is not clear that all mental disorders lead people to evaluate in skewed ways. Alternatively, there may be some conditions in my sense that are not properly thought of as mental disorders at all (much less brain disorders) even though they might reasonably be thought to temporarily undermine DMC for evaluative reasons.

My framework provides a way of drawing distinctions within the category of mental disorder and explaining why only certain diagnoses might be relevant to a particular assessment of capacity. They are relevant because some mental disorders cause people to be worse than usual at prudential decision-making.

My framework also allows us to acknowledge that there may be some psychological conditions that radically affect a person's evaluative outlook, but which are not disorders. The primary example I have in mind is extreme grief, though I suspect there may be others. There is, of course, disagreement among psychiatrists over whether grief is a mental disorder. Recent re-classifications have made it into one. But I think this is a mistake. Moreover, I suspect that on this point Kim would agree with me, since he is attracted to the idea that mental disorders are brain disorders and I doubt anyone would be tempted to see grief as a form of brain malfunction. In the immediate aftermath of a significant loss, a person may be in a condition where she is genuinely unable to make good decisions for herself. Not only that, she may be much more likely than ordinary people (and much more likely than herself ordinarily) to make a prudential mistake.

The other condition Kim proposes is an authenticity requirement. For reasons of space I will not say much about it here. I simply wish to point out that the authenticity requirement faces problems similar to those faced by reliance on brain malfunction; namely, we want a better account of why a failure to judge authentically really *matters*. Inauthentic judgments are (relative to the individual) unusual, but why are they a sign of a lack of decisional capacity? It seems plausible to me that if authenticity matters, it matters because of a link to poor prudential judgment.

7. Concluding Remarks

It is important to emphasize that despite the focus of this essay—which after all is supposed to be a critical commentary—I am really in agreement with Kim about quite a bit. I have tried to use my preferred framework to develop friendly amendments to Kim's account. However, Kim may well *not* wish to adopt my framework because it is admittedly controversial. My framework will, no doubt, strike many as unappealing because of its talk about personal good, and the fact that it allows capacity assessors to consider whether there is any reason to think the individual is making a poor choice.

However, discussions of DMC have all too frequently tried to avoid talking about things that in my opinion we cannot really avoid. Many perennial problems in understanding capacity assessment stem from the fact that we do not typically acknowledge that the end of medical decisions is the individual's own good, and that decisional capacity needs to be assessed relative to the aim of decision-making. Things that make people worse than usual at this aim are things that undermine capacity. Without such a move we can only point to "formal" flaws in the process of decision-making, and with that limitation it will indeed be hard to explain how evaluative states can be part of the problem. There are few if any formal requirements on evaluative states beyond consistency.

In bioethics people worry all the time about paternalism, seeing instances of it everywhere. Some will no doubt view my proposal as objectionably paternalistic. But this is too hasty. First, insofar as I rely on the notion of personal good, I emphasize that good is relative to individuals. I am not adopting some substantive view of what is good for others and then trying to impose such a view. Nor am I recommending that others do so. Second, on my view no one could ever be declared lacking decisional capacity simply on the basis of our assumption that she is making a prudential mistake. The only role for such judgments is very minor. Such judgments can tip the balance when we are already certain that the individual is in a condition that typically undermines prudential decision-making in significant ways. That sort of highly limited use is, I think, compatible with acknowledging that we can never be certain about such judgments, as well as compatible with recognizing the right of most ordinary adults to make prudential mistakes.

I therefore hope that Kim in particular, and those interested in capacity assessment generally, will see something useful in this approach. It needs much work, but it strikes me as worth developing.

8a

Fragments of the Self

Dissociation, Agency, and Integration

Franklin Worrell and Alison Denham

> The ultimate aim with DID therapy, which is not always possible and sometimes too risky to attempt, is for the patient's mind to reintegrate and become whole. Does Patricia want to integrate? She shakes her head. "My attitude is: how can I get a memory? I wasn't there. I was not in that room when that happened."
>
> (Amanda Mitchison, 2011, "Kim Noble: The Woman with 100 Personalities")

> [W]hat justifies the judgment that certain of your beliefs are irrational might not also justify the judgment that it would be rational for you to act in such a way as to eradicate those beliefs. Suppose you learn of a kind of psycho-surgery that enables people to bring all of their beliefs about their positive and negative attributes into line with the facts. Suppose you also learn that only this psycho-surgery would eliminate all of your biased beliefs about yourself, that it is very expensive, and that it would probably cut ten years off your life. Would it be rational for you to sign up for the surgery? Obviously not.
>
> (Alfred Mele, 2004, "Rational Irrationality")

1. Introduction

Dissociative identity disorder (DID) is a natural process gone awry. In dissociation, psychological functions that normally act in concert become segregated, yielding a "disruption of and/or discontinuity in the normal integration of consciousness, memory, identity, emotion, perception, body representation, motor control, and behavior" (APA 2013, 291). Thus characterized, dissociation is neither maladaptive nor unhealthy. Indeed, it plays an important role in everyday functioning, permitting us to segment our targets of conscious awareness and so to perform one task while attending to another. Anyone who has driven some distance while deep in thought, only to arrive at his destination with no memories of the journey, has dissociated. Similarly, anyone whose thoughts have been sidetracked while reading a book, and then realized that they have "read" several pages without registering them, has also had a dissociative episode.

In these everyday cases, certain of the subject's psychological sub-systems—for instance, his perceptual and motor systems—have disengaged from conscious awareness, monitoring, and control, continuing to operate independently of his occurrent experience. DID is a pathological development of similar processes, in which the subject's dis-integration is both more extreme and more persistent, compromising his ability to function as a practical agent. The disorder typically emerges as a coping mechanism in the face of extreme trauma and/or abuse. In treating DID, therapists normally attempt to reintegrate what has fragmented—to reintegrate the various identities, personalities, or alters into a unified self.

Our aims in this paper are to understand what such integration consists in and to examine the values upon which this therapeutic goal is based. These will require us to investigate some murky conceptual issues surrounding the nature of the patient's alternate personalities. Section 2 outlines the clinical presentation of DID, its causal origins, and the prevailing idea that integration is the proper end of clinical treatment. In Sections 3 and 4, we examine the metaphysical status of alternative personality states; we address in particular their standing as persons and agents and dispute the classic interpretations of DID subjects as, one and all, comprising either multiple or single identities. Section 5 returns to the therapeutic goal of integration and its normative significance. Why do we value agentive integration? We reject the proposal that the value of rational agency itself constitutes an independent justifier. Section 6 argues that fragmented agency may be preferable to fully integrated, maximally consistent agency—even in non-pathological cases.

2. DID: Causes, Characteristics, and Cure

2.1 The *DSM-5* describes DID in terms of identifying symptoms and etiological constraints, two of which are of special interest here. The first is the "disruption of identity characterized by two or more distinct personality states," involving "marked discontinuity in sense of self and sense of agency, accompanied by related alterations in affect, behavior, consciousness, memory, perception, cognition, and/or sensory-motor functioning" (APA 2013, 292). The second criterion is amnesia, defined as "recurrent gaps in the recall of everyday events, important personal information, and/or traumatic events that are inconsistent with ordinary forgetting" (APA 2013, 292).[1] The *DSM*'s two key diagnostic criteria for DID—multiple personality states and autobiographical amnesia—can be summarized in the following manner:

> DID reflects a failure to integrate various aspects of identity, memory and consciousness in a single multidimensional consciousness. Usually, a primary identity carries the individual's given name and is passive, dependent, guilty and depressed. When in control, each personality state, or alter, may be experienced as if it

> has a distinct history, self-image and identity. The alters' characteristics—including name, reported age and gender, vocabulary, general knowledge, and predominant mood—contrast with those of the primary identity. Certain circumstances or stressors can cause a particular alter to emerge. The various identities may deny knowledge of one another, be critical of one another or appear to be in open conflict.[2]

DID patients also frequently present with some of the Schneiderian first-rank symptoms of schizophrenia, such as experiences of thought insertion, involuntary volitions and movement, auditory hallucinations (often voices arguing), visual hallucinations, and withdrawal. DID is very often co-morbid with other disorders, including depression and borderline personality disorder (Dell 2006; APA 2013, 298); one review of the literature found no instance of DID without co-occurring psychopathology (Dorahy *et al.* 2014, 405). Due to this array of symptoms, patients are functionally impaired with respect to their social roles, finding it difficult to fulfill familial, personal, and professional responsibilities. As Paul Dell puts it, in DID "the phenomena of pathological dissociation are recurrent, jarring intrusions into executive functioning and sense of self, and … pathological dissociative phenomena affect every aspect of human experience" (Dell 2006, 123).

Despite DID's complex profile, the *DSM*'s emphasis on the features of multiple personality states and amnestic states is neither arbitrary nor misplaced. These are not merely two markers alongside others; they are intermediate causal conditions, and many of the subject's other difficulties issue from them. More importantly, accessing and mitigating multiplicity and amnesia are regarded as causally necessary for cure. Privileging multiplicity and amnesia as source conditions does not, of course, suggest that they are not the product of a prior, experiential cause. The widely accepted developmental view is that they result from early, disorganized attachment coupled with childhood trauma, typically abuse (and usually sexual abuse) at the hands of a caregiver. As the *Guidelines for Treating Dissociative Identity Disorder* explain:

> [E]xperts … hypothesize that alternate identities result from the inability of a traumatized child to develop a unified sense of self that is maintained across various behavioral states, particularly if the traumatic exposure first occurs before the age of 5. These difficulties often occur in the context of relational or attachment disruption that may precede and set the stage for abuse and the development of dissociative coping.
>
> *(ISSTD 2011, 122)*

Key to this developmental picture, DID is *not* presented as a deviation from a previously mature, unified self—a pre-existing core personality that has fractured. Rather, the subject is viewed as developmentally incomplete, her cognitive trajectory arrested *en route* to its destination. Specifically, she has failed to achieve the requisite *integration* of various psychological functions. Conceptualized in this way, it is tempting to conceive of therapeutic treatment as taking up where the child's early experiences left off, that is, to effect an integration of the dissociated parts of the subject's mental economy. The criterion of success for this enterprise is to achieve "fusion" of the subject's alternate identities, and thereby also relieve his amnestic symptoms. Most clinicians use the term "integration" to refer to the longer-term therapeutic gains that are made in addressing all dissociative processes, while "fusion" refers more specifically to the bringing together of two or more alternate identities, and "final fusion" or "unification" to the achievement of a unified and unitary self. We will use the terms "integration" and "fusion" interchangeably; both aptly label a combinatorial process whereby distinct entities are transformed in a single item.

2.2 This is, in outline, the conception of DID and its proper treatment prevailing among clinicians who countenance it as a distinctive disorder. The conception combines a traumagenic description of its origins and a therapeutic prescription of integration for its cure. It should be noted that this conception itself is by no means unanimously endorsed within the psychiatric community. Challenging the description, many researchers have argued that DID is a socio-cognitive phenomenon with iatrogenic origins.[3] That is, it is a construction born of the therapeutic process itself—the subject creates alter identities at the suggestion of the therapist, perhaps influenced by popular media depictions.[4] The socio-cognitive model thus questions the etiology of the patient's experience of multiple identities. For the purposes of this paper we focus solely on the traumagenic conception. Numerous case studies and interviews with clinicians provide powerful evidence of the spontaneity and trauma-related origins of the disorder.[5] We will here assume the genuineness of the phenomena of multiplicity and amnestic discontinuities that distinguish DID from other disorders.

The prescription for integration seems to flow naturally from the traumagenic model in at least two ways. First, the model invites us to see integration as *reparative* or *restorative*, fulfilling the clinician's *telos* of reclaiming for a damaged system its proper functions. Second, the traumagenic description recommends integration as subserving cherished ideals of autonomy and self-governance. While "trauma" is itself a contested concept, almost all definitions recognize as traumatic aversive experiences that severely threaten a subject's physical or psychological integrity—that overwhelm his ability to coherently unify his cognitive and affective responses.[6] The construction of alters is a mechanism of conflict avoidance in which these dis-integrated responses are assigned to distinct autobiographical "tracks." While this strategy may spare the subject the distress of internal dissonance, it does so at a cost: Insofar as the agentive powers—choosing, intending, and acting—in any one persona are vulnerable to disruption by an alter, DID places those powers out of reach. Even if it is granted that the multiple is a person or persons, his status as an agent will be tragically compromised unless and until his integrity is restored.

We will later challenge both of these evaluative inferences. We do not deny that integration can be, and often is, a legitimate therapeutic end; nonetheless, we will question whether it is in *every* case a proper therapeutic goal. First, however, it is necessary to look more closely at just what integration is. For the value of integration depends on just who or what is being integrated—the nature of the "identity states" that are its therapeutic target.

3. "Personal Identity States": Multiple Persons or Fragmented Selves

3.1 Both the *DSM* and the clinical literature under-determine the cycling personality states that are the distinguishing mark of DID. What exactly are they individually, and what do they jointly comprise? When we call them separate personalities, are we merely speaking metaphorically of radically divergent aspects of one person's character? Are they a kind of proto-person, a one-dimensional element that the patient has come to believe is a distinct personality? Or are they fully-fledged persons? If so, are they different persons or different manifestations of the same person?[7] These are, at least at the outset, straightforwardly philosophical questions, requiring the theorist to demarcate conceptual categories (e.g., "person") and to supply accurate criteria for identifying and individuating their members. At the same time, the target entities—DID alters—constitute a specific empirical phenomenon, which must also be properly characterized.

The philosophical literature addressing DID has been remarkably myopic in its consideration of the clinical evidence: Theorists typically content themselves with examining one or a handful of famous multiples and neglect the radical divergence of clinical presentations in DID, particularly with respect to the number, complexity, and robustness of alters in play. From limited evidence, they often draw hasty, general conclusions from unrepresentative samples. Alters vary too much in depth and complexity to judge *a priori* the status of all cases, or indeed any specific case. The clinical presentation of DID is not uniform, and nor should our metaphysical verdicts be.

Philosophers most often defend either the view that a DID subject contains multiple persons or the view that she is a single person suffering from deep psychological division. We will refer to these as the Multiple Person Thesis (MPT) and the Single Person Thesis (SPT) respectively.[8] We begin by outlining what might be thought of as the classic presentation of DID: a relatively low number of well-developed alters. Later, we incorporate less familiar research and case studies to test the generalizability of the MTP and STP. Both of these universal pronouncements, we argue, are inadequate.

3. 2 Therapist Morton Prince's (1913) account of his patient Christine L. Beauchamp has served as a paradigm in the philosophical literature on DID. During approximately six years of treatment (1898–1904), Prince identified four personalities in the Beauchamp multiple; he labeled them B1, Sally, B4, and B2. B1, Sally, and B4 were all distinct in their outlooks and personalities, as well as how they spoke and carried themselves. Prince thought of each personality as being of a different type. He called B1 "The Saint" and described her as exceptionally morally high-minded. "The Woman," B4, was a paradigm of human frailty, driven by egoistic desires. Sally was dubbed "The Devil" because Prince thought her to be "a mischievous imp, one of that kind which we might imagine would take pleasure in thwarting the aspirations of humanity" (1913, 16–17).[9] Each personality was well developed and able to function when regnant. Furthermore, at various points in Beauchamp's treatment, the alters actively worked to thwart each other's purposes and plans (e.g., after initially becoming regnant, Sally embarked upon a one-sided prank war with B1).

The amnesiac relationships between Beauchamp's alters were complicated. All other alters were amnesiac for Sally's periods of regnancy—indeed, they were completely ignorant of her existence until informed by Prince—and no other alter had access to Sally's thoughts and actions; however, Sally could at least "watch" the actions of the other three personalities and was aware of B1's and B2's thoughts even when they were regnant. B4 was ignorant of the past several years of Beauchamp's life, and she was not aware of either B1 or Sally. B1 had no knowledge of B4.

The "real" Beauchamp eluded Prince for some time. Initially, Prince took B1—the personality who presented for treatment in his office—as the host identity; however, after B4 arrived on the scene, he reconsidered and took B4 to be the original identity. B4 was more "normal" than B1, which he hypothesized broke off as the result of some trauma "as some quasi-somnambulistic personage" (1913, 213). Prince's therapeutic agenda took a third sharp turn when he realized that particular hypnotic states of both B1 and B4 were actually one and the same. This personality, B2, was not amnesiac—she had the memories available to both B1 and B4. Furthermore, B2 identified herself as being both B1 and B4. Prince decided B2 was the real Christine Beauchamp, and he decided to put this personality in charge. His decision prompted Sally and B4 to begin a life-and-death battle for supremacy, with B4 blocking Prince's hypnotic access to B2.

Supporting the traumagenic view of DID, all the personalities eventually told Prince of a traumatic event involving a male friend of Beauchamp's that occurred in 1893, which caused changes to Beauchamp's character.[10] B4's amnesia for the past several years seemed to begin on that night in 1893, and Prince inferred from this that Beauchamp dissociated into a type of fugue state in which the passive, reticent B1 took over.

Prince seems to have stereotyped Beauchamp's alters in ways that conform to familiar traumagenic categories. According to the traumagenic account, alters emerge as ways for a child to emotionally and cognitively deal with extreme forms of abuse. Ross, for instance, describes common types of alters including child, protector, persecutor, and opposite sex alters (1989, 111–18). Each alter emerges to serve a different function in the fractured multiple. For example, alters of the opposite sex can be ways of coping with homosexual desire with which the patient does not identify (Ross 1989, 116) or they can emerge because the child thinks she might escape sexual abuse if she were male (Kluft 1999, 5). Protector personalities emerge from the desire to have someone strong enough and powerful enough to resist the abuse and fight off the abuser (Kluft 1999, 5). Each of these types of personalities may display a full range of affect, character, and so on. All of them, however, develop for a specific purpose. Further, they tend to become regnant based on situations that they were designed to cope with and that call for the skills that specific alter possesses. Thus, homosexual attraction may elicit a same-sex alter, while the threat of violence may call forth a protector alter.

Confer and Ables' (1983, esp. 53–59) account of Rene, a woman housing six personalities, reinforces both the traumagenic model of DID and the descriptions of typical alters provided by Ross and Kluft. Each of Rene's alters fulfilled a role like those outlined above. Bobby, an angry 20-year-old man, wanted only to take revenge for the abuse heaped on Rene as a child. Jeane was a sort of protector who could remember the abusive episodes for which Rene was amnesiac—it also seems that Jeane had some sort of awareness of the other alters. Stella was the seat of Rene's sexual desires, whereas Sissy Gail—a four-year-old girl—compartmentalized Rene's terror in the face of her abuse; Mary was Rene's capacity for forgiveness and peace.

Cases like these have been the central focus of philosophical attention, and they have certain key features in common. Dissociation occurred as a result of trauma, apparently sexual in nature. Alters were amnesiac of times in which others were regnant, and alters manifested almost contradictory characters and traits. The multiple housed only a few alters that were rather well developed—a characteristic typical for early twentieth-century cases, if less typical now (Spanos 1996, 2; see also Goff and Simms 1993, 597–98). Based on cases such as these, some philosophers have argued that a multiple genuinely is multiple and contains more than one person. As Sinnott-Armstrong and Behnke note, the most common way for an argument about the metaphysical status of alters to progress is to point to certain plausible criteria of personhood and argue that the alters either do or do not meet these criteria; typical arguments on both sides of the MPT/SPT debate proceed along these lines (2000, 306). We consider each in turn.

3.3 Dennett's six criteria for personhood provide a good starting point. These criteria focus primarily on the *capacities* of the entity in question. Specifically, to count as a person it must (1) be rational, (2) be the type of thing to which we ascribe intentional predicates, (3) be the type of thing toward which we adopt a certain stance, (4) be able to reciprocate this stance, (5) be able to use language, and (6) be self-conscious (Dennett 1976, 177–78). Kathleen Wilkes utilizes these criteria and supplements them with four further conditions for *individuating* the alters as persons. These are that (1) alters have characters or personalities, (2) alters have the ability to make do when in control of the body for prolonged periods, (3) it may not be initially clear which personality is dominant,[11] (4) plurality can be both diachronic and synchronic, and (5) imagining the case from the first-person perspective elicits the intuition of multiplicity (1988, 120–27).

Do the alters of DID subjects fulfill these criteria? It is clear that some do. Wilkes uses the Beauchamp case as her paradigm, concluding that Beauchamp's alters satisfied Dennett's criteria, with only minor qualifications (1988, 120–23). This seems correct. We ascribe intentional predicates to all four personalities. Each personality is something toward which we take the intentional stance and something that can reciprocate that stance.[12] Each personality can use language effectively. Further, each personality is a rational agent and is self-conscious. These observations are repeated with consideration of Rene's alters. Wilkes goes on to consider her own individuating criteria for the distinctness of alters. She finds that these favor a judgment of multiplicity in the Beauchamp case (1988, 123–27). Again, this seems correct. The first requirement that each alter have its own distinct personality appears to be fulfilled: as Prince describes the case, B1 was prudish and reserved; Sally was flamboyant and charming; B4 was snarky and afraid of the dark. Second, each Beauchamp alter actually did function successfully when regnant for an extended period. Third, given the type of therapeutic intervention Prince pursued, it was not clear which personality he would pick to survive as Christine Beauchamp: he changed his mind at least twice. Fourth, Sally claimed to observe the perceptions and actions of Beauchamp's other personalities third-personally as not her own. The Beauchamp multiple's plurality was synchronic and diachronic. Finally, Wilkes argues that it is difficult to deny multiplicity if we imagine ourselves as one of the Beauchamp alters—each alter was different and most were amnesiac when not regnant.[13]

Wilkes' case for multiplicity rests on Dennett's criteria for identifying an alter as a person, supplemented with her own criteria for distinguishing them as different, individual persons. But other criteria, including those favored by narrative conceptions of the self, may yield similar conclusions.[14] So, for instance, Hardcastle and Flanagan argue that multiples contain multiple persons, because each alter has its own self-narrative, and (importantly) these narratives cannot, as presented, be consistently unified into a *single* narrative. The DID subject presenting with these incompatible yet individually complete self-narratives therefore presents multiple persons (1999, 651–52). Whatever one may think of narrative conceptions of the self, it is true that each Beauchamp alter had different interests, pursued different activities, manifested different evaluative judgments, and supported different practical agendas. For example, B1 went to church regularly and engaged in charitable enterprises—activities that Sally and B4 despised. Furthermore, each alter demonstrated diachronic unity and its personality and traits persisted through multiple appearances.

What conclusion can we draw from these arguments? Both give good reason to suppose that the Beauchamp multiple was, in fact, multiple. It housed no less than four persons. From here, it is an easy step to endorsing the MPT. If one could also show that *other* DID cases are relevantly like the Beauchamp case, one might then abstract from these cases and claim that DID patients quite generally house multiple persons. Since cases like Confer and Ables' Rene are relevantly like the Beauchamp multiple, the generalization seems to have some basis. The major evidence adduced in favor of the MPT is psychological: Alters have different experiential memories, demonstrate amnesia when another alter is regnant, have different goals and personalities, and understand themselves in terms of a self-narrative that is distinct from and inconsistent with the narratives of the subject's other alters. So the question is, do all, or even most, cases of clinically diagnosed DID lend support to the MPT by the same standards? Or does the SPT more aptly accommodate some further evidence?

3.4 The SPT maintains that alters and host are all just parts of *one person*. Dividing a person is like dividing a cake: it does not give you multiple people. The act of dividing simply results in diminished parts of a person—person "slices"—none of which constitutes a complete person in itself. The analogy is plausible in the case of imagining some division of the psychologies of ordinary, non-pathological subjects: You and I, after all, seem to have just one operative memory system, related to one retrieval system, related to one affective system, and so forth. Whatever could count as a "dividing" of our unified, psychological systems that was not simply taking a "slice" of the unitary individuals that we are? How might we be divided to yield two, or three, or more people? The correct answer seems to be that no division of the self could have that result. How, then, could the MPT be true?

Proponents of the SPT argue that multiples do not house more than one individual. Two considerations support this view. First, the psychological discontinuity allegedly demarcating alters is not, in fact, sufficient to adequately individuate them. Second, the parts comprising alters fail to properly constitute persons: they are incomplete. We examine each consideration in turn.

What individuates alters, each from the other? A key individuating criterion on which MPT theorists rely is differences in memory contents. There are, however, different kinds of memory. Experiential memory delivers a record of events and objects from a first-personal point of view—representations of past events as experienced by the subject, *that* thus and such occurred. Procedural memory or "know-how," by contrast, need not be represented: Once you have learned how to ride a bicycle the procedure is available to you on command, independent of any explicit experiential record of the learning process. Likewise, alters do not need to relearn language or how to tie their shoes or how to perform other acquired skills available to the DID primary identity. Perhaps, then, the amnesia between various personalities is more limited than we have supposed, while the psychological continuity between them is really quite high. As Kennett and Matthews remark:

> [I]t seems that the continuity-of-self problem the DID patient has is in a sense monothematic. Only those bits of information directly or indirectly associated with experiential memory are lost; the rest is preserved. This fact seems far more compatible with the Single Person thesis than its alternatives. It suggests that, in addition to the preservation of bodily continuity, there is a significant degree of psychological continuity across altered states.
>
> *(Kennett and Matthews 2002, 512)*

This observation does indeed seem to apply to the Beauchamp multiple. Each alter knew English and could function quite highly in many other respects. The memory gaps were experiential in nature. Granted, Sally claimed not to know French even though B1 and B4 did, but this gap is explained by Sally "not paying attention" during Beauchamp's school lesson. It is unclear whether Sally suffered a gap in genuine "know-how," or in experiential memory.

Elsewhere, Kennett and Matthews have argued that alters are not individual persons because they lack the *unity of agency* required for personal identity.[15] The thought is that a capacity for sustained practical reasoning—making choices, forming intentions and plans, initiating deliberated actions—is a necessary (and perhaps sufficient) criterion of personhood. This idea is familiar from neo-Kantian accounts of personhood such as those of Korsgaard and Rovane. As Kennett and Matthews put the point:

> Effective agency … requires a unity of purpose both at a time, in order that we may eliminate conflict among our motives and do one thing rather than another, and over time, because many of the things we do form part of longer-term projects and make sense only in the light of these projects and life plans.
>
> *(Kennett and Matthews 2003, 307)*

Specifically, Kennett and Matthews argue that the metaphysics of identity is constrained by the requirement that personhood entails accountability to standards of practical rationality and the sustained and developed values that are its foundation:

> The unity of agency thesis thus provides a normative constraint on personal identity: the proper constitution of selves over time is required to enable the accomplishment of projects and the occupation of roles that have an independent moral and social value.
>
> *(Kennett and Matthews 2003, 308)*

On this view, for an entity to count as a person it must be sufficiently psychologically complex to participate in certain relationships and long-term commitments that manifest its values. These underpin our ability to set practical principles for ourselves as autonomous agents, capable of choosing and implementing our choices in actions (Kennett and Matthews 2003, 307).

Many DID subjects, by contrast, are severely compromised in their abilities to develop meaningful relationships or create and follow through with sustained projects. Alters are often characterized by amnestic gaps that prohibit ongoing engagement with other persons, even those encountered while that alter was regnant. Moreover, most alters are likely to be regnant for too little time to significantly develop any relationships that might be forged. Finally, they have a very limited ability to sustain projects and goals because the other personalities sharing the body cannot be relied upon to pursue them (Kennett and Matthews 2003, 308–10). Thus, alters are too incomplete in their *practical* identities to develop the level of agency required by the MPT. Again, these worries find a ready home in the details of the Beauchamp case. When Beauchamp went through a period of frequent cycling, B1, B4, and Sally all made commitments that the others disregarded. B1's finances were constantly in disarray because of B4 and Sally's trickery and contrary impulses. The activities and projects each alter cared about were difficult to pursue, and carrying long-term goals and projects through to the end was next to impossible.

To sum, the arguments against the MPT derive from two observations. First, the advertised psychological discontinuity between alters is not thorough-going and is restricted to distortions in experiential memory. Second, alters lack the agentive characteristics necessary for practical reasoning and, hence, for personhood. Specifically, alters cannot develop the projects, commitments, and relationships required for unified agency. Thus, a DID subject *must* be singular because the alters within it are too diminished to be persons in their own right—they do not count as persons at all and so cannot constitute multiple persons.[16]

It is worth noting that the second consideration might equally support skepticism that a DID subject contains any subject at all—a No Person Thesis. Some multiples might be so divided and fractured, and their regnancy so transient and episodic, that no identity possesses sufficiently sustained and complete agentive powers to qualify it as a person. Indeed, Kennett and Matthews go so far as to say of a DID patient that "at the most general level there are just too few of those psychological connections between different stages of the agent that are needed to effect diachronic self-control" (Kennett and Matthews 2003, 310). Matthews has independently indicated the possibility that in the case of some hypothetical multiples the No Person Thesis would be the only plausible one:

> At the other end of the spectrum, consider a logically possible case of an individual with a thousand or so different alter personalities, who frequently switch. In such a case the reason the single person thesis no longer applies is that we no longer have any person at all, so *a fortiori*, we do not have a single one. The individual has not reached the threshold for personal identity because we are not satisfied that aspects of personhood have been assigned in either the right quantity or the right fit.
>
> *(Matthews 2003, 171–72)*

As we shall see, some researchers suggest that such fracture is not merely logically possible, but has *actually occurred*. The substantial breakdown of the abilities of the multiple may entail that the multiple contains no persons. There is no agential capacity working in any substantially developed way. Thus, if one accepts that rational agency is a requirement of personhood, there is no person. Similarly, we can conceive of possible brain injury and dementia cases wherein radical personality change occurs and dissolves the formerly present person without replacing it with another (Radden 1996, 61). It is at least possible that when some alters become regnant, a non-person has taken control of the body. When that alter is no longer regnant, a person returns. Furthermore, DID may so undermine the capacities of the multiple that the original person who fractured is no longer there and has been replaced by a non-person or a collection of non-persons.

4. How Many Persons? It Depends...

4.1. We have canvassed two plausible interpretations of the phenomena associated with DID. And each interpretation seems correct in certain cases of DID; however, none of them will apply across the board without exception. Both the MPT and the SPT fail because they implicitly assume a uniformity in the clinical presentations of DID cases. This uniformity does not exist. Different cases of DID demonstrate alters of widely divergent complexity and psychological capability—there are even extensive differences between alters within the same patient. Though cases like Beauchamp and Rene have proven themselves paradigmatic to (both psychiatric and philosophical) DID research, they do not exhaust the clinical literature. These cases are frequently taken to be typical; however, "typical" is a loose term when we are dealing with a disease as controversial and multifaceted as DID. While some alters meet all the conditions laid out by philosophers like Wilkes, other alters are not nearly as complex and developed in functionality, mental capacity, psychological unity, or personality. These cases are the more controversial ones, granted; but they have been described by leading researchers in the field.

For example, Kluft (1988) has described two cases in which each multiple contained over 4,000 alters.[17] It is extremely improbable (if not impossible) for each of the 4,000 alters to be regnant long enough to develop the capacities and characteristics required to fulfill the conditions laid out by multiplicity proponents. For example, they clearly could not develop sustained projects, their being competent in handling prolonged regnant periods would be very unlikely, and the likelihood that all of their personalities would be substantially different or substantially developed seems unlikely. Kluft describes such patients:

> As children they had been so bombarded with outrages that they had not been able to develop a cohesive and comprehensive system of alters within which their further traumata could be managed. Instead, new alters were formed frequently on an ad hoc basis, and many persisted, some becoming major, some highly specialized, and some fairly inactive.
>
> *(1988, 49–50)*

He goes on to describe such alters, and it seems apparent that they will not live up to the criteria discussed above:

> Many formed a high percentage of their alters in direct response to traumatic events; the more traumata, the more alters. These alters contained the memories of these events and/or their associated perceptions and affects. They persisted as vehicles of memory, but rarely played major roles in day-to-day life unless events analogous to their unique experiences occurred. They were rarely invested in separateness and often integrated immediately or with little help after being allowed to tell their stories.
>
> *(Kluft 1988, 50)*

The alters in such cases are minimal in the memories they contain and situations they are designed to respond to—they're extremely specialized. In short, such cases exemplify the concerns put forward by Kennett and Matthews: Some alters are simply too fragmentary to be persons. The proponents of the MPT implicitly assume that all alters are substantially developed personalities that can and do take regular possession of the body.

4.2 There are, therefore, good reasons to be suspicious of the conjecture that all alters demonstrate a level of complexity and development sufficient to meet the criteria of personhood that proponents of the MPT endorse. However, the variations in clinical presentation of DID cut both ways. The existence of radically underdeveloped alters threatens to undermine the MPT, but the existence of well-developed alters poses a similar threat to proponents of the SPT. As we have been pressing, Beauchamp's Sally is an excellent example of an alter that strikes us as a fully developed and complicated person. She meets many of the criteria surveyed above. Furthermore, she demonstrates a level of complexity and awareness (in part allowed by her access to the thoughts and actions of the other personalities) that permits her the sustained development of projects and cultivation of relationships, which could plausibly qualify her for the unity of agency that Kennett and Matthews appeal to. Additionally, it is important to remember in this context that Prince considered B1—the personality that presented for treatment—to be an alter, and B1 *had been regnant and functional for approximately five years.* There is even some evidence from the Beauchamp case to suggest that not all alters are totally parasitic on the abilities of the host. It appeared to Prince as though Sally had to learn how to use the body when she first became regnant: "It was as if she had not yet learned to co-ordinate her newly acquired muscles, and had general ataxia in consequence. This too disappeared later" (1913, 34). Since some alters are developed enough to meet such criteria, the SPT will not extend to all cases.

Some alters seem to be complete persons unto themselves with full personalities, unique outlooks, and a perspective claimed to be completely independent of the primary or host identity. Other alters are extremely fragmentary and mere cartoons of single traits or characteristics that have never actually held executive control of the multiple's body outside the therapist's office. It is a relatively simple matter to make a strong case that Sally was a person. It is much more difficult to make a case that shallow and transitory animal personalities are persons. Thus, there is reason to think that some alters should count as persons while others should not. The MPT and SPT both fail because each creates a hard-and-fast rule for whether a multiple is a single person or a collection of persons—making such a judgment requires empirical inspection of the actual complexity of the alters present in a multiple. Alters exist along a spectrum of complexity that resists a uniform judgment of their metaphysical status. Diversity of clinical presentation yields diversity of metaphysical standings.[18]

5. Integration: Homicide or Healing?

5.1 The clinician charged with treating a DID subject, we have argued, faces a question concerning the metaphysics of identity: Is his patient properly defined as multiple persons inhabiting a single body or as a single person whose identity has fragmented? The preceding section argued that any answer to this question depends in part on one's criteria for identifying and re-identifying persons. Such criteria are contested; we chose to focus, as have others, on criteria of psychological continuity, including continuities in memories, temperament, dispositions, and agential goals. We surveyed how these criteria do and do not apply to different cases and how they can be differently applied to one and the same case, and we concluded that the question ultimately admits of no general answer. DID subjects constitute a disparate set, some members of which are good candidates for judgments of multiplicity, others better candidates for singularity.

This may seem an unsatisfying result from both a philosophical and a clinical point of view. Philosophically, it reveals tensions within our criteria for identifying and re-identifying persons; clinically, it recommends different judgments to different theorists, not only of the general category of DID subjects, but even of an individual case such as Beauchamp. Indeed, our conclusion will suggest to some that the philosophical criteria are not fit for clinical purposes: they leave too much to the clinician's personal judgment, failing to provide determinate guidance as to how he should conceive of his patient's fundamental identity. Of course, if the answer makes no difference to the clinician's therapeutic aims and methods, then that might not much matter. Does indeterminacy regarding the DID patient's metaphysical status matter in this way?

5.2 We noted earlier that the professional guidelines for DID treatment endorse the overall goal of integration, and that the traumagenic etiology of DID reinforces the prescription for integration as natural, as reparative, as welfare-maximizing, and as a condition of restoring lost autonomy. The *Guidelines for Treating Dissociative Identity Disorder* support this general conception, asserting that "treatment should move the patient toward better integrated functioning" and observing that "a fundamental tenet of the psychotherapy of patients with DID is to bring about an increased degree of communication and coordination among the identities" (ISSTD 2011, 132). Most clinicians will, in practice, take the "fusion" of alternate identities to be central to this process—their "joining together with a complete loss of subjective separateness" (ISSTD 2011, 13). Finally, many regard the "gold standard" of successful treatment, and the outcome that is most stable, to be "final fusion" or "unification"—"complete integration, merger, and loss of separateness … of all identity states" (ISSTD 2011, 133). In sum, clinical treatment of DID aims, to varying degrees, to restore unity to the patient's first-personal experience and its behavioral manifestations—to integrate the multiple identities into a single cognitive and motivational system.

Why is integration so confidently affirmed as the proper goal of treatment for DID patients? On what grounds is it valued? We should expect the clinician's view of his patient's standing as multiple persons or a single person to matter to the treatment he prescribes for two reasons. First, the treatment methods appropriate to treating multiple persons with conflicting interests is presumably very different from those appropriate to a single person who manifests several fictitious identities. Second, and more importantly, the normative implications of integration are very different for multiple-persons subjects and single-person subjects.

Carol Rovane, acknowledging that the data can be interpreted in either way, notes that "the first interpretation would entail that the integrative cure of dissociative identity disorder would amount to a sort of homicide, while the second interpretation would make integrative cure a kind of rational imperative" (Rovane 2004,186–87). A committed MPT theorist will, or should, find integration ethically controversial. Even if he resists Rovane's suggestion that it constitutes "a sort of homicide," it is difficult to avoid the conclusion that, in at least many cases, it brings about the willful extinction or obliteration of a person.[19] That should surely suffice to motivate some ethical reservations about the value of integration. It is perhaps unsurprising, then, that the *Guidelines*' profile of the DID subject does not seriously contemplate the MPT. They instead state confidently that "the DID patient is a single person who experiences himself or herself as having separate alternate identities"—a single person whose "subjective identities may take executive control of the person's body and behavior and/or influence his or her experience and behavior from 'within'" (ISSTD 2011, 120). Perhaps unfortunately, the *Guidelines* also go on to say that "taken together, all of the alternate identities make up the identity or personality of the human being with DID" (ISSTD 2011, 120). It is less than obvious how these claims can all be true—how the patient can be a "single person" whilst at the same time existing as a composite of all of his identities "taken together."

Be that as it may, practicing clinicians seldom question the wider aim of integration as a treatment imperative. Why, given the moral risk associated with extinguishing well-developed, complex alters, is this imperative so widely accepted? In the clinical record of the Beauchamp case, for instance, her therapist speaks without compunction of "choosing which identity will survive," even after recognizing that he had previously misjudged just which identity was the "real" Christine Beauchamp. Given the clinician's precarious epistemic position regarding multiplicity and singularity in any particular case, he is arguably obliged at least to justify the agenda of integration. The question of what grounds its value cannot be evaded. Let us consider some alternative rationales.

One simple rationale justifies integration in terms of the clinician's professional role and its incumbent duties. On this view, the clinician's remit is to effect psychological health, conceived of in terms of successful functioning. It is clearly difficult, if not impossible, for many DID patients to function successfully; the episodic and unpredictable switching of alters disrupts their ability to sustain personal relationships, fulfill employment obligations, safeguard their health and finances, and pursue personal projects. Only a relatively stable and persisting agent can do those things. So the argument is this: Unity is a condition of functionality, which is a condition of health, the promotion of which in turn defines the clinician's professional duties.

This rationale is ultimately uncompelling, relying as it does on a narrow and contestable conception of proper functioning, and the equation of that with good health. Worse yet, it fails entirely to address the moral challenge posed by the extinction of alters. The clinician offering this rationale must either be assuming the truth of the SPT, in which case he may be mistaken, or ignoring the moral claims of the patient's alter identities. In either case, the rationale fails to justify integration.

5.3 A deeper rationale appeals to considerations adduced earlier relating to the conditions of agency (Sec. 3). It is these considerations that Rovane has in mind when she speaks of integration as a "rational imperative." For Rovane, it is not psychological continuity qua continuity of conscious states or phenomenology that constitutes a person's identity. It is rather the unity of her actions—her "practical unity." If you are a person, then you are nothing more, but also nothing less, than an agent—you are able to chart a course through the world in which your choices, intentions, and behaviors are linked together over time, connecting your past, present, and future. Moreover, that connection is not merely causal, but rational. You deliberate between options and choose between alternative courses on the basis of reasons; having chosen, you form intentions that you have reason to think will achieve your ends; your intentions are then implemented in actions that are rationally motivated. On this view, to be a person/agent is at once to be governed by an aim of overall rational unity in what one chooses and what one does:

> Insofar as an agent is something that deliberates and chooses from a first person point of view, it is something that is committed to meeting certain normative requirements of rationality. Here are some examples of such specific requirements: to be consistent in one's beliefs; to rank one's preferences transitively; to accept the deductive and inductive consequences of one's attitudes; to evaluate one's ends by reference to the means that must [be] employed in order to achieve them; to evaluate one's ends by reference to the foreseeable consequences of achieving them.
>
> *(Rovane 2004, 183)*

Now suppose that DID alters generally are incapable of self-governance of this kind, owing to their episodic switches. Suppose further that the hypothesized "single person" of the *Guidelines* also is incapable of such self-governance, being ever vulnerable to the persistent and unpredictable disruptions of his alter(s). This is likely enough in many cases, given that DID subjects lack continuities of memory (because they are amnestic) and of volition (because their alters realize different motivational sets). Without these continuities, the basic trajectory of rational agency is unavailable to the DID subject: the trajectory of deliberating, choosing, intending, and implementing a course of action. It is not difficult to see why, on this view, integration should be the clinician's goal. For to the extent that no integrated, rationally unified agent inhabits the patient's body, he otherwise fails to be a person at all. The clinician's remit for integration is, on this view, to reconstitute (or even to create) a fully fledged person out of dis-integrated fragments.

5.4 This Rovanean rationale relies on an equation of agentive unity and personhood. Even if one rejects that equation, however, the independent value of the former surely recommends "[moving] the patient toward better integrated functioning" and bringing about "an increased degree of communication and coordination among the identities" (ISSTD 2011, 132).

Or does it? There are at least three reasons to suppose that it does not. First, this rationale in no way relieves the clinician of the burden of deciding between multiplicity and singularity in a particular case; it merely introduces a different criterion—agentive unity—by which to do that. The idea that integration creates a person "out of fragments" assumes that none of the individual alters themselves already constitute well-formed agents. But, as Rovane herself argues, we cannot simply dismiss the possibility that a single "human-sized" entity (a single body) might contain multiple, independently operating agents. In such cases,

> Multiple agents ... are agents in exactly the same sense that human agents are. All of them have first person points of view from which they deliberate and act in accordance with the same normative requirements of rationality that by definition apply to all individual agents.
>
> (*Rovane 2004, 193*)

If this is true of a DID alter or alters in a particular case, then the clinician has a new justificatory burden: He must justify his preference for the goal of creating just *one* center of agency—one person—rather than preserving the many. He may, of course, adduce independent reasons for that preference, but the burden of argument still falls to him.

A second doubt about the Rovanean rationale for integration targets the premise that agentive self-governance—governance by rational authority—is valuable. If we reject the equation of agency and personhood, then the value of personhood does not automatically transfer to rational agency. True enough, agentive self-governance is in fact a ubiquitous ideal: it is something that most people in most circumstances find valuable, and its value is vividly enshrined in political manifestos and constitutions the world over. DID subjects, however, are very unlike the statistically normal person. Self-governance may be the least of their concerns, particularly in view of the many modes of distress typically co-morbid with dissociative disorders—depression, hallucinations, inattention, fearfulness, and anger, to mention a few. The value of rational unity and the self-governance it confers may not be valued by the DID patient *himself* relative to certain other ends. DID patients often present as intelligent, articulate, empathic, and resourceful; they are by no means globally impoverished in either cognitive or emotional capacities. The very fact that such a patient's psychological system has disengaged certain memories, affects, and dispositions should perhaps signal to us that the value of unitary self-governance is already under pressure from other, competing demands. It is at least conceivable that the dis-integrated multiple has developed as *the best person(s) he can be*—perhaps by standards that are, in some sense, authentically his own. Just what that might mean and how it might be judged or decided is unclear; we do not propose to settle those questions here. The point is that it is presumptuous to suppose that DID patients generally *ought* to maximize their capacity for agentive unification, whatever other interests they may have.

Third, and more tellingly, we might wonder about the ideal of agentive unification even as it applies to ordinary, non-pathological subjects. Jennifer Radden has expressed skepticism about the evaluative supremacy Rovane accords it:

> As an ideal, perfect self-unity of this kind, whether sought by one self or several sub-selves, seems to bespeak something more akin to divine or artificial than to human intelligence. The confusion and complexity found in the usual psyche are a valuable part of human nature, suited to the moral categories and social institutions we cherish—and encompassed, I believe, within less stringent conceptions of rationality. The individual variation between those who knit up their lives with long-term projects, and those who live life in a more picaresque or episodic fashion, enriches human experience, as does that between lives devoted to a single goal and those involving many different ones.
>
> *(Radden 2011, 9)*

Radden here voices two concerns. The first is that, by holding ourselves accountable to too pure a conception of rational unity, we will become alienated from certain historical "moral categories and social institutions"—values and conventions which have developed in response to our less-than-ideally-rational psychologies. This may be so. However, if we have outgrown, or could profitably outgrow, those categories and institutions—as we have outgrown the category of witchcraft and the institution of slavery—this need be no bad thing. All change involves loss, some of it for the best.

Radden's second worry is more compelling. It is that the bearer of value is not our ideal natures, but our actual, imperfectly rational ones. This strikes nearer to the heart of the Rovanean justification for seeking integration. We surely do appreciate in some ways the "individual variation" imposed on us by personal temperament, taste, impulse, and the indefinitely many other non-rational "inclinations" that draw us away from the ideal of Kantian unity. However, by emphasizing the charm and interest of these personal diversities, Radden arguably misses a related, but deeper and more interesting point. The Rovanean rationale ties the value of integration to rational unity, as a condition of agency. But does agency in fact require unity of this kind? Or are there forms of human agency more befitting to the imperfectly rational beings that we are?

We suggest that in the case of the DID subject—and even in our own more ordinary selves—the value of integration should be measured against the claims of the individual's other psychological imperatives—his fears, his desires, his convictions and ideals. It may be that agentive authority for human beings consists as much in accepting and respecting our given natures as in ruling them. To see what this might mean, let us digress briefly to a different, pre-modern illustration of dis-integrated agency: the tragic narrative.

6. Necessity, Integration, and Sopoclean Agency

6.1 No genre of literature has been more preoccupied with divided and dissociated selves, nor portrayed them more vividly and painfully, than the classical Greek tragedies. Sometimes the immediate catalyst for the tragic protagonist's internal schism is a moral dilemma—a traumatic situation in which he or she must choose a course between impossibly bad options, as when Agamemnon must sacrifice either his daughter or his honor, or Antigone must choose either to respect her duty to bury her brother or her duty to obey the law. At other times, the forces dividing the protagonist are those of destiny—as when Oedipus is fated to murder his father and marry his mother, or when his sons, Eteocles and Polynices, are fated by their father's curse to die by one another's hands. In a third kind of case, divine forces invade a character's first-personal psychology, altering his motivating reasons by manipulating his beliefs, desires, or intentions—Clytemnestra is possessed by the *Alastor's* spirit of revenge, Pentheus is bewitched by Bacchus, Ajax's psyche is invaded and deluded by Athena. A theme connecting all of these cases is that the tragic hero is psychologically poised between, on one hand, the legitimate demands of his personal will and, on the other, various fearful necessities that he is powerless to control. Modern psychology did not invent the notion of trauma, or its divisive effects.

The tragedian's worldview delivers a psychology of action very different from our own. The sources of trauma and internal disintegration were not, for the Greeks, something to be overcome and left behind. Human beings were, in their ethical worldview, not only occasionally and accidentally divided against themselves. Rather, their position was *essentially* a conflicted one in which they were both capable of autonomous self-determination and driven by arbitrary, unbidden, and irrational powers. Practical agency was a matter of steering a course between those aspects of one's nature that were compelled and those that were deliberated and chosen. Integration into a coherent, reason-governed whole was not an option.

6.2 This perspective, we suggest, offers some insight into the position of the DID subject, and the ways in which integration is (and is not) valuable to him. Many DID patients affirm that they do not wish their alters to be fully fused. Kim Noble, the subject of our first epigraph, is one such (Mitchison 2011). Noble contains perhaps a hundred or more alters, but only a handful of these are normally regnant. She switches several times a day between the dominant identities; and, like many DID subjects, she relies on different ones to take responsibility for different functions: tracking the finances, cleaning the house, even taking a bath are all managed by distinct alters. Noble's switches are accompanied by amnesia; she cannot cook or drive, for instance, because she might switch and leave the oven on or lose track of where she has parked the car. However, she is partially integrated; she is aware of the existence and characters of her dominant alters, and some patchy memory continuity obtains between them. She is also keenly aware of the abuse she suffered as a small child, although her memories tend to come in sporadic flashbacks: The first-personal, subjective memories of trauma and her own hostile reactions are enacted by alters who appear only occasionally. Noble accepts her alters as jointly constituting who she is and as together managing an autobiography that, if unified, she would find overwhelming and painful. She remains in therapy as a stabilizing strategy, but has no desire to fuse her identities. She does not consider them "alien" or "external"; she accepts her multiplicity as who she is. Nobel exemplifies a "stable" DID subject.

Multiples such as Noble, we suggest, may be regarded as having negotiated a balance between inconsistent parts of their natures and biographies. They are not unified, but neither do they repudiate those dimensions of their inner lives that fail to cohere. Their self-conceptions include the inheritance of their personal histories, and are consonant with their fragmented natures. It is true that no one identity is wholly self-governing, insofar as it is subject to the episodic authority of other alters. But we should not deny that these subjects fail to be *agents* in some robust sense of that term. After all, they willingly live out and respect the natures they have been given, and their identities have connected, internally coherent trajectories. Consider the fact that even in ordinary, non-pathological experience, agency does not require the absence of necessity. Indeed, doing as one wills, in many cases, *requires* responding to and affirming certain necessities. The standard conception of romantic love, for instance, is that of a state in which one's attitude to the beloved is non-optional: "He could love no other," we say, and, "It had to be," and, "It was fated." Other kinds of love have the same structure: A mother may realize that she has no good reason to love and care for her particular child as she does; he is, in himself, unremarkable enough. But she does love him like no other and could not do otherwise; she is *compelled* to devote her attentions only to the son that is her own—and she bears no regrets about that.[20]

Likewise, creative artists often describe their aesthetic judgments as a response to what the work demands—how the story must unfold, how the legato passage must be played, just which colors the painting requires. Collaborative musical performance, too, offers a particularly vivid case: Success in playing a Bartok quartet depends crucially on each party coordinating his actions with and even subordinating them to those of the other players. This kind of deference is essential to the end of producing a coordinated action of which no one player is capable on his own. Responding to necessity in all of these cases is not experienced as a *loss* of agency so much as a discovery of how best to exercise it in order to achieve one's aims. We might call it "Sophoclean agency," in recognition of its affinity to the agentive profile of that writer's great tragic protagonists.[21]

6.3 To better understand the structure of Sophoclean agency, it is helpful to consider cases in which we experience ourselves as subject to external control in ways that are threatening, oppressive, or just unwelcome. Such experience is typically characterized by either or both of two features, each of which may occur independently of the others: alienation and repudiation. "Alienation," as we use it here, refers not to the place of a motivation in the structure of an agent's will—his desires, values, or plans. Rather, it refers to a particular way of experiencing such a motivation—the associated first-personal phenomenology. Imagine Samuel, a committed meat-eater who feels disdain and contempt for vegetarians. Samuel visits a slaughterhouse one day in his capacity as a school chaperone. He is made uneasy by what he sees and finds himself relieved when the tour comes to an end. However, Samuel in no way changes his views of the virtues of his diet, and the disturbing slaughterhouse scenes make no difference to his decisive judgment that the very best meals feature a good steak. Afterwards, however, he finds himself experiencing an aversion to such meals. His aversion surprises him, and he *viscerally feels* as if it comes from outside of him—unwelcome, incomprehensible, alien.

Repudiation is a quite different phenomenon. Repudiation is not a visceral feeling; it is an evaluative response registering the proper place of the unbidden motivation in one's psychological economy—namely, that it has no place there at all. When we repudiate a motivation, we disavow or disown it; we may form a commitment to repress or defeat it. Repudiation, unlike alienation, is a property of the structure of a person's desires, values, or plans. Imagine now Sarah, a committed vegetarian and animal-rights enthusiast who is well-informed about the procedures by which meat products are produced. Sarah's deliberations have led her to the unequivocal conclusion that eating meat is wrong, and she acts accordingly. Unfortunately, she is Samuel's daughter and was raised on a hearty carnivorous diet. She often feels a longing for more of the same; the aroma of a Sunday roast is almost more than she can bear. Sarah is accustomed to these longings; she recognizes that they are a part of who she is and has been since before she can recall. Sarah's longings do not feel alien or strange to her; they are all too familiar. But she repudiates them: They are contrary to her values and practical convictions, and she refuses to be ruled by them.

The responses of alienation and repudiation are the experiential marks of *externality*, perhaps, but they need not accompany every experience of necessity. When we are beset by motivations that elicit responses of alienation and repudiation, we then are likely to perceive ourselves as compelled or constrained, or even invaded. It is not, we think, the other way around. That is, it is not when we *judge* a motivation to be compelled or constrained or imposed by necessity that we experience it as external, as meriting alienation and repudiation. This is evident in the examples of the lover who is compelled to seek out the company of his beloved, or the mother who feels she has no choice but to respond to her child's needs, or the musician constrained by the demands of a composition's style and structure. None of these experiences elicit either alienation or repudiation of the demands made upon them. The lover, the mother, and the artist act as free and willing agents *and* do so in response to demands they experience as necessary. Necessity and compulsion are one thing; loss of agency is another. They need not go hand in hand. In these instances of tragic agency, the subjects have not *defeated* or *extinguished* the powers that govern their actions. Rather, they have ceased to feel that these powers are alien or that they must be repudiated.

6.4 Suppose that a stable DID subject could get that far, reconciling his identities to co-existence and cooperation. Suppose, that is, he could become a Sophoclean, rather than a rationally unified, agent. Even this much would surely require him to acknowledge or recognize the psychic forces within himself *as* necessities—to understand their traumatic origins and the role they play within his psychological economy. It would depend, too, on his ability to accept rather than repudiate them and to defuse his visceral sense of their externality. The rationale for such Sophoclean integration is obvious and uncontroversial: It allows the subject to lead a life and, to use Havel's famous phrase, to "live in truth." It is akin to what the *Guidelines* refer to as the "reconciliation" of identities. In reconciliation, alters survive, but they survive as Sophoclean agents, recognizing their dependence upon and determination by psychological necessities beyond their control, and according the agentive manifestations of those necessities—the alters with which they co-exist—the acknowledgement and respect they are due.

Final fusion of a DID subject's multiples—complete integration—requires something more. In final fusion a patient internalizes his identities: He experiences them first-personally as parts of a single, coherent self. Is this level of integration therapeutically ideal? In at least some cases it may be less valuable than is often assumed. As Rovane observes:

> [I]f the circumstances of a human being are sufficiently fragmented, that will make it less feasible for the human being to retain a unified deliberative perspective as it moves from one circumstance to another. In fact, striving to do so will simply underscore for the human being the ways in which its two lives don't and can't make rational sense together. That is why it may be rational for the human being to forego the project of leading a unified human life and to opt instead for fragmentation into two independent agents, each of whom can coherently pursue a life of its own.
>
> *(Rovane 2004, 193–94)*

Rovane may be right about the *possibility* of independent agents inhabiting a single physical being, "each of whom can coherently pursue a life of its own." But how does one judge when to bow to necessity and embrace the alternative of fragmentation, and when to aspire to harmonious unity? Suppose that a clinician accepts that the MPT is true in a particular case. On what grounds should he decide to encourage his patient towards final fusion, rather than, say, reconciliation as we have outlined it above? These questions return us to the metaphysical issues with which we began and to their ethical implications. We cannot do justice to them here. If we could, however, our answer would take seriously the possibility that a better, more authentic, and even richer life may be had by multiple agents than by one who persists in reaching for a form of unity that lies beyond his grasp. It may be that not only in the case of DID, but also in our own everyday, often fragmented lives, Sophoclean agency is sometimes the better option.

Notes

1 The remaining three are: (1) the disruption of identity and amnesia must cause distress or impairment, (2) the interruptions of identity and memory must not occur as part of a culturally sanctioned religious practice or as part of childhood play, and (3) neither a substance nor another medical problem can explain the disruptions (APA 2013, 292).
2 Quoted from Diagnosis Dictionary, "Dissociative Identity Disorder (Multiple Personality Disorder)," *Psychology Today*. Available at https://www.psychologytoday.com/conditions/dissociative-identity-disorder-multiple-personality-disorder.
3 For example, Spanos 1996.
4 Proponents of the sociocognitive model do not deny that some pathology or other is present—only that its distinguishing feature has the origins claimed for it. That is, the presentation of multiple identities is simply a florid, socially constructed expression of other, related ailments. This model can account for the undue proliferation of DID diagnoses in the United States in the 1970s and 1980s—a several-thousand-fold increase over the preceding century. For instance, it is now widely agreed that "Sybil" was iatrogenically created—if not a hoax (e.g., Rieber 1999). It is also undoubtedly the best explanation for some, even many, self-reports of DID.
5 See, for example, Lewis *et al.* 1997, Dorahy *et al.* 2014, Cohen 2004.
6 Psychological trauma is the unique individual experience of an event or enduring conditions, in which:

> 1. The individual's ability to integrate his/her emotional experience is overwhelmed, or
> 2. The individual experiences (subjectively) a threat to life, bodily integrity, or sanity.
>
> (Pearlman and Saakvitne 1995, 60)

7 Clinical issues aside, these questions have independent interest for the metaphysics of personal identity. DID has been posited as a counterexample to psychological theories of identity and personhood (e.g., Brown 2001; Bayne 2002). Additionally, in answering questions of the moral and legal responsibility of DID patients, our opinion might be swayed if we determined that these personalities were or were not persons in their own right (e.g., Sinnott-Armstrong and Behnke 2000).
8 We follow Kennett and Matthews in this convention.
9 B2 is omitted, because at that point in his treatment of Beauchamp B2's presence had not been revealed.
10 The nature of the incident is unclear in Prince's text. He seems to think that Beauchamp, as a result of her rather reserved character, overreacted to it (Prince 1913, 215). Wilkes interprets the passage to mean that Beauchamp thought of it as nearly being a rape (1988, 112).
11 We have taken a liberty with this condition. Wilkes applies it only to the Beauchamp case in which elimination was the treatment used by the therapist; thus, this consideration may be completely irrelevant when considering other methods of treatment.
12 Wilkes actually takes the stance conditions here as moral conditions, so her verdict is somewhat ambiguous on the stance we take towards alters. This type of stance, however, is not what Dennett is concerned with. We are unclear as to why Wilkes handles these conditions in this manner.
13 Wilkes ultimately does not endorse the MPT on grounds that appeal to normative considerations.
14 According to such views, personal identity consists in having a self-narrative, a story about oneself, that situates your life within your own perspective and gives you a framework for understanding yourself.
15 Hardcastle and Flanagan also noticed that each alter was a diminished person in that it only contained part of what a whole person should contain and noticed that DID patients could not be whole people on their own (1999, 652). However, they did not see that this concession threatens their endorsement of the MPT.

16 One may dispute Kennett and Matthews' claim that the unity of agency is a condition of personhood. However, plausible psychological understandings of personhood make use of many of the characteristics that collectively constitute the unity of agency. Thus, their arguments can be taken as indicative even though we might hold a different view of the connection between personhood and the unity of agency.
17 As Piper and Merskey point out, skepticism about this claim is warranted (2004, 597).
18 Graham hints at, but does not pursue, something close to our critique of the MPT and SPT: "[T]he most germane question is how many selves occur in a particular case of [DID]" (1999, 172).
19 Bayne 2002 and Shoemaker 2009 have also pointed out this problem.
20 See Arpaly 2006, p. 7
21 See Denham 2014.

References

American Psychiatric Association (APA). 2013. *DSM-5: Diagnostic and Statistical Manuel of Mental Disorders, 5th ed.* Washington, DC: American Psychiatric Publishing.

Arpaly, N. 2006. *Merit, Meaning and Human Bondage: An Essay on Free Will.* Princeton, NJ: Princeton University Press,

Bayne, T. J. 2002. "Moral Status and the Treatment of Dissociative Identity Disorder." *Journal of Medicine and Philosophy* 27: 87–105.

Brown, M. T. 2001. "Multiple Personality and Personal Identity." *Philosophical Psychology* 14: 435–47.

Cohen, A. 2004. "Dissociative Identity Disorder: Perspectives and Alternatives." *Ethical Human Psychology and Psychiatry* 6: 217–30.

Confer, W. N. and B. S. Ables. 1983. *Multiple Personality: Etiology, Diagnosis, and Treatment.* New York: Human Sciences Press.

Dell, P. F. 2006. "A New Model of Dissociative Identity Disorder." *Psychiatric Clinics of North America* 29: 1–26.

Denham, A. E. 2014 "Tragedy Without the Gods: Autonomy, Necessity and the Real Self." *British Journal of Aesthetics* 54 (2):141–59.

Dennett, D. 1976. "Conditions of Personhood." In A. O. Rorty, ed. *The Identities of Persons.* Berkeley, CA: University of California Press, 175–96.

Dorahy, M. J., B. L. Brand, V. Şar, C. Krüger, P. Stavropoulos, A. Martínez-Taboas, R. Lewis-Fernández, and W. Middleton. 2014. "Dissociative Identity Disorder: An Empirical Overview." *Australian and New Zealand Journal of Psychiatry* 48: 402–17.

Goff, D. G. and C. A. Simms. 1993. "Has Multiple Personality Disorder Remained Consistent Over Time? A Comparison of Past and Recent Cases." *The Journal of Nervous and Mental Disease* 181: 595–600.

Graham, G. 1999. "Fuzzy Fault Lines: Selves in Multiple Personality Disorder." *Philosophical Explorations* 3: 159–74.

Hardcastle, V. G. and O. Flanagan. 1999. "Multiplex vs. Multiple Selves: Distinguishing Dissociative Disorders." *The Monist* 82: 645–57.

International Society for the Study of Trauma and Dissociation (ISSTD). 2011. "Guidelines for Treating Dissociative Identity Disorder in Adults, Third Revision." *Journal of Trauma & Dissociation* 12: 115–87.

Kennett, J. and S. Matthews. 2002. "Identity, Control and Responsibility: The Case of Dissociative Identity Disorder." *Philosophical Psychology* 15: 509–26.

——. 2003. "The Unity and Disunity of Agency." *Philosophy, Psychiatry, and Psychology* 10: 305–12.

Kluft, R. P. 1988. "The Phenomenology and Treatment of Extremely Complex Multiple Personality Disorder." *Dissociation* 1 (4): 47–58.

——. 1999. "Current Issues in Dissociative Identity Disorder." *Journal of Practical Psychiatry and Behavioral Health* 7: 3–19.

Lewis, D. O., C. A. Yeager, Y. Swica, J. H. Pincus, and M. Lewis. 1997. "Objective Documentation of Child Abuse and Dissociation in 12 Murderers with Dissociative Identity Disorder." *American Journal of Psychiatry* 154: 1703–10.

Matthews, S. 2003. "Blaming Agents and Excusing Persons: The Case of DID." *Philosophy, Psychiatry, and Psychology* 10: 169–74.

Mele, A. 2004. "Rational Irrationality." *The Philosophers' Magazine* 26: 31–32.

Mitchison, A. 2011, September 30. "Kim Noble: The Woman with 100 Personalities." *The Guardian*. Retrieved from www.theguardian.com/lifeandstyle/2011/sep/30/kim-noble-woman-with-100-personalities. Last accessed April 29, 2015.

Pearlman, L. A. and K. W. Saakvitne. 1995. *Trauma and the Therapist*. New York: Norton.

Piper, A. and H. Merskey. 2004. "The Persistence of Folly: A Critical Examination of Dissociative Identity Disorder. Part I. The Excesses of an Improbable Concept." *The Canadian Journal of Psychiatry* 49: 592–600.

Prince, M. 1913. *The Dissociation of a Personality: A Biographical Study in Abnormal Psychology*. 2nd ed. New York: Longman, Green, and Co.

Radden, J. 1996. *Divided Minds and Successive Selves: Ethical Issues in Disorders of Identity and Personality*. Cambridge, MA: The MIT Press.

——. 2011. "Multiple Selves" in S. Gallagher, ed. *Oxford Handbook of the Self*. New York: Oxford University Press, pp. 547–70.

Rieber, R. W. 1999. "Hypnosis, False Memory and Multiple Personality: A Trinity of Affinity." *History of Psychiatry* 10: 3–11.

Ross, C. A. 1989. *Multiple Personality Disorder: Diagnosis, Clinical Features, and Treatment*. New York: John Wiley and Sons.

Rovane, C. 2004. "What Is an Agent?" *Synthese* 140: 181–98.

Shoemaker, D. 2009. *Personal Identity and Ethics: A Brief Introduction*. Buffalo, NY: Broadview Press.

Sinnott-Armstrong, W. and S. Behnke. 2000. "Responsibility in Cases of Multiple Personality Disorder." *Philosophical Perspectives* 14: 301–23.

Spanos, N. P. 1996. *Multiple Identities and False Memories: A Sociocognitive Perspective*. Washington, DC: American Psychological Association.

Wilkes, K. V. 1988. *Real People: Personal Identity without Thought Experiments*. New York: Clarendon Press.

8b

Commentary on Worrell and Denham: The Fragmented Sense of Self is an Epiphenomenon in Dissociative Disorders

Deactivation of Dissociative Processes in the Relationship with Self and Others Informs Clinical Trajectories

Richard A. Chefetz

> Certainly psychopathology might well be measured by degrees of dissociation of important versions of self. Yet it seems mistaken to assume that a digestion and blending of different versions of self is preferable to the capacity to contain shifting and conflictual versions of self. Mixing colors together does not increase their intensity or beauty; it washes them out into a featureless gray. Discontinuities in self-organization is part of what enriches life, enabling conflicted domains of experience to be developed without the pressure of continual moderation and integration.
>
> (Mitchell 1993: 105)

Stephen Mitchell's words reflect some of the sentiment of Worrell and Denham, but he was referencing a theory in relational psychoanalysis about the human mind in general, and not specifically addressing the profound impairments in living that afflict people with robust dissociative disorders, such as a high incidence of suicidality (Foote et al. 2008). Variety may be the spice of life, but disaggregate mentation due to dissociative process is more like arsenic than oregano. The science behind claims regarding the need for integration and fusion of the diverse self-states of what was formerly called multiple personality disorder and is now known as dissociative identity disorder (DID) favors the needs for integration and fusion as a logical outcome based upon what was originally 33 collected case studies (Kluft 1984b), but now is in the hundreds. What I describe below is a relational approach to the psychotherapy of dissociative identity disorder that has a sound psychotherapeutic basis, but does not have, as yet, the cumulative case studies to argue that it is superior to the outcomes reported by Kluft. It does echo some of the concerns of Worrell and Denham, but from a relational psychodynamic perspective and multiple self-state model of the human mind.

Dissociative disorders are not about what happens to an individual's personality as a result of trauma, they're about what happens to a person's mind when healthy capacities to modulate adverse human experience are exceeded. The understanding of these disorders has gone far beyond what Morton Prince and Pierre Janet could offer us regarding the science that underlies the psychological presentation of the dissociative disorders. The neurobiological context is of a modular brain that is prone to synaptic, neurohumoral, and biochemical disruption and disconnection when severely stressed (Yehuda 1998; Yehuda et al. 2014; Yin et al. 2011; Shin and Liberzon 2010; Phelps et al. 2001). There is dissociation (unlinking) of ordinarily integrated neural functions regarding such areas as implicit and explicit memory, medial prefrontal cortical modulation of fear (Rauch et al. 1996), somatic experience (depersonalization related to temporo-parietal junction dysfunction (Michal et al. 2007; Phillips et al. 2001; Michal et al. 2013), and so on, and disrupted psychological functions along dimensions such as cognitive, affective, somatosensory, and behavioural (Braun 1988; Loewenstein 1991; Holmes et al. 2005). The kinds of neural and psychological disturbances as a result of chronic verbal abuse alone (not physical or sexual), bullying, are profound, and include altered developmental trajectories and impaired activity of the hippocampus (working memory), corpus callosum (interhemispheric communication), and precuneus (executive function) (Teicher and Samson 2013; Teicher et al. 2010), as well as other areas of dysfunction related to traumatic experience (Bremner et al. 2003; Bremner et al. 1996; Vermetten et al. 2006; Rauch et al. 1996; Shin et al. 2006). Dissociative disorders are about how such a neurally and psychologically compromised person then adapts to distortions in perception that are both subtle and profound as they influence the capacity to accurately contextualize experience while a person still tries to live a life.

Not only are dissociative processes phenomenologically visible in infancy, as shown by infant attachment studies (Type D), but the relational nature of being human is clearly paramount in the human failures that make activation of dissociation more likely (Main and Hesse 1990; Ogawa et al. 1997; Lyons-Ruth 2003). Human relatedness later triumphs when it facilitates the relief of dissociative processes gone awry in psychotherapy (Brand et al. 2012). Let's be clear at the outset of this discussion that the dissociative disorders have a rock-solid scientific basis upon which they can be understood. The clinical focus on the dissociative disorders (formerly multiple personality disorders) has been on the dramatic nature of the presence of alternate personalities, identity alteration (Steinberg 1993; American Psychiatric Association 2013), and this has been a distraction from the important underlying ubiquitous dissociative processes that run the show, so to speak.

Worrell and Denham make an implicit assertion that human dignity be paramount in regard to the treatment of psychiatric problems like dissociative identity disorder. I support the idea. They challenge the idea of trying to integrate or fuse his plural identities "into a single cognitive and motivational system" (p. 227), an over-valuing of "rational unity." They suggest that "fragmented agency may be preferable to fully integrated, maximally consistent agency—even in non-pathological cases" (p. 215). They don't really present any clinical data to back up their assertions and rely on archaic case histories for some of their perspective. They present data regarding socio-cognitive rebuttals to dissociative disorders but don't cite more recent responses to those contentions such as the elaborate responses of Dalenberg et al. (2012) and Brand, Loewenstein, and Spiegel (2014). Regardless, it behooves a thoughtful person to respond seriously to their concerns about personal agency, identity, and freedom in psychotherapy. A relational psychotherapy may be consistent with those concerns (Bromberg 1998).

Dissociative processes are multi-dimensional, ubiquitous, and essential to the normal function of the human mind. These processes calmly erase their tracks as they mercifully deprive us of what might devastate us if we knew about it. This is a problem that is often invisible to the affected person who then may not notice the fleeting discontinuities in their experience. The problem with dissociation isn't that it occurs during stress. The problem is that it doesn't turn off when the stress has ended. People often live in a world of perceiving constant threat consistent with the failure of the extinction of traumatic memory noted in posttraumatic stress disorder (PTSD) (Milad et al. 2009; Milad et al. 2006). It's as if the past is still present[1] and there is no room for living without preoccupation.

On one level, dissociative processes should be considered as one part of a dialectic of unconscious and conscious sorting of experience; the mind's effort to create meaningful coherence through a balance between connecting what is salient (association) and discarding what is not (dissociation). However, on a more complex level such as dissociative identity disorder, the tension between associative linking and dissociative unlinking manifest as depersonalization, derealization, amnesia, identify confusion, and identity alteration (Steinberg 1993). Depersonalization is typically described as somehow feeling unreal, while with derealization it's the world that feels odd, phony, or unreal. Amnesia in the dissociative disorders may extend for years, and it's also true that evidence for amnesia mostly shows up in psychotherapy as micro-amnesias; a kind of "swiss cheese" memory (Kluft 1984a) where five minutes after discussing something there is a shift in consciousness and lack of crisp awareness of the discussion. There may be a vague sense of "knowing what was talked about" but the feeling of having been present for the conversation may be absent. Identity confusion resembles the foggy state typical in the immediate aftermath of an automobile accident where personal knowledge seems to have evaporated, but then suddenly returns some minutes or hours later. The return of this knowledge in DID generally rests upon a change of self-state and access to state-dependent memory (Eich 1980, 1987, 1995). Self-states have also been called an alternate personality, or alter (Kluft 1984b; 1984a). The most salient characteristic of self-states is related to the compartmentalization of mental content (Holmes et al. 2005), thoughts, feelings, ideas, sensations, knowledge (Braun 1988), world-view, sense of self, and so on.

Dissociative experience is just that—something that is lived. It's not just a curious idea. Listen to the description of dissociative experience by a young woman with depersonalization and amnesia:

> I hear myself talk in my mind and analyze myself as I'm talking, which is distracting. I worry about how I'm coming across and comment on things I'm doing. This is mainly at work. Actually no, it happens with friends too. My hands feel like they're not attached sometimes. Mainly when I notice them, am looking down at them. When I'm typing for work, when I wash my hands after going to the bathroom or cooking. When I wash them and rub them together with the soap they look distant. I want to remember things when I see a picture of them. [My girlfriend] said that the [old] picture [of me and my girlfriends] on facebook from [the school play] was from junior year of high school. I want to remember that.
>
> *(Chefetz 2015)*

Bowlby's initial conceptualizations about attachment (Bowlby 1969/1982, 1980), combined with the subsequent work by collaborators and other researchers (Ainsworth et al. 1978; Main 1993, 1995, 2000; Main and Hesse 1990; Main and Morgan 1996; Solomon and George 1999a, 1999b; Solomon and Siegel 2003; Schore and Schore 2008; IJzendoorn 1995) and partly summarized by Bretherton (1992) shows the dramatic extent to which dissociative processes are active as defensive exclusion, deactivation, and segregated subsystems. Main, and others, above, showed how Type D disorganized/disoriented infant attachment consists of an infant's responsiveness to the return of a caretaker in the Strange Situation of Ainsworth and represents the simultaneous contradictory internal working models of a child who cannot determine if they will be confronted with the frightened vs. the frightening behaviors of their caretaker. We know from longitudinal studies with 25-year follow up that Type D disorganization is transmissible between generations (Ogawa et al. 1997; Lyons-Ruth 2008). Thus, the mental structures that generate Type D infant attachment are sustained such that Type D adults demonstrate high levels of dissociation. I would offer that the implicit self-state structure from early in life seems to be maintained, though this is a retrospective view based upon reports of patients recalling their childhood, not infancy, and may be subject to distortion.

Worrell and Denham offer this summary regarding the alternate self-states of DID:

> The construction of alters is a mechanism of conflict avoidance in which these dis-integrated responses are assigned to distinct autobiographical "tracks." While this strategy may spare the subject the distress of internal dissonance, it does so at a cost: Insofar as the agentive powers—choosing, intending, and acting—in any one persona are vulnerable to disruption by an alter, DID places those powers out of reach. Even if it is granted that the multiple is a person or persons, his status as an agent will be tragically compromised unless and until his integrity is restored.
>
> *(p. 217)*

The less knowledgeable reader may read this as a process of some conscious intention for an affected person. There's no clinical data to support that contention. Clinical wisdom suggests that active dissociation wards off things like the experience of terror, physical pain and brutality, threat of death, or abject shaming or humiliation, not simply conflict. There is also no clinical data to support the multiple person hypothesis regarding the alter system of DID. There is the face-value evidence of a person coming to treatment and having the subjective experience of changing states. One person with DID reported that as they led a high-level meeting in their organization, they were suddenly struck by the sensation of feeling like their legs weren't long enough for their feet to touch the floor. Disoriented by this, but finally realizing they'd had a state change, they quietly asked the colleague next to them to run the meeting while they internally worked out the issues related to feeling like a child. People with dissociative identity disorder aren't occupied by many people; they are plagued by not having enough internally integrated experience to feel like a whole person. They are neither multiple nor a whole singleton; they have the subjective experience of feeling incomplete and not real. It is true that there are people with dissociative identity disorder who believe there are other people living inside them, and it's also true that this is the description of a technical term: the delusion of separateness (Loewenstein 1991). There are numerous potential psychodynamic advantages to believing in the physical separateness of mental self-states, for example, not being the person who was abused. However, this delusion is a central treatment issue rather than a reality. There is only one body. There is the experience of having more than one sense of self. And then there is the reality that no sense of self feels complete in DID even if there is the initial assertion otherwise.

Given that there are multiple self-states in DID and that the feeling central to typical depersonalization is profound, feeling unreal, how does this and other dissociative processes resolve? Does there need to be a formal process of integration or fusion? There are several pertinent responses. First, the failures of extinction of trauma memory, noted above, must resolve through trauma-focused work via psychotherapeutic exploration of the past in detailed conversation, or with eye movement desensitization and reprocessing (EMDR), hypnosis, or other similar special techniques which help a person tolerate the terror of recollection of what was previously unbearable. However, no technique, in and of itself, can create a sense of interpersonal safety in which a person can explore what's painful after achieving stabilization (Steele, van der Hart, and Nijenhuis 2005). That's partly the job of the relationship in psychotherapy. Relational traumas, interpersonal betrayals such as incest, or more complex scenes such as object-coercive doubting (Kramer 1983) often make themselves known to the clinical dyad via enactment (Bromberg 2006; Levenkron 2006; Stern 2010; McLaughlin 1991; Chused 1991) and require delicate and skillful exploration to allow resolution of old behavioral and emotional scripts (Tomkins 1995).

In the end, how can the reader integrate and fuse this knowledge to make a coherent explication of dissociative identity disorder? There are so many pieces and perspectives to connect. Consider the dilemma of the person who comes to therapy and discovers their mind has been the overarching container for some ten to twenty incomplete "ways of being me" (Chefetz 2013) who through a complex psychotherapy have come to be little different, one from the other. As I put it to the person with the boardroom experience of having legs that didn't reach the floor:

> I can tell you what the literature says about the course of treatment and notions about how a mind is, and I can tell you what integration and fusion are about, but in the end, it's your choice about how you want to live. It's part of my job to advise you about what the advantages and disadvantages of some of these choices might theoretically be. But, regardless of what I know, and what I've read, this is still your life and you get to decide how you want to live it.

As we talked about what the literature said, and clarified as we went along, he suddenly stopped and looked at me in surprise:

> It's started. I feel somewhat shocked by what's happening, even though I've had the sense for the last few minutes that I knew what I wanted to do. But, the guys are kind of lining up. As I watch them in my mind I can see them merging into me and disappearing. In fact, it's almost done, at least the physical part, because I don't see anybody inside my mind anymore, just me.

It took several more weeks before he had a sense of stability about how he felt and what it was like to think in a single-minded way, without additional input from another sense of self. The psychotherapy continued as we explored his experience of work, family, friends, and so on, from a new vantage point and worked on unresolved issues that were part of his ongoing therapy.

The perspective Worrell and Dehnam bring to the issue of integration and fusion is what a psychoanalyst might call a one-person psychology—the psychology of the objective and wise clinician who is well versed in a subject area and can advise a patient with wise counsel about their illness and treatment. The two-person psychology of which I've spoken is a relational and interpersonal psychodynamic perspective that doesn't privilege the knowledge of the clinician over that of the patient. What has privilege in the two-person psychology is the relationship; a living and breathing creation of the two participants in the psychotherapeutic endeavor. Even in the two-person psychology, it is the responsibility of the clinician to know the science behind the psychotherapy issues and to put them on the psychotherapeutic table for review. In that context, we have gone a distance beyond issues related to the dictation of how a person ought to live their life, and how they ought to craft their mind, to whatever extent that might be a choice.

A multiple self-state model of mind is a robust concept for all of us and works very well as an over-arching model of the human mind (Howell 2005; Chefetz 2015; Mitchell 1991, 1993; Bromberg 2011; Stern 1997). Think about it. When was the last time you said something like the following after a faux pas: "I'm so sorry, that's not like me. I don't know what got into me." Nothing got into you. It was already there. Just another way of being you—a "not-me" aspect of you. My hope is that all the different ways of being me (or you) can live flexibly and creatively, together, without dissociative disruption of the flow of thought, feeling, behavior, and while feeling vitally alive in a body and having a mind of my own.

Notes

1 The most comprehensive and cogent description of dissociative processes is Loewenstein (1991).

References

Ainsworth, Mary D.S., M.C. Blehar, Everett Waters, and S. Wall. 1978. *Patterns of attachment: A psychological study of the strange situation*. Hillsdale, NJ: Lawrence Erlbaum.

American Psychiatric Association. 2013. *Diagnostic and statistical manual of mental disorders*. Washington, DC: American Psychiatric Press.

Bowlby, John. 1969/1982. *Attachment (second edition)*. New York: Basic Books.

——1980. *Attachment and loss: Volume III. Loss: Sadness and depression*. New York: Basic Books.

Brand, Bethany L., R.J. Loewenstein, and D. Spiegel. 2014. "Dispelling myths about dissociative identity disorder in treatment: An empirically based approach." *Psychiatry* 77 (2): 169–89.

Brand, Bethany L., S.W. McNary, A.C. Myrick, C.C. Classen, R. Lanius, R.J. Loewenstein, C. Pain, and F.W. Putnam. 2012. "A longitudinal naturalistic study of patients with dissociative disorders treated by community clinicians." *Psychological Trauma: Theory, Research, Practice, and Policy* 5 (4): 301–8.

Braun, Bennett G. 1988. "The BASK model of dissociation." *Dissociation* 1 (1): 4–23.

Bremner, J.D., J.H. Krystal, D.S. Charney, and S.M. Southwick. 1996. "Neural mechanisms in dissociative amnesia for childhood abuse: Relevance to the current controversy surrounding 'false memory syndrome'." *Amercian Journal of Psychiatry* 153 (7): 71–82.

Bremner, J.D., M. Vythilingam, E. Vermetten, S.M. Southwick, T. McGlashan, A. Nazeer, S. Khan, L.V. Vaccarino, R. Soufer, P.K. Garg, C.K. Ng, L.H. Staib, J.S. Duncan, and D.S. Charney. 2003. "MRI and PET study of deficits in hippocampal structure and function in women with childhood sexual abuse and posttraumatic stress disorder." *American Journal of Psychiatry* 160: 924–32.

Bretherton, Inge. 1992. "The origins of attachment theory: John Bowlby and Mary Ainsworth." *Developmental psychology* 28 (5): 759.

Bromberg, Philip M. 1998. *Standing in the spaces*. Hillsdale, NJ: The Analytic Press.

——2006. *Awakening the dreamer: Clinical journeys*. Mahwah, NJ: Analytic Press.

——2011. *The shadow of the tsunami and the growth of the relational mind*. New York: Routledge.

Chefetz, Richard A. 2013. "A fluctuating capacity to mentalize: Affect scripts and self-state systems as (not so) 'strange attractors': A discussion of Margy Sperry's 'Putting our heads together: Mentalizing systems'." *Psychoanalytic Dialogues* 23 (6): 708–14.

——2015. *Intensive psychotherapy for persistent dissociative processes: The fear of feeling real*. Edited by Allan N. Schore, *Interpersonal Neurobiology Series*. New York: W.W. Norton.

Chused, Judith F. 1991. "The evocative power of enactments." *Journal of the American Psychoanalytic Association* 39: 615–39.

Dalenberg, C., B. Brand, D. Gleaves, M. Dorahy, R. Loewenstein, E. Cardena, E. Carlson, and D. Spiegel. 2012. " Evaluation of the evidence for the trauma and fantasy models of dissociation." *Psychological Bulletin* 138 (3): 550–88.

Eich, J. E. 1980. "The cue-dependent nature of state-dependent retrieval." *Memory & Cognition* 8 (2): 157–73.

——1987. "Theoretical issues in state-dependent memory." In *Varieties of memory and consciousness: Essays in honour of Endel Tulving*, edited by H.L. Roediger and F.I.M. Craik, 331–54. Hillsdale, NJ: Erlbaum.

——1995. "Searching for mood dependent memory." *Psychological Science* 6: 65–75.

Foote, Brad, Yvette Smolin, Deborah I. Neft, and Deborah Lipschitz. 2008. "Dissociative disorders and suicidality in psychiatric outpatients." *The Journal of Nervous and Mental Disease* 196 (1): 29–36.

Holmes, E.A., R.J. Brown, W. Manselld, R.P. Fearon, E.C.M. Hunter, F. Frasquilho, and D.A. Oakley. 2005. "Are there two qualitatively distinct forms of dissociation? A review of some clinical implications." *Clinical Psychology Review* 25: 1–23.

Howell, Elizabeth F. 2005. *The dissociative mind.* Hillsdale, NJ: Analytic Press.

IJzendoorn, Marinus H. van. 1995. "Adult attachment representations, parental responsiveness, and infant attachment: A meta-analysis on the predictive validity of the adult attachment interview." *Psychological Bulletin* 117 (3): 387–403.

Kluft, Richard P. 1984a. "An introduction to multiple personality disorder." *Psychiatric Annals* 14 (1): 19–24.

——1984b. "Treatment of multiple personality disorder: A study of 33 cases." *Psychiatric Clinics of North America* 7 (1): 9–29.

Kramer, Selma. 1983. "Object-coercive doubting: A pathological defensive response to maternal incest." *Journal of the American Psychoanalytic Association* 31S: 325–51.

Levenkron, Holly. 2006. "Love (and hate) with the proper stranger: Affective honesty and enactment." *Psychoanalytic Inquiry* 26 (2): 157–81.

Loewenstein, Richard J. 1991. "An office mental status examination for complex chronic dissociative symptoms and multiple personality disorder." In *Psychiatric Clinics of North America*, edited by Richard J. Loewenstein, 567–604. Philadelphia: W.B. Saunders Company.

Lyons-Ruth, Karlen. 2003. "Dissociation and the parent-infant dialogue: A longitudinal perspective from attachment research." *Journal of the American Psychoanalytic Association* 51 (3): 883–911.

——2008. "Contributions of the mother-infant relationship to dissociative, borderline, and conduct symptoms in young adulthood." *Infant Mental Health Journal* 29 (3): 203–18.

Main, Mary. 1993. "Discourse, prediction, and recent studies in attachment: Implications for psychoanalysis." *Journal of the American Psychoanalytic Association* 41: 209–42.

——1995. "Recent studies in attachment: Overview, with selected implications for clinical work." In *Attachment theory: Social, developmental, and clinical perspectives*, edited by Roy Muir Susan Goldberg, and John Kerr, 407–74. Hillsdale, NJ: The Analytic Press.

——2000. "The organized categories of infant, child, and adult attachment: Flexible vs. inflexible attention under attachment-related stress." *Journal of the American Psychoanalytic Association* 48: 1055–95.

——, and Erik Hesse. 1990. "Parents' unresolved traumatic experiences are related to infant disorganized attachment status: Is frightened and/or frightening parental behavior the linking mechanism?" In *Attachment in the preschool years: Theory, research, and intervention*, edited by Mark T. Greenberg, Dante Ciccheti, and E. Mark Cummings, 161–82. Chicago: The University of Chicago Press.

——, and Hillary Morgan. 1996. "Disorganization and disorientation in infant strange situation behavior: Phenotypic resemblance to dissociative states." In *Handbook of dissociation: Theoretical, empirical, and clinical perspectives*, edited by Larry K. Michelson and William J. Ray, 107–38. New York: Plenum Press.

McLaughlin, James. 1991. "Clinical and theoretical aspects of enactment." *Journal of the American Psychoanalytic Association* 39: 595–614.

Michal, M., M.E. Beutel, J. Jordan, M. Zimmerman, S. Wolters, and T. Heindenreich. 2007. "Depersonalization, mindfulness, and childhood trauma." *Journal of Nervous and Mental Disease* 195: 693–96.

Michal, M., A. Koechel, M. Canterino, J. Adler, I. Reiner, G. Vossel, M.E. Beutel, and M. Gamner. 2013. "Depersonalization disorder: Disconnection of cognitive evaluation from autonomic responses to emotional stimuli." *PlosOne* 8 (9): e74331 (1–12).

Milad, M.R., R.K. Pitman, C.B. Ellis, A.L. Gold, L.M. Shin, N.B. Lasko, M.A. Zeidan, K. Handwerger, S.P. Orr, and S.L. Rauch. 2009. "Neurobiological basis of failure to recall extinction memory in posttraumatic stress disorder." *Biological Psychiatry* 66 (12): 1075–82.

Milad, M.R., S.L. Rauch, R.K. Pitman, and G.J. Quirk. 2006. "Fear extinction in rats: Implications for human brain imaging and anxiety disorders." *Biological Psychiatry* 73: 61–71.

Mitchell, Stephen A. 1991. "Contemporary perspectives on self: Toward an integration." *Psychoanalytic Dialogues* 1: 121–47.

——1993. *Hope and dread in psychoanalysis.* New York: Basic Books.

Ogawa, J.R., L.A. Sroufe, N.S. Weinfield, E.A. Carlson, and B. Egelend. 1997. "Development and the fragmented self: Longitudinal study of dissociative symptomatology in a nonclinical sample." *Development and Psychopathology* 9: 855–79.

Phelps, Elizabeth A., K.J. O'Connor, J.C. Gatenby, J.C. Gore, C. Grillon, and M. Davis. 2001. "Activation of the left amygdala to a cognitive representation of fear." *Nature Neuroscience* 4: 437–41.

Phillips, M.L., N. Medford, C. Senior, E.T. Bullmore, J. Suckling, M.J. Brammer, A. Chris, M. Sierra, S.C.R. William, and A.S. David. 2001. "Depersonalization disorder: Thinking without feeling." *Psychiatry Research: Neuroimaging Section* 108: 145–60.

Rauch, Scott L., B.A. van der Kolk, R.E. Fisler, N.M. Alpert, S.P. Orr, C.R. Savage, A.J. Fischman, M.A Jenike, and R.K. Pitman. 1996. "A symptom provocation study of post-traumatic stress disorder using positron emission tomography and script driven imagery." *Archives of General Psychiatry* 53: 380–87.

Schore, J.R., and A.N. Schore. 2008. "Modern attachment theory: The central role of affect regulation in development and treatment." *Clinical Social Work Journal* 36: 9–20.

Shin, Lisa M., and I. Liberzon. 2010. "The neurocircuitry of fear, stress, and anxiety disorders." *Neuropsychopharmacology REVIEWS* 35: 169–91.

Shin, L.M., Rauch, S.L., and Pitman, R.K. 2006. "Amygdala, medial prefrontal cortex, and hippocampal function in PTSD." *Annals of the New York Academy of Sciences* 1071: 67–79.

Solomon, Judith, and Carol George. 1999a. *Attachment disorganization.* New York: Guilford Press.

——1999b. "The place of disorganization in attachment theory." In *Attachment disorganization,* edited by Judith Solomon and Carol George, 3–32. New York: Guilford Press.

Solomon, Marion F., and D.J. Siegel, eds. 2003. *Healing trauma: Attachment, mind, body, and brain.* Edited by Daniel J. Siegel, *The Norton Series on Interpersonal Neurobiology.* New York: W.W. Norton & Company.

Steele, Kathy, O. van der Hart, and E.R.S. Nijenhuis. 2005. "Phase-oriented treatment of structural dissociation in complex traumatization: Overcoming trauma-related phobias." *Journal of Trauma & Dissociation* 6 (3): 11–53.

Steinberg, Marlene. 1993. *Structured clinical interview for DSM-IV dissociative disorders.* Washington, DC: American Psychiatric Press.

Stern, Donnel B. 1997. *Unformulated experience: From dissociation to imagination in psychoanalysis.* Hillsdale, NJ: The Analytic Press.

——2010. *Partners in thought: Working with unformulated experience, dissociation, and enactment.* London: Routledge.

Teicher, Martin H., and J.A. Samson. 2013. "Childhood maltreatment and psychopathology: A case for ecophenotypic variants as clinically and neurobiologically distinct subtypes." *American Journal of Psychiatry* 170: 1114–33.

Teicher, Martin H., Jacqueline A. Samson, Yi-Shin Sheu, Ann Polcari, and Cynthia E. McGreenery. 2010. "Hurtful words: Association of exposure of peer verbal abuse with elevated psychiatric symptom scores and corpus callosum abnormalities." *American Journal of Psychiatry* 167 (12): 1464–71.

Tomkins, Silvan S. 1995. "Script theory." In *Exploring affect: The selected writings of Silvan S. Tomkins,* edited by E. Virginia Demos, 312–88. New York: Cambridge University Press.

Vermetten, Eric, C. Schmahl, S. Lindner, R.J. Loewenstein, and J.D. Bremner. 2006. "Hippocampal and amygdalar volumes in dissociative identity disorder." *American Journal of Psychiatry* 163: 630–36.

Yehuda, Rachel. 1998. "Psychoneuroendocrinology of post-traumatic stress disorder." In *Psychoneuroendocrinology*, edited by Charles B. Nemeroff, 359–79. Philadelphia: W.B. Saunders.

——, N.P. Daskalakis, A. Lehrner, F. Desarnaud, H.N. Bader, I. Makotkine, J.D. Flory, L.M. Bierer, and M.J. Meaney. 2014. "Influences of maternal and paternal PTSD on epigenetic regulation of the glucocorticoid receptor gene in holocaust survivor offspring." *American Journal of Psychiatry* 171: 872–80.

Yin, Yan, C. Jin, X. Hu, L. Duan, Z. Li, M. Song, H. Chen, B. Feng, T. Jiang, H. Jin, C. Wong, Q. Gong, and L. Li. 2011. "Altered resting-state functional connectivity of thalamus in earthquake-induced posttraumatic stress disorder: A functional magnetic resonance imaging study." *Brain Research* 1411: 98–107

Part 3
Philosophy Out of Psychiatry

9a

Reproductive Steroids and Depression

The Brain in Context

David R. Rubinow

1. Introduction

It's great to be able to write about my favorite topic: sex and the brain. In this chapter, I will address how reproductive steroids can provide spectacular insights into the mechanisms underlying affective regulation and dysregulation and help us address what is arguably the most important question in psychiatry and medicine in general: "Why do different people respond differently to the same stimulus?" Now I warn you that I am going to assault you with details, so let me ask only that you abstract the big picture concepts. And those concepts are differential sensitivity, susceptibility, and context. Ultimately, everything in physiology is context-dependent, and failure to ignore context results in inappropriate inferences about how biology works and about how behavior works.

The reproductive endocrine-related mood disorders that I will examine are characterized by an enormous amount of morbidity and even mortality. Premenstrual dysphoria has a prevalence of about 5 percent and has been associated with 14.5 million disability adjusted life years (a measure from the World Health Organization) annually (Halbreich et al. 2003). Postpartum depression (PPD) has a prevalence of somewhere between 8–14 percent depending on whether you include minor depression. Additionally in the Confidential Inquiries into Maternal Health study, which was carried out about seven years ago in the UK, PPD was identified as the major source of maternal death, more than hemorrhage or sepsis. It was depression associated with pregnancy. And then finally, although the prevalence of perimenopausal depression is uncertain, if you are depressed and in your perimenopausal years, you've got a 50 percent greater chance of dying from cardiovascular reasons. So the question then is:

What do reproductive steroids have to do with these disorders, other than perhaps the coincidental appearance of depressive symptoms during periods of reproductive endocrine change? Why would reproductive steroids have a role in affective regulation?

2. Reproductive Steroids Influence the Pathophysiological Substrates of Depression

One answer is that estradiol touches virtually every system that has ever been implicated as causal in depression. So just running through a couple of obvious ones: estradiol regulates the synthetic and metabolic enzymes for all the neurotransmitters of the biogenic *amines* and *gaba* and regulates the synthesis of the receptor proteins and signal transduction proteins by which they influence the nucleus. Reproductive steroids like estrogen can regulate stress, and in fact the CRH gene has several estrogen response elements on it. Estradiol regulates synaptic plasticity and dendritic spine density and is neuroprotective against a variety of insults such as hypoxia, inflammation, and glutamate excess. Additionally, estradiol regulates the metabolism of the amyloid precursor protein in such a way as to prevent metabolism to the toxic beta amyloid protein. Estradiol regulates mitochondrial respiratory efficiency in such a way as to prevent the formation of free radicals, the reactive oxygen species that are toxic to DNA and many cellular proteins. Finally, if you examine the chronic illnesses that kill most people in this country – cardiovascular disease, diabetes, obesity, depression, and stress-related illnesses – you see that all of them are associated with increases in the "inflammatory" cytokines, such as MCP-1, IL-6, TNF-a, and reduced insulin sensitivity; estradiol has an opposite effect on all these presumed biomarkers for chronic disease.

3. Molecular Actions of Reproductive Steroids: Staring into the Jaws of Biological Diversity

If estrogen appears to have all of these beneficial effects, how can we understand the variance in response to gonadal steroids? All steroid hormones share a common precursor: cholesterol. Once cholesterol enters the mitochondria, the energy factory of the cell, a six-carbon side chain is cleaved, producing a compound called pregnenolone, and the pregnenolone is acted on in such as way as to create all of the biologically active steroids: estrogen, progesterone, testosterone, cortisol, and aldosterone.

The biological diversity at one level then is determined by how the steroid precursors are metabolized. For example, testosterone can be reduced to produce dihydrotestosterone, which is a much more powerful androgen than testosterone and is necessary to sustain the male reproductive tract tissues such as the prostate and seminal vesicles. Testosterone can be acted on by other enzymes to produce androsterone, which is a neurosteroid acting at the membrane to acutely change cellular effects. And testosterone can be metabolized by still another enzyme, aromatase, to produce estradiol, which acts through its receptors to initiate a whole other series of biological effects. It is noteworthy that this process can take place in the brain, independent of peripheral steroid synthesis.

Variability is further seen as a function of local context and biological interactions. For example, Yue et al. (2005) studied plaque development in brains of mice with a genetic predisposition to Alzheimer's disease-like lesions. If the ovaries were removed (thus eliminating the main peripheral source of E2), plaque development was unaffected, but if the E2 synthetic enzyme aromatase was inhibited (including in the brain), a premature explosion of the plaques occurred. So there you have reproductive steroids in the brain affecting the expression of a genetic vulnerability to experience a neurodegenerative disease. It's one mechanism by which reproductive steroids can influence the disease process.

How does it go about doing this? Jensen and Jacobson (1962) identified an intracellular protein, which turned out to be the estrogen receptor (ER). The estrogen receptor, like all steroid receptors and unlike growth factor or other hormone receptors, exists within the cell, not on the cell membrane, the site of neurotransmitter receptors. Steroid hormones, because they are fats, go into the cell and bind to the estrogen receptor, which binds to a so-called response element on the DNA, causes transcription of a message, which gets translated into a protein, and then you're on your way because all these proteins regulate cellular function. The problem is, it's a tiny bit more complicated than that.

Let's examine a number of elements. First, estradiol can bind to membrane-binding receptors, including the classical estrogen receptors which exist on the membrane, and then initiate signal transduction. What is signal transduction? It is largely this promiscuous exchange of phosphate groups. And these phosphate groups, for reasons I don't pretend to understand, are associated with activation of enzymes, gene transcription factors, and with changes of conformations of proteins in ways that are of great physiologic relevance.

Now these intracellular proteins, these steroid receptors, are themselves transcription factors that can bind to DNA, but they also represent the point of convergence of multiple signal transduction pathways, so neurotransmitters such as dopamine or insulin or growth factors can directly phosphorylate the intracytoplasmic receptor in such a way as to activate it and produce the effects of that steroid receptor *in the absence of a hormone.* Further, there are at least two types of estrogen receptors, and that's a whole other paper, estrogen receptors alpha and beta, coded for in different chromosomes, 6 & 14, and they largely have antagonistic effects. This is very important for understanding why estrogen can cause breast cancer, or endometrial cancer, and yet protect against the development of vascular disease. Indeed, manipulation of the agonists for these receptor variants produces dramatically different physiologic effects, which offers great therapeutic potential.

As an added layer of complexity, the effect of an activated hormone receptor is entirely dependent on its interaction with other proteins called coregulators. Coregulators can be coactivators or coinhibitors. When the ER is bound by the hormone, it changes its shape, it flexes in such a way as to expose new binding sites and attract these coregulators, and, depending upon which ones are present and attracted, the net effect will be to turn genes on or off. The coregulator, then, is really the business end of an activated receptor, and the same hormone binding the same receptor in different tissues will have entirely different genetic effects as a product of the nature and concentration of the coregulators in that tissue.

So everything in biology is about what dance partners a particular molecule winds up selecting to go to the dance with. That's all that matters. It gets worse: The coregulator is not really a single coregulator, but usually is a collection of six or more of the 350 known coregulators. So when you think about why a hormone does different things, it does different things in different tissues because of these coregulators. Similarly, since the shape of the hormone influences the shape of the receptor that recruits the coregulators, hormones with slightly different structures can have similar effects in one tissue but quite different effects in another tissue. Case in point is the class of pharmacologic agents called selective ER modulators, or SERMS. When SERMS bind ER, they flex it differently from estradiol so as to actually shut off ER effects by attracting coinhibitors rather than coactivators. That's why, in part, these SERMS can act like an ER antagonist in tissues such as breast and uterus, where you want to block estrogen activity, and act like an estrogen agonist in bone or brain, where you want it to. To repeat: The shape of the hormone determines the shape of the receptor, which then specifies the binding partners, the coregulators, which determine what the gene does. This same "shape-determined" selection of binding partners occurs at the DNA and further regulates gene transcription: The DNA specifies the conformation of the receptor and hence what transcription factors get recruited in the same way that the hormone agonist does. So you're always twisting these things to create new biological actions. These differences in shape explain in part why estradiol, which is the physiologically active part of estrogen, is not the same as conjugated estrogen, which is a mix of about 16 different estrogen-like compounds taken from horse urine, but actually contain less than 1 percent estradiol. It makes a difference.

So what are the sources of variation? You've got levels of hormones, levels of receptor proteins, how the hormones are metabolized, genetic differences in the enzymes that lead to different metabolites, intracellular modulators like coregulators, and now DNA structure. Structural differences in DNA can code for different proteins, can dictate a change in gene expression (more or less of the messenger RNA), can dictate a change in processing so the message lives for a longer period of time or not (mRNA stability), can produce different effects through epistasis (which refers to the ability of a mutation in one gene to affect the mutation in another gene [so there is co-operativity that can produce very significant biologic effects]), and finally can influence sensitivity to environment. And this last point is really incredibly important because it suggests that *genetic differences can determine how we respond to psychosocioeconomic stressors.* There's this wonderful study done by Steve Cole et al. (2010) that goes as follows. There are a number of chronic diseases that are associated with immune system changes and that are associated with increased IL6. Those include cardiovascular disease, many neurodegenerative changes, as well as some cancers. So they performed this Macarthur successful aging study: They looked at ostensibly healthy people who were 70–80 years old, and they followed them for 12 years. Next, they assumed that adverse, stressful social effects, for which they took depression as a proxy, would influence the activation of IL6. The idea was that stress activates the sympathetic nervous system, releases norepinephrine, acts through the beta adrenergic receptor, which increases the transcription factor of GATA1, which binds to the IL6 gene to promote IL6 secretion, leading to chronic IL6 exposure, which they inferred was bad for you. Then they used this wonderful computational biological process to identify a single nucleotide, a single building block of the DNA, that was largely responsible for GATA1 binding. And then they said: If we look at the health of individuals who appear depressed over the course of this study, will the presence of this mutation, which prevents GATA1 binding, have any relevance to disease outcomes? And remarkably, they found that it absolutely did.

In the group as a whole, the depressed individuals died at a much more rapid rate. However, in those individuals who had the C-allele, which is responsible for decreasing GATA1 binding to IL6, *there was absolutely no effect of depression on their deaths – they looked just like those who were not depressed.* So this is really an incredible example of how just a single genetic mutation can take a relatively opaque concept such as stress sensitivity or stress resilience and turn it into something that is meaningful in terms of the specific pathways by which stress may adversely affect health or not.

Another level of variation is seen in the translation of environmental events into marked differences in genetic expression – a process called epigenesis. Every cell in your body has the same genome, but some cells become myocytes, some become neurons, some become bones, or osteocytes. What is it that causes that? It's simply which genes get read and which genes don't get read. That's all that determines the difference. And the expression of genes is powerfully regulated by the addition of chemical groups – acetyl, methyl, phosphate, and so on – to the DNA and to the proteins around which the DNA is wrapped (histones). Add one type of chemical and the DNA opens up to be read; add another group and the DNA closes up, thus silencing the genes. Michael Meany has demonstrated that stressful events during critical periods of development alters the so-called post-translational modifications of these histone proteins in such a way as to change genetic expression for the rest of the life of the individual. In some instances, these can even be passed from generation to generation. Again, this is a way in which the environment gets transduced not into irreversible changes in gene structure, but rather to potentially irreversible changes in gene expression.

The whole point of this is that we're taught a very simple DNA to RNA to protein to biochemicals to the comfy seat of the shrink, but in fact it's really the state and level of genetic expression that influences most of the processes that are of relevance to behavior. Eric Nestler and colleagues (Tsankova et al. 2006) have demonstrated that antidepressants, at least in animal studies, work by inhibiting a specific kind of histone modifier (deacetylase). So these differences in genetic expression can actually have an impact on the diseases we study, the drugs we use, and the level of stress adaptation. Timing of the environmental event also critically determines the impact on genetic expression and behavior. Exposure, for example, of a pregnant dam (female rat) to a high-fat diet will ever after change the genetic expression – and structure – in the pup's brain so as to program the brain for different responses to food. The offspring will prefer high-fat food, eat to excess, and develop a metabolic syndrome despite being exposed to a normal diet throughout their lives. Further, the genetic susceptibility to develop obesity can be completely reversed by replacing the colonic contents of animals during youth, even if you expose them to high-fat diets subsequently. The micro-biome, the trillions of bacteria in our body, can actually co-opt the host genetic machinery in such a way as to lead to very different physiological responses to the very same environmental stimuli, in this case food.

The take home: Not all hormones are the same; it's about how these things interact with each other. The effects of hormones are *ubiquitous*, *tissue-specific*, and *context-dependent*. Now we know that they're context-dependent when we look at the biology, but we've forgotten about that when we talk about behavior. That's because we still tend to think of the brain as a bunch of wires and circuits instead of being a context-dependent organ. It's a non-linear transformation, in which you don't know what the response to a stimulus is going to be absent an understanding of what the past history was and what the current physiologic state is.

4. Context-Dependent Physiology: Aging and Perimenopausal Depression

In fact, all of physiology is context-dependent. It's developmental stage-dependent; that is, the effect depends on when an animal or a human sees whatever it sees. That's the concept of a *critical period*. As an example, Piferrer et al. (1993) were able to transform a genetic female Chinook salmon into a fully functional male simply by exposing the eggs to an aromatase inhibitor, which prevents the conversion of testosterone to estradiol, for 2 hours during development.

Reproductive steroids, then, also create a context that influences development. Sex differences can be observed across the whole neuroaxis, from the pattern of synapses to the structure of some nuclei to the response of cells to the same stimulus. Male prefrontal cortical neurons look pretty asthenic compared with those from females, but after three days of culture with progesterone, the male neurons get really happy and start putting out neurites and the female neurons involute – absent any differential exposure. They're getting the same thing, but they're programmed to respond differently, even with the same stimulus.

Age is a context – there are cognitive changes that occur with aging, and affective changes have been reported as well to accompany reproductive aging, as described by William Conklin, over 100 years ago:

> The peculiar nervous instability of the climacteric woman is aptly described by that word. … Neurasthenia, the symptoms of which are so variable and ill defined as almost to defeat the attempt to marshal them into order. Sunshine and shadow rapidly chase each other over her daily life. She is self-sacrificing in the performance of duty at one time and again, is querulous, vacillating in purpose and capricious in temper. She is oppressed by fears of impending evils, and grows moody, when she becomes a veritable Jacques, with a melancholia of her own, compounded of many simples, extracted from many objects. She is tortured by bodily pains equally hard to bear. There is scarcely an arrow in the armory of pain that is not unsheathed at this period.
>
> *(Conklin, 1889)*

The elegance of the prose aside, the question is really: Do the mood changes with aging have anything to do with the reproductive changes? Fifteen years ago, Peter Schmidt and I demonstrated that women with depression during the perimenopause experienced alleviation of their symptoms after several weeks of double blind, placebo-controlled estradiol administration, with improvement seen even in those women who did not experience hot flashes (which might otherwise have compromised the blind) (Schmidt et al. 2000). We recently replicated these findings, so it looks like estradiol has some significant therapeutic benefit.

Despite being effective in *peri*menopausal women, E2 is not effective in *post*-menopausal women, as Mary Morrison et al. (2004) demonstrated. This is important to remember when one examines the findings of the Women's Health Initiative. This study took 17,000 "apparently healthy" postmenopausal women – I say "apparently healthy" because 8 percent of them had already had heart attacks, 34 percent were obese, 36 percent were hypertensive, and 49 percent were current or former smokers, but ok, "apparently healthy" – aged 50–79, 10 percent of whom were between the ages of 50 and 60. They gave them Prempro, and they examined coronary heart disease as the primary outcome, because the vast majority of the observational studies suggested that hormone-replacement therapy will decrease the risk of heart attacks by 50 percent. The adverse outcome was invasive breast cancer because the majority of studies had shown that if you take hormone replacement therapy for more than four years your risk of developing breast cancer goes up by 30 percent. They found that the risk of coronary heart disease went up instead of down, as did the risk of breast cancer (Rossouw et al 2002). Science magazine reported, "[T]his is the final nail in the coffin for hormone replacement therapy" – and it was for a while with research that involved estrogen (Couzin 2004). So if estrogen is so "good for you," why are they saying such horrible things about it?

Let's go back to the context again. Timing is critically important, not only developmentally, but also because during this period we are talking about aging. Phyllis Wise (Suzuki et al. 2007), in a wonderful study, took 19-week-old animals, removed their ovaries, and then gave them either oil or estrogen for one week, tied off their middle cerebral arteries, sacrificed them, and then looked at their brains. So the animal that got oil had most of its cortex wiped out, and the brain of the animal that got estrogen was largely protected. But what was particularly interesting was what came next: She again performed the oophorectomy, this time at 9 weeks, waited for 10 weeks, then compared the effects of oil or estradiol for one week. She found that the estrogen did nothing. Absolutely no neuroprotective effect if you give it at a distance from the elimination of estrogen. This recapitulates what Mikkola and Clarkson (2002) showed with heart disease – exactly the same thing. Give the hormone close to the removal of estrogen, it's protective on the cardiovasculature. Give it at a distance, it's actually harmful (Sophonsritsuk et al. 2013).

Zhang et al. (2011) performed another study showing the same thing in the brain. You take animals, remove their ovaries, and you either treat them for 10 weeks with placebo or estrogen – that's one group. The other group, you remove their ovaries, you let them go for 10 weeks, and then you give them a week of placebo or estrogen. In their data, you don't need statistics to see that if you give estrogen proximate to removal of the ovaries, the neurons are intact, and if you give it 10 weeks later, the neurons die off. And this is exactly what happens with aging. Why does this happen? Because with prolonged absence of estrogen, there is an increased interaction of the estrogen receptor with a protein called CHIP, which results in the degradation of the estrogen receptor. Translated to humans, this means that if you're giving estrogen to a 79-year-old woman, you are giving estrogen to someone with dramatically reduced estrogen receptors in her brain, but the peripheral effects remain intact. So the estrogen receptor in the uterus does not go away, and it doesn't go away in the vascular plaques or in the macrophages, so you're exposing her to all the toxic effects of estradiol with none of the beneficial effects.

So this led to what Robberta Diaz Brinton calls the Healthy Cell Hypothesis: Give estrogen to a healthy cell, good things happen; give estrogen to a diseased cell, bad things happen, either by causing excessive calcium accumulation in the cell, which for a neuron that is exposed to excessive amounts of glutamate will kill it, or in your cardiovasculature, you give it to someone who already has atherosclerotic plaques, because they are 60 or 70, and you destabilize the plaque and increase the risk of stroke and heart attacks. (Paracelsus said in the 16th century, "A drug can be an inert substance, a poison, or a therapeutic agent dependent upon how it is used and the dosage in which is it given." Talk about having to relearn what we already know.)

And then finally, the Women's Health Initiative failed to consider individual differences in steroid sensitivity. Let me give you several examples of this, because this is what reproductive mood disorders are all about, and we can prove it. (1) Does estradiol withdrawal precipitate depressive symptoms in perimenopausal women, and (2) does it have a differential effect in women with vs. those without a history of perimenopausal depression? In a recently completed study, Peter Schmidt took women who had a history of being on hormone replacement therapy, put them back on estrogen blindly, and then either withdrew them by substituting placebo or maintained them on estradiol (Schmidt et al. unpublished manuscript). He performed the same study in women with no history of perimenopausal depression. He observed that the euthymic women with a past history of perimenopausal depression who were put on hormone replacement became depressed when blindly withdrawn from estradiol, while the women lacking the history of perimenopausal depression had absolutely no effect of estradiol withdrawal on their mood at all. This is one example of what I mean by differential sensitivity – same stimulus, very different phenotypic response.

This differential sensitivity can be revealed under different hormonal states, which themselves determine how the brain functions in response to a stimulus. We began a series of studies that involved putting women on Lupron, which is a GNRH agonist, which shuts off the pituitary secretion of the hormones that stimulate the ovaries. So what you're doing is creating a medical menopause. Then we added back estrogen or progesterone to see if we could in isolation determine what the effects of estrogen or progesterone are when the brain performs a cognitive task – in this case a prefrontal task called the Wisconsin Card Sort.

If you have progesterone on board, or if you have estrogen on board, you see the normal activation pattern. If you shut off reproductive function with Lupron, you shut off the dorsolateral prefrontal cortex. Similarly, there are regions, the precuneus and the prefrontal cortex, that are involved in the so-called "default network" and that are differentially processed by reproductive hormones. These regions are increased by estradiol and decreased by the other two conditions (Lupron alone or progesterone alone). This default network is what you are doing when you are not solving a task; it's your associations, if you will. Your associations are critical for information processing, and it tells you a lot about your affective state.

Beyond regional activational patterns, what is important is how the brain regions fit together: their connectivity. The top-down model of affective processing suggests that the prefrontal cortex is responsible for dampening the excessive limbic activity. These brain regions are connected during estrogen administration, connected during progesterone administration, and disconnected during hypogonadism. In effect what you have done, then, is taken the prefrontal cortex offline, so it's no longer able to influence this critical limbic brain region. Protopopescu et al. (2005) observed that the medial pre-frontal cortex has greater activity in the follicular phase of the menstrual cycle than the luteal phase. But what they found that is much more interesting is that in the follicular phase of the menstrual cycle, the prefrontal cortex responds only to positive stimuli, while in the luteal phase, it responds only to negative stimuli. So the hormones have altered the way the brain will respond to events in the environment that clearly are linked to both perception and affective response.

Finally, we also looked at the effects of reproductive hormones on reward circuitry in the brain. We found that several brain regions that are critical for affect and critical for reward show greater activity in the follicular phase than the luteal phase, with the degree of activation significantly related to the levels of estradiol and progesterone – again further suggesting that these hormones are regulating reward circuitry. Using the Lupron paradigm, activation in these same regions was preferentially observed during the estradiol replacement phase. So estradiol at least regulates the reward circuitry as well as the connectivity of the prefrontal cortex with the limbic system.

5. Premenstrual Dysphoria and Differential Sensitivity

Finally, I want to focus on how premenstrual dysphoria can serve as a model for affective regulation, demonstrating differential sensitivity, how symptoms get triggered, but also how one can understand the susceptibility that allows these triggers to operate (because the trigger is inoperative in certain women and it's clearly operative in others, again demonstrating *differential sensitivity*). Premenstrual dysphoria is a time-related diagnosis, not a symptom-related diagnosis, so all that matters is when symptoms appear in relation to the menstrual cycle phase. And so if someone says, "I have PMS symptoms all month long," that's a tip off that this is not PMDD. The symptoms of PMDD must appear, by definition, during the latter part of the luteal phase of the menstrual cycle, the approximately 14 days between ovulation and the onset of menses, the shedding of the uterine lining that marks the start of the next menstrual cycle.

Once you select a group of individuals in whom you can prospectively demonstrate the confinement of symptoms to the luteal phase, the first question is: Are luteal phase-related symptoms associated with luteal phase-specific physiologic abnormalities? And the answer is no. There is nothing wrong with the reproductive system, there are no hormonal changes, there is nothing you can find that appears only in the luteal phase that you can associate with symptoms. You could next ask: Well do you even need the luteal phase? This is a study we did 20 years ago, and we used a compound called RU486, which is a progesterone receptor and antagonist called mifepristone now. If you give RU486, it does two things: It blocks uterine progesterone receptors, which causes menses; and it interferes with the corpus luteum, which is the part of the ovary that remains after the egg is extruded – that's a hormone factory. We used a combination of RU486 (to terminate the luteal phase), RU486 + HCG (which preserves the luteal phase despite an initial menses due to blockade of the uterine progesterone receptors) and placebo to blind women to where they were in their menstrual cycle. After this first menses, women didn't know whether they were advanced into the follicular phase of the next cycle or remained in the preserved luteal phase of the first cycle. And what we found is that women who were in the next phase of the cycle went ahead and had their symptoms anyway. So we eliminated the mid-to-late luteal phase and it didn't influence symptom onset at all (Schmidt et al. 1991). So you don't need the luteal phase, which suggests one of two things. One, the symptoms may be linked to or choreographed to the menstrual cycle, or, two, it could be that you have to eliminate the whole menstrual cycle to see an effect.

That's the next study we did. Peter Schmidt again used Lupron to eliminate ovarian function and compared results with those getting placebo. After two to three months of ovarian suppression, the group getting Lupron had no symptoms at all. The group that got placebo maintained symptom severity and cyclicity. *Shut off the menstrual cycle, symptoms go away.* What happens if you take these women, and you add back estrogen and you add back progesterone? What you see is that the oppressive symptoms return. So it looks like estrogen and progesterone in this group are causing these symptoms. It does cause symptoms, but again, when you do the exact same manipulation creating the exact same hormonal levels in women without a history of premenstrual dysphoria, you see no effect on mood (Schmidt et al. 1998). So yes, the hormones are triggering this, but no, that's not a *sufficient* explanation for why they are. Note, by the way, that the symptoms go away by themselves over time, so that raised the possibility that the symptoms could be related to the change in hormones, or they could simply require an obligatory level of hormone in order for a CNS infradian (approximately monthly) driver of mood monthly cycle to express itself.

So is it the level of the hormone or the change in the level of the hormone that is relevant? What we did is took women with premenstrual dysphoria and put them on Lupron steadily for three months, and then we added back estrogen and progesterone. If symptoms were due to a change in hormones, you would see that the symptoms return, after which you would see no more symptoms; if symptoms were due to the obligatory presence of hormones at a certain level, the symptoms would appear, then disappear, then a month later reappear. We observed that under conditions of stable hormone replacement, symptoms appeared soon after replacement, disappeared within several weeks, and then failed to reappear for the remainder of the three months. Further, the hormone elevations appeared coincident with or slightly anticipated the appearance of dysphoric symptoms. It is, then, clearly the change in hormones that triggers the onset of symptoms in women with premenstrual dysphoria.

Why do these hormone-precipitated affective symptoms occur only in certain people – what causes the susceptibility? One possible answer is the genome. There are a number of ways of thinking about genetic influence, and I am just going to mention one. We decided to do gene-based haplotyping to look at a variety of potential sites across four genes of interest that we thought might be associated with stress reactivity in women with premenstrual dysphoria: estrogen receptor alpha, estrogen receptor beta, progesterone receptor, and the GABAa receptor delta subunit. To our surprise, there were four significant hits, all in the fourth intronic region of estrogen receptor alpha, that were predictive of premenstrual dysphoria (Huo et al. 2007). Further, these single nucleotide polymorphisms (SNPs) were also associated with symptoms that differentiate women with premenstrual dysphoria from the control group. Finally, this association was only seen in the group of women who had the catecholamine O methyl transferase (COMT) VAL/VAL polymorphism. COMT breaks down dopamine, and in the prefrontal brain region, there is no other means of dopamine metabolism (because of the absence there of dopamine transporters). If you have the VAL/VAL form of the gene, it results in excessive enzymatic activity and decreased dopamine levels. Remember that our imaging studies demonstrate that estradiol regulates prefrontal cortical activity and connectivity, the COMT gene has an estrogen response element, and COMT is responsible for estrogen metabolism. So here you have this clustering of data that are pointing to altered estrogen receptor alpha, dopamine regulation, and prefrontal cortical activity in premenstrual dysphoria. And indeed, when we looked at PET scanning and FMRI scanning, in women with PMDD vs. controls, under the three conditions described above – Lupron induced hypogonadism, estradiol, and progesterone – we found over-activation of the dorsolateral prefrontal cortex irrespective of hormone condition or of the modality used to study these women (Baller et al. 2013). And this increased activity was highly associated with the severity ratings of the individual patient. This suggests a trait difference in PFC activity in women with PMDD. We have, however, also demonstrated differential cortical activation as a function of hormone condition in women with PMDD. In two brain regions identified as critical for affective regulation – the subgenual anterior cingulate and the medial prefrontal cortex – women without PMDD show no difference in activation across induced hormonal states, but women with PMDD show increased activity during hypogonadism and the lowest activity during the administration of progesterone, which is often the major symptomatic culprit in premenstrual dysphoria. So yes there are trait differences, and there are also differential responses to reproductive steroids.

6. Context: The Biological "Interactome"

And that simply underscores my last point, which is that *one cannot understand the effects of either genome or environment by examining them separately*. You'll get very false conclusions, and I have an illustrative example. We examined the effects of COMT genotype on cognitive-stimulated activity in the dorsolateral prefrontal cortex. Under hypogonadal conditions, those with a VAL/VAL genotype (leading to decreased prefrontal cortical dopamine) show increased activity – a measure of cortical inefficiency – compared with those with the MET/MET genotype. Under conditions of estradiol administration however, the VAL/VAL individuals do better (lower activation) and the MET/MET individuals do worse. This mirrors exactly what Bruce McEwen and others have shown in the animal literature when they study cognitive function. You see estrus cycle effects on cognition and behavior, you see effects of the BDNF and COMT genotypes, but you also see an interaction between hormonal state and genotype. If you look at either one in isolation, you'll reach very erroneous conclusions about the likely behavioral phenotype, and, as a consequence, you're going to wind up missing tremendous opportunities for understanding the variance in behavior. In the example above, the failure to consider hormonal state when examining the effects of genotype (or the inverse) would lead to the false conclusion that there was no effect. Although dauntingly complex, my main point is that this is as relevant for your work with patients as it is for your efforts to understand the underlying neurobiology of the disorders – that is, everything is context-dependent. The point at which something occurs developmentally, for example, determines to a major extent the biological and behavioral impact (and residua). We are the products of a continual dialogue between our internal and external environments, inextricably linked in shaping their interdependent responses. We create our world in the same way that our world creates us.

This suggests the malignant irresponsibility of those who dictate the nature of our healthcare system, which completely disregards behavior and treats people as diseases rather than as persons, each of whom has undergone a very unique process to get where they are. Part of what we do when we work with our patients is to try to figure out what that process is to enable them to change their experience. How does this occur? Why can it lead to a sustained difference if somebody responds with empathic understanding?

I'd argue that you're changing the brain, you're changing gene expression, you're changing network consolidation and, consequently, perception. Why should reproductive steroids play a major role in this process? Because at the end of the day, it's about food and sex. That's all that's required for the prolongation of the species; the rest is commentary. So if reproductive steroids can't change behavior, we are in big trouble as a species.

The bottom line is that dissecting how the brain works and understanding how differential response and context get encoded are critical activities that may have value simply in enabling our patients to better understand what is happening to them. Daunting complexity notwithstanding, this dialogue that exists between basic science and clinical science is what makes our field the most exciting, the most interesting field in medicine. As such, the complexity is well worth embracing.

References

Baller, E.B., Wei, S.M, Kohn, P.D., Rubinow, D.R., Alarcón, G., Schmidt, P.J., Berman, K. F. "Abnormalities of dorsolateral prefrontal function in women with premenstrual dysphoric disorder: a multimodal neuroimaging study." *The American Journal of Psychiatry*. 2013 Mar 1;170(3):305–14. doi: 10.1176/appi.ajp.2012.12030385. Review. PubMed PMID: 23361612; PubMed Central PMCID: PMC3968942.

Cole, S.W., Arevalo, J.M., Takahashi, R., Sloan, E.K., Lutgendorf, S.K., Sood, A.K., Sheridan, J.F., Seeman, T.E. "Computational identification of gene-social environment interaction at the human IL6 locus." *Proceedings of the National Academy of Sciences USA*. 2010 Mar 23;107 (12):5681–86. doi: 10.1073/pnas.0911515107. Epub 2010 Feb 22. PubMed PMID: 20176930; PubMed Central PMCID: PMC2851818.

Conklin, W. J. "Some neuroses of the menopause." *Transactions of the American Association of Obstetricians and Gynecologists*. 1889;2:301–11.

Couzin, Jennifer. "NIH ends estrogen study." *Science*. 2004 March 5:1449.

Halbreich, U., Borenstein, J., Pearlstein, T., Kahn, L.S. "The prevalence, impairment, impact, and burden of premenstrual dysphoric disorder (PMS/PMDD)." *Psychoneuroendocrinology*. 2003 Aug;28 Suppl 3: 1–23. Review. PubMed PMID: 12892987.

Huo, L., Straub, R.E., Roca, C., Schmidt, P.J., Shi, K., Vakkalanka, R., Weinberger, D.R., Rubinow, D.R. "Risk for premenstrual dysphoric disorder is associated with genetic variation in ESR1, the estrogen receptor alpha gene." *Biological Psychiatry*. 2007 Oct 15;62(8):925–33. Epub 2007 Jun 27. PubMed PMID: 17599809; PubMed Central PMCID: PMC2762203.

Jensen, E.V., and H.I. Jacobson. "Basic guides to the mechanism of estrogen action." *Recent Progress in Hormone Research*. 1962;18:387–414.

Mikkola, T.S., Clarkson, T.B. "Estrogen replacement therapy, atherosclerosis, and vascular function." *Cardiovascular Research* 2002;53:605–19.

Morrison, M.F., Kallan, M.J., Ten Have, T., Katz, I., Tweedy, K., Battistini, M. "Lack of efficacy of estradiol for depression in postmenopausal women: a randomized, controlled trial." *Biological Psychiatry*. 2004 Feb 15;55(4):406–12. PubMed PMID: 14960294.

Piferrer, F., Baker,.I.J., Donaldson, E.M. "Effects of natural, synthetic, aromatizable, and non-aromatizable androgens in inducing male sex differentiation in genotypic female chinook salmon (Oncorhynchus tshawytscha)." *General and Comparative Endocrinology*. 1993 Jul;91 (1):59–65. PubMed PMID: 8405891.

Protopopescu, X., Pan, H., Altemus, M., Tuescher, O., Polanecsky, M., McEwen, B., Silbersweig, D., Stern, E. "Orbitofrontal cortex activity related to emotional processing changes across the menstrual cycle." *Proceedings of the National Academy of Sciences USA*. 2005 Nov 1;102(44):16060–65. Epub 2005 Oct 24. PubMed PMID: 16247013; PubMed Central PMCID: PMC1276043.

Rossouw, J.E., Anderson, G.L., Prentice, R.L., LaCroix, A.Z., Kooperberg, C., Stefanick, M. L., Jackson, R.D., Beresford, S.A., Howard, B.V., Johnson, K.C., Kotchen, J.M., Ockene, J. "Writing Group for the Women's Health Initiative Investigators. Risks and benefits of estrogen plus progestin in healthy postmenopausal women: Principal results from the Women's Health Initiative randomized controlled trial." *Journal of the American Medical Association*. 2002 Jul 17;288(3):321–33. PubMed PMID: 12117397.

Schmidt, P.J., Nieman, L., Danaceau, M.A., Tobin, M.B., Roca, C.A., Murphy, J.H., Rubinow, D.R. "Estrogen replacement in perimenopause-related depression: A preliminary report." *American Journal of Obstetrics and Gynecology*. 2000 Aug;183(2):414–20. PubMed PMID: 10942479.

Schmidt, P.J., Nieman, L.K., Danaceau, M.A., Adams, L.F., Rubinow, D.R. "Differential behavioral effects of gonadal steroids in women with and in those without premenstrual syndrome." *New England Journal of Medicine*. 1998 Jan 22;338(4):209–16. PubMed PMID: 9435325.

Schmidt, P.J., Nieman, L.K., Grover, G.N., Muller, K.L., Merriam, G.R., Rubinow, D.R. "Lack of effect of induced menses on symptoms in women with premenstrual syndrome." *New England Journal of Medicine*. 1991 Apr 25;324(17):1174–79. PubMed PMID: 2011161.

Sophonsritsuk, A., Appt, S.E., Clarkson, T.B., Shively, C.A., Espeland, M.A., Register, T. C. "Differential effects of estradiol on carotid artery inflammation when administered early versus late after surgical menopause." *Menopause*. 2013 May;20(5):540–47. doi: 10.1097/GME.0b013e31827461e0. PubMed PMID: 23615645.

Suzuki, S., Brown, C.M., De la Cruz, C.D., Yang, E., Bridwell, D.A., Wise, P.M. "Timing of estrogen therapy after ovariectomy dictates the efficacy of its neuroprotective and anti-inflammatory actions." *Proceedings of the National Academy of Sciences USA*. 2007 Apr 3;104 (14):6013–18. Epub 2007 Mar 26. PubMed PMID: 17389368; PubMed Central PMCID: PMC1851608.

Tsankova, N.M., Berton, O., Renthal, W., Kumar, A., Neve, R.L., Nestler, E.J. "Sustained hippocampal chromatin regulation in a mouse model of depression and antidepressant action." *Nature Neuroscience*. 2006 Apr;9(4):519–25. Epub 2006 Feb 26. PubMed PMID: 16501568.

Yue, X., Lu, M., Lancaster, T., Cao, P., Honda, S., Staufenbiel, M., Harada, N., Zhong, Z., Shen, Y., Li, R. "Brain estrogen deficiency accelerates Abeta plaque formation in an Alzheimer's disease animal model." *Proceedings of the National Academy of Sciences USA*. 2005 Dec 27;102 (52):19198–203. Epub 2005 Dec 19. PubMed PMID: 16365303; PubMed Central PMCID: PMC1323154.

Zhang, Q.G., Han, D., Wang, R.M., Dong, Y., Yang, F., Vadlamudi, R.K., Brann, D.W. "C terminus of Hsc70-interacting protein (CHIP)-mediated degradation of hippocampal estrogen receptor-alpha and the critical period hypothesis of estrogen neuroprotection." *Proceedings of the National Academy of Sciences USA*. 2011 Aug 30;108(35):E617–24. doi: 10.1073/pnas.1104391108. Epub 2011 Aug 1. PubMed PMID: 21808025; PubMed Central PMCID: PMC3167560.

9b

Commentary on Rubinow: Seeing the Forest

The Social Determinants of Mental Health

Valerie Hardcastle

1. Introduction

In "Reproductive Steroids and Depression: The Brain in Context," David Rubinow makes three large and important points about how to understand human illness, mental disorders, and suffering. First and most important: context matters. Generalizations in biology or medicine will only get you so far, and they will not even get you there if you do not understand the details behind the generalizations. (Rubinow also talks about differential cells sensitivity and differential disease susceptibility, but that is just another way of talking about context. Some contextual elements are external, and some are internal.) Second: hormones touch just about every aspect of our brains' functioning and are causally implicated in most of the chronic diseases of the Western world. Third: genetic differences explain differences in our physiological and psychological responses to a variety of stressors.

Rubinow goes small in his analysis; I want to go large. Rubinow discusses the correlation between the presence of a single nucleotide and increased mortality in depressed individuals. If you have one form of a gene, then depression can kill you; if you have another, then it will not. He draws the moral that "genetic differences can determine how we respond to psychosocioeconomic stressors" (p. 254). He puts this moral in italics to demonstrate how important it is. And he is right; this is an important insight and it should be in italics.

However, I grow concerned that Rubinow and others in psychiatry can at times focus on the trees to the exclusion of the forest. I completely agree with his conclusion that context matters more than most believe. But contexts can be large things as well as very tiny things. I want to discuss the perhaps surprising influences that larger contexts can have on illness, mental disorders, and basic human suffering. In particular, I shall discuss the social determinants of health and health outcomes. One change in one gene can make someone die from depression; so can one's neighborhood. The unequal distribution of finance, power, knowledge, and support structures taken together are the social determinants of health, and their impact on disease and mental health are as powerful as our genes.

Many believed that the Human Genome Project (1990–2003) would help scientists and doctors to understand and cure our deadliest diseases. But, more than a decade later, those high expectations are unrealized: we have not substantially reduced the health impact of the major diseases of the 21st century – cardiovascular disease, hypertension, cancer, and diabetes. How and where we live, what we know, and whom we live beside makes a tremendous difference in health outcomes, and these disparities have little to do with our basic genetic makeup and everything to do with our society and culture.

2. Health Disparities

Typically, research on health disparities and differential life expectancies focuses on race, gender, and ethnicity, with a particular emphasis on the differences between African Americans and white Americans. The gap between African-American and white life expectancy in the United States is over five years, a fact much discussed in the popular press and elsewhere. But once we dig below this surface difference, we find even larger disparities. For example, the gap between life expectancy between an African-American man (68.7 years) and an Asian-American woman (86.7 years) is almost 20 years. Inner-city African-American men in the United States have about the same life expectancy as citizens of Belarus and Uzbekistan, both low-income developing nations, while Asian women's life expectancy exceeds that of Japanese women by three years, which has the highest national life expectancy for women in the world (World Health Organization 2002).

And these differences pale in comparison with differences between counties and by combination of race and county. Native American males living in several counties located in South Dakota have a life expectancy of less than 60 years, while Asian females in Bergen County, New Jersey, have a life expectancy of over 90 years – a gap of over 30 years. Indeed, the gap between the highest and lowest life expectancies for race–county combinations in the United States is over 35 years (Murray et al. 2006)!

If we were able to do this sort of analysis in the United States at an even finer grain, taking into account other social factors, I am confident that not only would the gaps be larger, but also many of the racial differences would virtually disappear. For example, looking just at the white population in the United States, we see that the life expectancy of low-income whites from rural areas in the upper Midwest exceeds that of middle-income urban and suburban white Americans by a substantial amount, even though the middle-income Americans have the advantages of greater wealth. And low-income whites in rural Appalachia and the Mississippi Valley, whose income level is similar to that of the low-income rural whites in the Midwest, have a much lower life expectancy, similar to what we see in Mexico or Panama (Murray et al. 2006).

Injuries and chronic diseases explain most of these gaps. If we focus on the disparities in life expectancies for adults under the age of 65, we find that African Americans living in high-risk urban areas have a mortality rate similar to that of sub-Saharan Africa. Perhaps surprisingly, these high rates persist even after controlling for the effect of HIV/AIDS and homicides. Instead, the higher death rates are due largely to injuries, especially for the younger men, cardiovascular disease, diabetes, and other non-communicable diseases (Murray et al. 2006).

Why does where you live have such a potent effect on health outcomes? Rubinow points out that death from depression can in part be traced to a genetic mutation. How might the larger environment interact with, or override, one's genes? Let us look at the interaction among social factors, depression, and hypertension to see how this might occur.

3. The Social Determinants of Depression and Hypertension

Mental health, particularly depression, across the United States, and indeed around the globe, is an enormous problem. If we exclude those who are homeless, institutionalized, or incarcerated, about 21 percent of the general population in the United States has a mental disorder (U.S. Department of Health and Human Services 1999). By 2020, major depressive disorder is projected to be the second leading cause of disability in the world for all age groups (World Health Organization 2012). Between 1996 and 2005, antidepressants were the third most common prescription in the United States (Hsiao et al. 2010). After 2005, antidepressants, prescribed to approximately 27 million people, surpassed blood pressure medication to become the most commonly prescribed class of medications in the country (Olfson and Marcus 2009).

One challenge in treating mental disorders is that the majority of people experiencing psychiatric symptoms go to their primary care doctors for treatment (Mickus et al. 2000). But most primary care physicians receive very little training regarding mental illnesses and how best to treat them. For example, almost three-quarters of patients who are prescribed an antidepressant are not diagnosed with a psychiatric illness (Mojtabai and Olfson 2011).[1] In fact, just recognizing that a psychiatric disorder is present remains the biggest barrier to treating it successfully (Wun et al 2011; Cepoiu et al. 2008). Estimates are that at least 90 percent of patients who commit suicide have some psychiatric disorder (predominantly mood disorders), but more than 80 percent of them are not being treated for their mental disorders at the time of their deaths (Eisenberg et al. 2011; Henriksson et al. 2001; Lonnqvist et al. 1995; Mann et al. 2005). This is the case, even though fully three-quarters of people who end up committing suicide see a doctor in the year before their deaths. But less than a third see a professional with expertise in mental health, where more responsive diagnoses and treatments might be available (Luoma et al. 2002).

This failure to treat mental disorders effectively (or at all) is well known, but perhaps less well known is that this failure also interacts with the social determinants of health. Some of the barriers to mental health care are common across all America: cost, fragmentation or lack of services, and social stigmas toward mental illness (U.S. Department of Health and Human Services 1999). Others, however, are not. David

Satcher, the former Surgeon General of the United States, has pointed out that the differences in mental health care among the U.S. population is even more striking than for physical illnesses:

> Even more than other areas of health and medicine, the mental health field is plagued by disparities in the availability of and access to its services. These disparities are viewed readily through the lenses of racial and cultural diversity, age, and gender.
>
> *(U.S. Department of Health and Human Services 1999, p. vi)*

Probably not surprisingly, people in the lowest strata of income, education, and occupation are two to three times more likely to have a mental disorder than those in the highest strata. And, as a whole, underserved groups lack basic psychiatric care (Wang et al. 2005). They also have less access to mental health services. (To be sure, a lack of health insurance plays a role in this disparity, even though only about a quarter of the nation's underserved are uninsured.) In addition, "safety net" providers furnish a disproportionate share of mental health care to our poor, which ultimately translates into a lower quality of care (Lewin and Altman 2000). Less than half of urban patients with diagnosed clinical depression, panic disorder, generalized anxiety disorder, substance addictions, or who thought about committing suicide received any mental health treatment at all in the previous month (Olfson et al. 2000).

But, it is noteworthy that even with adequate private health insurance and good access, African Americans are still less likely to seek treatment or use services. There appears to be greater mistrust and fear of treatment among minorities for mental health disorders. As a result, African Americans collectively experience a greater disability burden from mental illness, even though the prevalence and severity of mental disorders among their communities is actually not greater than other neighborhoods (Satcher et al. 2001).

Even after controlling for socioeconomic status and differences in need, the percentage of African Americans receiving mental health treatment from any source is only about half that of whites (Swartz et al. 1998). Only about 12–15 percent of African Americans with mood or anxiety disorders see a mental health specialist, and less than a third see a provider of any kind. When African Americans do seek treatment, they are much more likely to go to their primary care provider than a mental health specialist (Pingitore et al. 2001). They often seek mental health care in emergency rooms and in psychiatric hospitals, largely because they delay pursuing treatment until symptoms are more severe.

Even setting aside these social and cultural differences, discrimination is alive and well against African Americans with mental disorders. Errors in diagnoses for schizophrenia and mood disorders are made more often with African Americans, especially in emergency rooms (Strakowski et al. 1997), and primary care physicians are less likely to diagnose African Americans accurately with depression (Borowsky et al. 2000). Finally, African Americans are less likely to receive care in accordance with professional treatment guidelines for depression or anxiety (Melfi et al. 2000; Young et al. 2001). Just over a quarter of African Americans received antidepressants when first diagnosed with depression, as compared with almost half of whites. And of those who did get medication, they were less likely to get an SSRI, the most effective medical treatment currently available for depression. Clearly, one's cultural background, as well as one's living conditions, directly influences not only one's mental health status, but also mental health treatments.

Now, here is the kicker: Being depressed means that one is more likely to have hypertension, especially for the urban poor (Pickering 2000). Why is this? The honest answer is that we do not really know. Doctors can identify the specific causes for hypertension in less than 5 percent of cases; the rest are labeled "essential hypertension," for which there is no known cause. Equally important for our discussion is the fact that depression also affects a patient's adherence to a drug regimen (DiMatteo et al. 2000; Ziegelstein et al. 2000; Dunbar-Jacob et al. 1998). In particular, depressed patients are three times more likely to ignore medical advice and recommendations for treatment (DiMatteo et al. 2000). And, of course, ignoring medical advice can have adverse consequences for controlling hypertension.

So, while it might turn out to be completely correct that a single gene mutation can determine whether depression can kill you, there is also a lot more that goes into that equation than who gets depressed with what genes. How that depression is treated, and how the depression interacts with other social determinants of health to impact physical health and chronic diseases, are surely just as fundamental to health outcomes.

To summarize: Those who live in urban areas are more likely to suffer from major depressive disorder, but are less likely to receive effective (or any) treatment for it. An increase in depression is tied to an increase in hypertension. Those who live in urban areas are more likely to have hypertension. Those with depression are less likely to follow medical advice or instruction. Finally, those who live in urban areas are much more likely to die prematurely from a chronic yet controllable health condition. It is no wonder at all that our urban communities have ongoing problems with health disparities and health outcomes. And it should be clear that alleviating these problems in these communities requires much more than understanding genetics.

In short: Rubinow is right in suggesting that we need to understand that complexity in order what is happening to our patients, and to us, and that this is a complexity "well worth embracing." It is also a complexity that is everywhere.

Acknowledgments

I would like to thank Rosalyn Stewart and Aaron Zelinsky for their collaborations on an earlier project, which fed into this commentary, and for the Weaver Institute for Law and Psychiatry for its ongoing support. In particular, Rosalyn's presentation on health disparities to the Weaver fellows launched this entire line of research for me.

Notes

1 Even if one is diagnosed appropriately, that is still no guarantee that appropriate treatment will follow. In one study, less than 13 percent of patients being seen by primary care

physicians who were diagnosed with mood, anxiety, impulse control, or substance-use disorders received minimally adequate care (Kessler et al. 2003).

References

Borowsky, S.J., Rubenstein, L.V., Meredith, L.S., Camp, P., Jackson-Triche, M., and Wells, K.B. 2000. "Who is at risk of nondetection of mental health problems in primary care?" *Journal of General Internal Medicine* 15: 381–88.

Cepoiu, M., McCusker, J., Cole, M.G., Martin, G., Sewitch, M., Belzile, W., and Ciampi, A. 2008. "Recognition of depression of non-psychiatric physicians – A systematic literature review and meta-analysis." *Journal of General Internal Medicine* 23: 25–36.

DiMatteo, M.R., Robin, M., Lepper, H.S., and Croghan, T.W. 2000. "Depression is a risk factor for noncompliance with medical treatment: Meta-analysis of the effects of anxiety and depression on patient adherence." *Archives of Internal Medicine* 160: 2101–7.

Dunbar-Jacob, J.M., Schlenk, E.A., Burke, L.E., and Matthews, J.T. 1998. "Predictors of patient adherence: Patient characteristics." In Shumaker, S.A., Schron, E.B., Ockene, J.K., McBee, W.L. (Eds) *The handbook of health behavior change. Second edition.* New York, NY: Springer Publishing Co, pp. 491–511.

Eisenberg, D., Hunt, J., Speer, N., and Zivin, K. 2011. "Mental health service utilization among college students in the United States." *Journal of Nervous and Mental Disorders* 99: 301–8.

Henriksson, S., Boëthius, G, and Isacsoon, G. 2001. "Suicides are seldom prescribed antidepressants: Findings from a prospective prescription database in Jämtland county, Sweden, 1985–95." *Acta Psychiatrica Scandinavica* 103: 301–6.

Hsiao, C.J., Cherry, D.K., Beatty, P.C., and Rechsteiner, E.A. 2010. "National ambulatory medical care survey: 2007 summary." *National Health Statistics Report.* Nov 3 (27): 1–32.

Kessler, R.C., Berglund, P., Demler, O., Jin, R., Koretz, D., Merikangas, K.R., Rush, A.J., Walters, E.E., Wang, P.S., National Comorbidity Survey Replication. 2003. "The epidemiology of major depressive disorder: Results from the National Comorbidity Survey Replication (NCS-R)." *Journal of the American Medical Association* 289: 3095–105.

Lewin, M.E., and Altman, S. (Eds.) 2000. "*American's Health Care Safety Net: Intact but Endangered.*" Washington, DC: National Academy Press.

Lonnqvist, J.K., Henriksson, M.M., Sisometsä, E.T., Marttunen, M.J., Heikkinen, M.E., Aro, H.M., Kuoppasalmi, K.I. 1995. "Mental disorders and suicide prevention." *Psychiatry and Clinical Neurosciences* 49: S111–S116.

Luoma, J.B., Martin, C.E., and Pearson, J.L. 2002. "Contact with mental health and primary care providers before suicide: A review of the evidence." *American Journal of Psychiatry* 159: 909–16.

Mann, J.J., Marusic, A., Mehlum, L., Patton, G., Phillips, M., Rutz, W., et al. 2005. "Suicide prevention strategies: A systematic review." *Journal of the American Medical Association* 294: 2064–74.

Melfi, C., Croghan, T., Hanna, M., and Robinson, R. 2000. "Racial variation in antidepressant treatment in a Medicaid population." *Journal of Clinical Psychiatry* 61: 16–21.

Mickus, M., Colenda, C.C., and Hogan, A.J. 2000. "Knowledge of mental health benefits and preferences for type of mental health providers among the general public." *Psychiatric Services* 51: 199–202.

Mojtabai, R., and Olfson, M. 2011. "Proportion of antidepressants prescribed without a psychiatric diagnosis is growing." *Health Affairs (Millwood)* 30: 1434–42.

Murray, C.J.L., Kulkarni, S.C., Michaud, C., Tomijima, N., Bulzacchelli, M.T., Iandiorio, T. J., and Ezzati, M. 2006. "Eight Americas: Investigating mortality disparities across races, counties, and race-counties in the United States." *PLoS Medicine*, 3: e260–1524.

Olfson, M., and Marcus, S.C. 2009. "National patterns in antidepressant medication treatment." *Archives of General Psychiatry* 66: 848–56.

Olfson, M., Shea, S., Feder, A., Fuentes, M., Nomura, Y., Gameroff, M., and Weissman, M. M. 2000. "Prevalence of anxiety, depression, and substance use disorders in an urban general medicine practice." *Archives of Family Medicine* 9: 876–83.

Pickering, T. 2000. "Depression, race, hypertension, and the heart." *Journal of Clinical Hypertension* 2: 410–12.
Pingitore, D., Snowden, L.R., Sansome, R., and Klinkman, M. 2001. "Persons with depression and the treatments they receive: A comparison of primary care physicians and psychiatrists." *International Journal of Psychiatry in Medicine* 31: 41–60.
Satcher, D. 2008. "Examining racial and ethnic disparities in health and hypertension control." *Annals of Family Medicine* 6: 482–85.
Strakowski, S.M., Hawkins, J.M., Keck, P.E., McElroy, S.L., West, S.A., Bourne, M.L., Sax, K.W., and Tugrul, K.C. 1997. "The effects of race and information variance on disagreement between psychiatric emergency service and research diagnoses in first-episode psychosis." *Journal of Clinical Psychiatry* 58: 457–63.
Swartz, M.S., Wagner, H.R, Swanson, J.W., Burns, B.J., George, L.K., and Padgett, D.K. 1998. "Comparing use of public and private mental health services: The enduring barriers of race and age." *Community Mental Health Journal* 34: 133–44.
U.S. Department of Health and Human Services. 1999. "*Mental health: A report of the surgeon General.*" Rockville, MD: Author.
Wang, P.S., Lane, M., Olfson, M., Pincus, H.A., Wells, K.B., and Kessler, R.C. 2005. "Twelve-month use of mental health services in the United States: Results from the National Comorbidity Survey Replication." *Archives of General Psychiatry* 62: 629–40.
World Health Organization. 2002. *The world health report 2002: Reducing risks, promoting healthy life.*" Geneva: World Health Organization.
——2012. *Depression.* http://www.who.int/mental_health/management/depression/definition/en/. Accessed November 6, 2011.
Wun, Y.T., Lam, T.P., Golderg, D., Lam, K.F., Li, K.T.D., and Yip, K.C. 2011. "Reasons for preferring a primary care physician for care if depressed." *Family Medicine* 43: 344–50.
Young, A.S., Klap, R., Sherbourne, C.D., and Wells, K.B. 2001. "The quality of care for depressive and anxiety disorders in the United States." *Archives of General Psychiatry* 52: 472–78.
Ziegelstein, R.C., Fauerbach, J.A., Stevens, S.S., Romanelli, J., Richter, D.P., and Bush, D.E. 2000. "Patients with depression are less likely to follow recommendations to reduce cardiac risk during recovery from a myocardial infarction." *Archives of Internal Medicine* 160: 1818–23.

10a

Replicant Love

Blade Runner Voight-Kampffed

C. D. C. Reeve

It is November 2019 and we are in the Los Angeles of Ridley Scott's *Blade Runner: The Director's Cut* (1992). Out of the vast industrial cityscape, an enormous Mayan-temple-like building comes into view. It is the Tyrell Corporation and its business is manufacturing Replicants—products "designed to copy human beings in every way except their emotions." The reason for the exception is soon clear. Pris is "a basic pleasure model. A standard item for military clubs in the out colonies." Imagine what it would be like if she had a rich array of human feelings. Or if Zhora, "trained for an off-world kick murder squad," did. Or Roy Batty, a "combat model" designed for "optimum self-sufficiency." With complex systems, though, you never know what they will do, given enough time: "The designers reckoned that after a few years, they might develop their own emotional responses. Hate, love, fear, anger, envy. So they built in a fail-safe device … Four-year lifespan."[1]

There they are, then, these short-lived Replicants, impassively and slavishly doing our degrading and violent dirty work far away in space. And what happens? They do develop emotions. Angry, envious, filled with hatred, and maybe in love with Pris, Roy leads her, Zhora, and Leon in revolt. They slaughter twenty-three people, jump a shuttle back to Earth, and head for the Tyrell Corporation. True, they will all self-destruct before long. Roy's "incept date" is 2016, Leon's is April 17, 2017. In the meantime, what they are is a problem.

That's where Blade Runners come in. A police squad trained to detect and "retire" Replicants who return to Earth, they are the first line of defense against the "machines" humans have made to be their slaves. The question is, will it be effective against those of the Nexus 6 generation, like Batty and the others? Maybe the detection method—the so-called Voight-Kampff test—won't work on them. Maybe Blade Runners won't be up to the task of "airing them out." When Holden, who is supposed to be good, runs into Leon, now an employee at Tyrell, he is the one that ends up on the critical list—"He can breathe okay, as long as nobody unplugs him." In desperation, Bryant, the squad leader, calls in the retired Rick Deckard. "This is a bad one. The worst yet. I need the old Blade Runner. I need your magic." It's a flattering appeal, but Deckard is deaf to it. Even he is daunted by what he would face. "I was quit when I came in here, Bryant," he says. "I'm twice as quit now." In the end, he has to be threatened to comply. "You know the score, pal. You're not cop, you're little people."

It is a threat that the whole atmosphere of the film makes real. "Is that why you're still on Earth?" Pris asks J. F. Sebastian, a genetic designer for Tyrell, when she learns he has a glandular disorder that ages him prematurely. "Yeah," he replies. "I couldn't pass the medical." We may be in the future, but we are not in the socially desirable part of it—the good neighborhood. Earth seems to have become one vast polluted industrial park, on which a brown drizzle endlessly falls. The owners and managers, like Eldon Tyrell, live high above it all, as close to off-world as they can get, while the workers (who for the most part really are little people) scurry around on crowded streets, under the ever-watchful eye of the authorities and their cameras. There is no visible vegetation. Natural species are largely extinct. "Do you think I'd be working in a place like this," Zhora asks Deckard, "if I could afford a *real* snake." Even cows are so rare that calfskin wallets are illegal. High culture, too, seems to have disappeared. What's left is fast Asian food from street vendors, artificial pets for those who can afford the high prices, and striptease and strong liquor at Taffy Lewis's. Sure, it's the demimonde typical of *film noir*, but it is also the wasteland Earth has become under human stewardship.

"Is this to be an empathy test?" Tyrell asks, when Deckard is sent by Bryant to see if Voight-Kampff works on a Nexus 6. "Capillary dilation of the so-called blush response? Fluctuation of the pupil. Involuntary dilation of the iris … I want to see it work on a person. I want to see a negative before I provide you with a positive." His candidate is Rachael. After a hundred or more questions (the normal is twenty or thirty), Tyrell sends her out of the room. Deckard, he sees, is coming to the conclusion that she is actually a positive.

DECKARD: She doesn't know?
TYRELL: She's beginning to suspect, I think.
DECKARD: Suspect! How can *it* not know what *it* is?

Tyrell's answer is revelatory—and in other than the intended way.

> Commerce is our goal here at Tyrell. "More human than human" is our motto. Rachael is an experiment. Nothing more. We began to recognize in them a strange obsession. After all, they are emotionally inexperienced, with only a few years to store up the experiences which you and I take for granted. If we gift them with a past, we create a cushion or a pillow for their emotions and consequently we can control them better.

Tyrell has not been keeping the police informed, we see, about Nexus 6s. What for Bryant is only a designer's projection—a maybe—is for him a certainty.

Replicants not only develop emotions, they do so quickly enough that a cushion is needed in addition to a fail-safe device. If the magnificent artificial owl presiding over Tyrell's office aerie is very expensive, what must Rachael or Pris or Roy Batty cost? Commercial viability requires a degree of longevity in a product—an adequate shelf life. But longevity comes with liabilities, which need then to be offset—cushioned. The business of the United States in 2019 may still be business, but the tensions between commercial interests and the commonweal are as real as ever.

"Memories," Deckard responds. "You're talking about memories." Well, *quasi-memories*[2] anyway—elements with a role in a Replicant's psychology like that of actual memories in a human's, but with an important difference. When I remember my first piano lesson, a causal chain connects the memory experience to the lesson via my perceptions of it. That's what makes it both a memory (rather than a fantasy) and mine. When Rachael "remembers" her first piano lesson, on the other hand, or playing doctor with her brother in an empty building, or the spider outside her bedroom window that gets eaten by its own babies, there are no causal links to her own past perceptions of these events. "Those aren't your memories," Deckard tells her. "They're somebody else's. They're Tyrell's niece's." They're "implants." Nevertheless, just as my sense of myself, of who and what I am, is a precipitate of my memories, so Rachael's is a precipitate of her quasi-memories. And what they tell her—like what her mirror and the reactions of others tell her—is that she's a human being. Had she been "gifted" with the superhuman strength, speed, and resilience of Batty, or the acrobatic skills and heat tolerance of Pris, the story might have been different. Rachael, however, wasn't designed for off-world dirty work. That's why she is a lot more like us than the others—a lot more human. Though it is implied that she is a Nexus 6, there is room for doubt about whether she really is one, and not some yet newer model. Batty and the others have four-year lifespans, but does she? It is important to the film that the question be left hanging.

"What do they risk coming back to Earth for?" Deckard asks Bryant as he is being briefed on Nexus 6s. "That's unusual. What do they want out of the Tyrell Corporation?" Quasi-memories answer both his questions. The emotional cushion or pillow they provide, as we see from the photographs Leon and Rachael both carry around like talismans, is a sense of home and family, of being loved and cherished, and the sense of self that comes with it. Nexus 6s return to the Tyrell Corporation for the same sorts of reasons we return home. And they are expected. "I'm surprised you didn't come here sooner," Tyrell tells Batty, when the two are at last face to face. "It's not an easy thing to meet your maker," he replies.

The ambiguity is intentional. Tyrell is a mixture of our earthly biological fathers and what we find it natural to call our heavenly father—God. At home, we are comforted and revitalized—reassured about who we are—by contact with the loving people and dear places of our childhood memories, precisely because they *are* the people and places of our childhood:

> There is no sense of ease like the ease we felt in those scenes where we were born, where objects had become dear to us before we had known the labour of choice, and where the outer world seemed only an extension of our own

> personality: we accepted and loved it as we loved and accepted our own sense of existence and our own limbs. Very commonplace, even ugly, that furniture of our early home might look if it were put up to auction; an improved taste in upholstery scorns it; and is not the striving after something better and better in our surroundings the grand characteristic that distinguishes man from the brute? ... But heaven knows where that striving might lead us, if our affections had not a trick of twining round those old familiar things—if the loves and sanctities of our life had no deep immovable roots in memory. One's delight in an elderberry bush overhanging the confused leafage of a hedgerow bank, as a more gladdening sight than the finest cistus or fuchsia spreading itself on the softest undulating turf, is an entirely unjustifiable preference to a nursery-gardener, or to any of those severely regulated minds who are free from the weakness of any attachment that does not rest on a demonstrable superiority of qualities. And there is no better reason for preferring this elderberry bush than that it stirs an early memory—that it is no novelty in my life, speaking to me merely through my present sensibilities to form and colour, but the long companion of my existence, that wove itself into my joys when joys were vivid.[3]

When Batty says, "I want more life ... Father," however, it isn't revitalizing and reassuring George Eliot-esque contact with vivid joys that he seeks. What he wants is what God alone can grant—the conquest of death. But death, as Tyrell admits, is "a little out of my jurisdiction."

We don't blame our fathers for not making us immortal. We know it isn't in their gift. We don't blame them for not giving us the genetic means to the greatest possible human life expectancy. That isn't theirs to give either (not yet, anyway). When Tyrell says that the "light that burns twice as bright, burns half as long. And you have burned so very brightly, Roy," we see the pertinence. The measure of a life's value is not its length alone. When Tyrell goes on to say, "You were made as well as we could make you," however, Batty is not deceived. "But *not to last*," he replies. A genetic "coding sequence" may indeed be unchangeable "*after* it has been established," but that doesn't mean that it could not have been established to code for a longer lifespan in the first place. Cold behind his thick, oversized glasses, Tyrell is impassive in the face of Batty's plight. Fatherly love isn't part of his equation. Trading stocks on the phone in the small hours, it is all commerce with him.

"I ought to be thy Adam," the creature Victor Frankenstein has created says to him, "but I am rather the fallen angel, whom thou drivest from joy for no misdeed ... I was benevolent and good; misery made me a fiend."[4] He has been made a fiend not by scalpel and electricity, but by lack of a father's love. When Batty transforms William Blake's line, "Fiery the angels rose," into "Fiery the angels *fell*," it is with this poor creature turned fiend that he identifies. When he realizes or confirms the grim truth about how and why he has been made as he is (he already knows about incept dates and longevity), he takes Tyrell's head between his hands, kisses him passionately on the mouth, and crushes his skull. The high wages of commerce only have been exacted. It is a nice irony that the poem from which Blake's line comes is "America, a Prophecy."

Judas betrayed Jesus to the Jewish and (ultimately) Roman authorities with a similarly passionate kiss.[5] Like that kiss, Batty's leads to the death of someone in whom both divine and human elements are mixed. To try to harm the divine, the source of all goodness is Satanic. "Evil, be thou my good," Milton's Satan says.[6] When Batty kills Chew, who designed his eyes, and Sebastian, who tried to help him, it is of that other fiery fallen angel we are reminded. We smell brimstone. Because Tyrell is neither God nor good, however, another odor is also present when he is killed—not of sanctity, to be sure, but of something sweet, all the same. Genius or not, Tyrell is very hard to like.

In the final exchange between father and son, with its biblical allusions and reference to heaven, the issue of immortality is subtly linked to those of freedom and moral responsibility.

TYRELL: You're the prodigal son. You're quite a prize.
BATTY: I've done questionable things.
TYRELL: Also extraordinary things. Revel in your time.
BATTY: Nothing the god of bio-mechanics wouldn't let you in heaven for.

Is he talking about himself? Maybe, he is. But he is also surely talking about Tyrell. The questionable things I, Batty, have done, he is saying, *you*, Tyrell, are responsible for, since you made me. Were we to bring a similar charge against our divine maker, he would respond, theologians tell us, by reminding us of our immortal souls and the freedom of will they enjoy as not wholly subject to the causal order. A machine or a soulless brute is not free, he would say, because factors over which it has no control determine its choices and actions. A soul is free, because there are no such factors. It can always choose and act otherwise than it does. Since immortal souls are outside his jurisdiction, Tyrell cannot respond in this way to Batty. The cushion quasi-memories provide for Replicant emotions, he says, allows them to be more effectively *controlled*. Perhaps, though, some other response is available. If control of Nexus 6s were perfect, after all, they would still be off-world doing the jobs they were designed to do, and Tyrell wouldn't be having the conversation that leads to his death.

When Rachael is Voight-Kampffed, a third traditional attribute of the soul—self-consciousness—is referred to: "How can *it* not know what *it* is?" At one level, the question is answered, as we saw, by the fact that Rachael's implanted memories are those of a human. There is another level involved, however, which only becomes explicit when Replicants discuss themselves:

BATTY: We're not computers, Sebastian. We're physical.
PRIS: I think, Sebastian, therefore I am.
BATTY: Very good, Pris. Now show him why.

In response she does a back-flip and reaches into a flask of boiling water to pull out an egg. They are tricks intended to appeal to the toy-loving Sebastian, whose assistance in reaching Tyrell she and Batty are trying to elicit. They are also philosophical jokes. The "I" whose existence Descartes hopes to establish by means of the so-called Cogito ("I think, therefore I am") is an entirely mental entity, which cannot perform such feats.[7] The fact remains that Pris seems to be able to establish her existence as Descartes thinks that we can establish ours. She may not have a soul, but she seems to have the self-consciousness that supposedly comes only with possessing one.

Impressive though this deep similarity between Pris and us undoubtedly is, Batty's instruction points to an equally impressive apparent difference. Pris knows *why* she exists. Her tricks are things she was designed to do, just as Sebastian's toys were designed to welcome him home. Her revealing clothes and sexy body are part of the repertoire of a basic pleasure model. But if Pris is a pleasure model, while Zhora is trained for a kick murder squad, why is it Zhora who is working as a snake dancer in a strip club? Why is it Pris who has the murderous legs? A Replicant's intended purpose, it seems, is one it can subvert. Design is not determining or freedom-destroying. It isn't fate. Replicants can thwart it.

In an extended comic scene, Deckard, masquerading as a representative of the Confidential Committee on Moral Abuses, interviews Zhora about her job. Did she feel exploited in any way by the club's management? To get the job, did she do or was she asked to do "anything that's lewd or unsavory or otherwise repulsive" to her person? Are there, perhaps, "little dirty holes" in her dressing-room walls through which men can watch her undress. "You'd be surprised," he says, "what a guy would go through to get a glimpse of a beautiful body." "No, I wouldn't," is her pointed reply. Zhora got her job, she is all too aware, not because she's a Replicant (no one knows she is one), but because men will pay for the sexual pleasure they get from watching women (real or Replicant) doing degrading things ("watch her take her pleasure from the serpent that once corrupted man"). Economic reality and male domination are not the same thing as universal causal determinism, to be sure, but the threat they pose to freedom is one the possession of a soul is a poor safeguard against—or no better a safeguard than rebellious Replicant slaves possess.

Though the freedom to which God appeals to defend himself against the charge of being responsible for our evil acts is incompatible with universal determinism, another conception of freedom exists that is compatible with it. Human beings are free, on this conception, not because they have souls that allow them to slip through nature's causal net, or because they can slip through it in some other way, but because they can often do what they want (and so have freedom of action), and also want what they want (and so have freedom of choice or will).[8] And that is all the freedom—defenders of this conception suggest—that is required for responsibility. What difference does it make, they ask, that someone could not have chosen or acted otherwise, if he would have chosen or acted in the same way in any case? Perhaps this is the sort of freedom that is within a Replicant's reach—the sort Tyrell might have appealed to in responding to Batty.

The issue here, to give a name to the relevant aspect of our sense of self, is that of *practical identity*. The will I have, we may suppose, is my own work. I have the wants and desires that cause or motivate the actions I perform because I—on the basis of experience and reflection—want to have them. What they constitute, as a result, is not just *a* will, but *my* will, my practical identity. If Rachael has the wants and desires she does because Tyrell's niece or someone else wanted them, however, the will she has may in some sense be free, but is it really *hers*?

In one scene in particular, the issue of practical identity seems explicitly in focus. Rachael has saved Deckard by shooting Leon and is with him in his apartment. We see him tend to his wounds, then drift off to sleep on the sofa. Rachael looks through the photos on his piano's music stand and begins to play. After a few bars, she stops and seems caught in a reverie. She reaches up and lets down her hair. Deckard awakes and joins her by the piano.

DECKARD: I dreamt music.
RACHAEL: I didn't know if I could play. I remember lessons. I don't know if it's me or Tyrell's niece.
DECKARD: You play beautifully.

He kisses her on the cheek and they gaze soulfully into one another's eyes. When he tries to kiss her on the mouth, however, Rachael pulls back. It's as if the doubts she has expressed about her identity as a pianist have made her uncertain about her identity as an agent. Am I the one who wants to return his kiss, her looks seems to say, or Tyrell's niece? She becomes agitated and tries to leave. Deckard blocks the doorway and kicks the door shut behind him. He grabs her by the shoulders and pushes her against the wall. There are many more violent scenes in the film, but few that are more disquieting. Then he pulls her to him and kisses her long and hard.

DECKARD: Now you kiss me.
RACHAEL: I can't rely on my mem...
DECKARD: Say, "kiss me."
RACHAEL: Kiss me.

Eventually, she begins to kiss him back. "I want you," he says. Her response is a low, uncertain echo: "I want you." "Again," he says. "I want you," she replies. This time her voice is stronger, the line seems hers, not his. Finally, she seems to speak entirely for herself, "Put your hands on me," she says. Ventriloquism no longer seems a live issue.

Rachael can play the piano. She can read music and strike the right notes. But does she do it as *she* would do it—expressing her own feelings, her own style—or as Tyrell's niece would? It is an odd sort of question, to be sure, but the film helps us give it sense. The way she is shown as first echoing Deckard and then more fully inhabiting her words and actions is emotionally convincing. Yet the question about her piano playing threatens our conviction. Ventriloquism may no longer *seem* to be an issue, but on what grounds exactly are we excluding it?

Physical pain has the capacity, apparently, to cut through the veneer of practical identity to what lies beneath.[9] When Deckard pushes her against the wall, the pain Rachael feels is hers not Tyrell's niece's, and nothing about memories can change that. Some sorts of pleasure may seem to have the same capacity—the pleasure of orgasm, for example, or of sexual excitement. The fact that Rachael becomes visibly more turned on as she comes to speak and act with greater apparent autonomy suggests that the film is trading in such ideas—intimating that a practical identity, previously questionable, can find in erotic love an authenticity which cannot be gainsaid by memory implants. That love can give the self a new center of gravity and lead us to remake our will is almost a commonplace. As the love of our parents gave us life, so our later loves can, within limits, make our life anew. What we see in the scene is the beginning of a new love, but also—we are invited to think—of new lives, new wills.

It is an invitation that, as gluttons for love stories with happy endings, we want to accept. Yet the film has again put obstacles in our way. Puzzled and upset after her Voight-Kampff test, Rachael goes to Tyrell. He refuses to see her. To him, as we know, she is "an experiment. Nothing more." To her, he seems much more than that—not a father, perhaps, but an admired employer, or a dear uncle, or something along those lines. In turmoil about her nature and sense of who or what she is, we can imagine her turning to her own memories and memorabilia for the comfort and reassurance he has denied her: "This is me with my mother." Then she visits Deckard and discovers that her memories and memorabilia are fakes. Not only does Tyrell not care about her, her loving mother never existed. She isn't loved by her now and was never loved by her.

Our mother's loving gaze and gentle touch, her suckling breast, her comforting embrace—all these are the life's blood of our emerging self and our sense of it. What pleasure and pain are for us is never—or never for long—simply a somatic matter. An inadequate mother may weave a thread of masochism into us, so that pain and love become knit together. Or she may weave in a different thread, one that makes pleasure of a certain sort crucial. As we develop and mature, we find, as a result, that nothing counts as love for us unless it involves violence or criticism or withholding or tantalization. This is, so to speak, the deep structure of our style of loving and being loved, like the personal style of a good pianist or a city's distinctive sense of place (the *there* that's there). In an intimate relationship it—usually unconsciously—is what is in operation. What if anything, we must wonder, plays this role in Rachael? If the answer is nothing, what does that imply about her? Is the new practical identity she is forming in falling in love with Deckard somehow compromised? Is it not really *hers* because it lacks a basis in a self that is certified, so to speak, by a mother's love? The film doesn't answer these questions, but it does allow them to cast a shadow of doubt on our romantic wishes for Deckard and Rachael.

When I feel empathy towards you, I stand in your shoes and *replicate* your thoughts and feelings. If I am good at it, I may be able to sense what is really going on with you in a way that even you yourself cannot. Thoughts and feelings are often inchoate and deeply buried. We don't always know what we are thinking or feeling. Sympathetic lovers can be a few steps ahead of us. They can know what is up with us when we are still in the dark. A good mother is like that with her child—sometimes, disconcertingly, even when he is grown up. We can disguise our thoughts and feelings, too, and often have to. The child's candor and guilelessness need to be replaced by adult discretion and discrimination. I don't *feel* grateful, but it would be callous not to at least pretend to be. I think your new dress is hideous, but it would be cruel not to dissimulate. To sustain our privacy we must sometimes hide, sometimes lie.

Most dissimulators are not skilled actors, so we can often see through them. We are quite good at detecting run-of-the-mill liars and fakes. Replicants, however, are not dissimulators. They aren't putting on an act. Their empathic or emotional responses to the scenarios Voight-Kampff deploys are sincere. There is a level of response, however, indicated by blushing, fluctuation of the pupil, involuntary dilation of the iris, that lies deeper not just than their capacity to simulate, but than anything that they could possibly have in their emotional repertoire, given their short lives and emotional inexperience. Voight-Kampff isn't, as it may at first seem, a lie-detector test, or a test for moral sentiments. It is more like a brief psychoanalytic session. We are clued into this at the beginning of the film when Holden is Voight-Kampffing Leon:

HOLDEN: Describe in single words only the good things that come into your mind about your mother.
LEON: My mother?
HOLDEN: Yeah.
LEON: I'll tell you about my mother. (He pulls out a gun and shoots Holden.)

But while psychoanalytic sessions explore an unconscious that is known to be there—a dark impress that is a residue of infantile experience and natural constitution—Voight-Kampff tests for the presence of an unconscious, and for the fine structure of feeling it betokens. Testing for it, as a result, is testing for the right sort of thing, given the aim. When Rachael fails the test, therefore, she fails something with consequences for her capacity really to empathize and love, and so for our own romantic wishes.

When we next see Deckard after his love scene with Rachael, he is parked in his car listening to Bryant telling him about the deaths of Tyrell and Sebastian. Replicant love may have taken root in him, but for now at least he is still the old Blade Runner, still in what he calls "the business." At Bryant's command, he is soon in Sebastian's apartment, his head being crushed between Pris's legs. When he manages to shoot her, her limbs thrash about so rapidly in her death throes that she seems more like a weird insect or an electric toy gone haywire than a human. The contrast with Batty's apparently noble and all-too-human end seems intentional. In deciding what to make of it, we are forced to factor Pris's into our decision. Would Batty thrash around insect-like, too, if his short life hadn't simply run its course—if his battery hadn't, so to speak, run down? Is he "like us" or not? As in the case of the romance between Deckard and Rachael, the film seems bent on preventing us from taking the easy way out.

"I have seen things you people wouldn't believe," Batty says as he breathes his last. "Attack ships on fire off the shoulder of Orion. I watched C-beams glitter in the dark near the Tannhäuser Gate. All these moments will be lost in time like tears in the rain." Indeed, they will. If the reason Batty wants more life is to prevent their loss, only immortality will serve his purpose. Immortality may not be something Tyrell can give, but implicitly, at least, it is what Batty seems in the end really to have wanted from him. When the philosopher Friedrich Schlegel writes that only "in relation to the infinite is there meaning and purpose,"[10] he speaks for much of philosophy and religion, but also it seems for Roy Batty. He speaks, too, for something deep inside all of us to which philosophy and religion give expression. We want to be immortal because we think that unless we are, nothing—not even ourselves—can have any ultimate value. Death devalues everything. Whether invented, discovered, or revealed, the soul is a relative of that deep-seated want.

That we humans have souls, we are confident. That mere brutes and mere machines do not, we are confident, too. Our value is assured; theirs, undermined or in jeopardy. What happens to us matters; what happens to them does not. Airing-out or retiring a Replicant, like slaughtering a cow or any other soulless brute, may be harder to watch than switching off a computer or unplugging a television set, but from the point of view of ultimate value, what is the difference? We can do what we like to the soulless. It is some such view, the film suggests, that explains the treatment meted out to Replicants by human beings. As Batty dies, the white dove he has been holding is released and flies off skyward. A traditional emblem of the soul leaving the body, it is here only a freed bird—and a wry comment on human values and what underwrites them.

In a short paper entitled "On Transience," written in 1916 in the midst of World War I, Sigmund Freud writes about a young poet with whom he once took a walk in the countryside:

> The poet admired the beauty of the scene around us but felt no joy in it. He was disturbed by the thought that all this beauty was fated to extinction, that it would vanish when winter came, like all human beauty and all the beauty and splendour that men have created or may create. All that he would otherwise have loved and admired seemed to him to be shorn of its worth by the transience which was its doom.

The poet, like Saint Augustine in his *Confessions*, thinks that only what cannot perish is worthy of love, so he refuses to love anything mortal. Freud is not convinced that this response is justified. Transience does not involve loss of worth, he thinks, but rather an increase: "Transience value is scarcity value in time. Limitation in the possibility of an enjoyment raises the value of the enjoyment."[11]

Whether we are convinced by Freud in this regard, we are even less likely to be convinced by the poet or the saint. Our love for things is independent of any beliefs we may have about their immortality. We love others before we know what they are or how long they will last. We are invested in advance and cannot withdraw our investment when we discover just how high the stakes are. We may believe that the ones we love are as immortal as we, but that may provide less comfort than we are typically inclined to think. First, we cannot ensure their salvation rather than their damnation, so that eternal separation—and with a cruel twist—may be our lot anyway. We cannot ensure the eternity of their love, so that even if they go on forever in the same place as ourselves, their love for us may not last. Love is mortal, even if lovers themselves are not. By making itself a love story, therefore, the film seems to side with mortality, with change.

When Deckard initially refuses to help with the Nexus 6s, Bryant's strange lieutenant, Gaff, places a small paper chicken on the desk. Later, when Deckard finds in

Leon's shower drain an artificial snake scale that leads him to Zhora, Gaff makes a matchstick man with what seems to be a large erection. In the film's closing scene, as Batty gives up the ghost, we hear Gaff's voice, then the man himself comes into view:

GAFF: You've done a man's job, sir. I guess you're through, huh?
DECKARD: Finished.

He throws Deckard his gun, dropped in the fight with Batty. The figures, we see, serve as a sort of commentary. Initially at risk of being a cowardly chicken, in the end Deckard shows himself to be a man. Gaff's final remark—"It's too bad she won't live. But then again, who does?"—takes us to the film's closing scene and to the third figure he produces.

We see Deckard entering his apartment, gun in hand, anxiously calling to Rachael. It's unclear at first whether what is on his bed covered head-to-toe by a sheet is she, her corpse, or something else. As he places his cheek next to hers, she awakens:

DECKARD: Do you love me?
RACHAEL: I love you.
DECKARD: Do you trust me?
RACHAEL: I trust you.

No question of ventriloquism this time, it seems. With Deckard in the lead, gun still in hand, the two make their way out into the corridor. As they do, Rachael's foot knocks over a small figure made of silver foil. Deckard picks it up. The camera focuses in on it until it fills the screen. We hear again Gaff's final words to Deckard, which now become the film's own final words: "It's too bad she won't live. But then again, who does?" As Deckard crushes the figure in his hand, he nods in assent. He accepts not just Rachael's mortality, it seems, but his own. It isn't only love that's mortal, the film seems to say, lovers—Replicant *and* human—are, too.

With the repetition of Gaff's words, death's dominion seems to have become universal, so that souls and the distinction they seem to legitimate between human and Replicant are at last abandoned. Everyone is in the same dark boat. The unicorn figure, however, destabilizes that thought. Deckard has told Rachael that her memories are implants. As he goes to get her a drink, she runs off. When we return to the scene, after watching the one in which Pris meets Sebastian, he is sitting at the piano, his head on the keyboard, his fingers picking out a fragmentary melody. As he seems to fall into a dream, we seem to see it with him. A white unicorn charges towards us, twisting its head to gore something with its horn. When the dream evaporates, the screen fills with a close-up of Deckard's family photographs. The message, apparently, is that his dream is an implant that is known to Gaff, his photographs, fakes. Like Rachael, he is a Replicant—mortal, but also soulless.

Well, that is one possible message, one way to read Gaff's final figure. But there is also another. In one of his notebooks, Leonardo da Vinci gives voice to some common lore about how unicorns finally get hunted and captured: "The unicorn, through its intemperance and not knowing how to control itself, for the love it bears to fair maidens forgets its ferocity and wildness; and laying aside all fear it will go up to a seated damsel and go to sleep in her lap, and thus the hunters take it."[12] Deckard knows this lore,[13] we may suppose, and dreams about a unicorn because he has already begun to fall for Rachael, and—subliminally—to register the consequences. In the business of hunting Replicants, by coming to love one, he has made himself prey to their hunters. "Would you come after me? Hunt me?" Rachael asks him after she has saved him from Leon. "No. No. I wouldn't," he replies. "I owe you one. But somebody would."

When Gaff says, "You've done a man's job, sir," he may simply be expressing in more refined—and more ironically ambiguous terms—what Bryant says more bluntly by calling Deckard "a goddamn one-man slaughterhouse." His remark about Rachael's longevity, however, suggests that he has something else in mind. It is a man's job to kill his enemies *and* to fall in love with the beautiful damsel—even if she is of enemy blood herself. By throwing him his gun, Gaff aligns himself as much with the love as with the slaughter. If he were simply Bryant's agent, he would hardly give a weapon to a man who declares himself "finished," before he has carried out all the boss's orders. "There's three to go," Deckard says when he has killed Zhora. "There's four," Bryant replies. "Now there's that skin-job you V-K'd at the Tyrell Corp. Rachael." On this reading, Gaff makes his final silver foil figure, as he does the others, to register what Deckard has become. He is not a chicken, not a macho phallic guy, but a real man.

By offering us these two ways of understanding Gaff's unicorn, *Blade Runner* leaves us with the question of what is at stake between them. Is the issue that of whether Deckard has a soul, or whether he is capable of empathy and love. "You know that Voight-Kampff test of yours," Rachael asks him, "did you ever take that test yourself?" If Replicant love is or can become real love, however, the question of who has a soul may not matter all that much.

Notes

1 Unless otherwise identified, quotations are from the soundtrack of the final cut of the film. The opening ones are from Bryant's first conversation with Deckard.
2 A notion first introduced into philosophy by Sydney Shoemaker, "Persons and Their Pasts," in his *Identity, Cause, and Mind* (Cambridge: Cambridge University Press, 1984).
3 George Eliot, *The Mill on the Floss* (London: Penguin Books, 2003), Book II Ch. 1, final paragraph.
4 Mary Shelley, *Frankenstein* (London: Penguin Books, 1992), Vol. II Ch. 2, p. 103.
5 The Greek verb that Matthew (26:47–50) and Mark (14:44–45) use to describe it is *kataphilein*, which means to kiss firmly, intensely, and passionately
6 John Milton, *Paradise Lost* (Oxford World's Classics: Oxford, 2008), Book IV, line 110.
7 René Descartes, *Meditations on First Philosophy* (Indianapolis: Hackett, 1993), Second Meditation, pp. 17–20.
8 The classic statement of the position is Harry G. Frankfurt, "Freedom of the Will and the Concept of a Person" and "Alternate Possibilities and Responsibility," in his *The Importance of What We Care About* (Cambridge: Cambridge University Press, 1988).

9 A view defended by Bernard Williams, "The Self and the Future," in his *Problems of the Self* (Cambridge: Cambridge University Press, 1973).
10 Friedrich Schlegel, *Lucinde and the Fragments* (Minneapolis: University of Minnesota Press, 1971), p. 241.
11 Sigmund Freud, "On Transience," in *The Standard Edition of the Complete Psychological Works of Sigmund Freud* (London: The Hogarth Press, 1957), pp. 305–7.
12 Leonardo da Vinci, *The Notebooks of Leonardo da Vinci* (Oxford: Oxford University Press, 1998).
13 Or Ridley Scott does.

Bibliography

Descartes, René. *Meditations on First Philosophy* (Indianapolis: Hackett, 1993).
Eliot, George. *The Mill on the Floss* (London: Penguin Books, 2003).
Frankfurt, Harry G. *The Importance of What We Care About* (Cambridge: Cambridge University Press, 1988).
Freud, Sigmund. "On Transience," in *The Standard Edition of the Complete Psychological Works of Sigmund Freud* (London: The Hogarth Press, 1957).
Milton, John. *Paradise Lost* (Oxford World's Classics: Oxford, 2008).
Schlegel, Friedrich. *Lucinde and the Fragments* (Minneapolis: University of Minnesota Press, 1971).
Shelley, Mary. *Frankenstein* (London: Penguin Books, 1992).
Shoemaker, Sydney. *Identity, Cause, and Mind* (Cambridge: Cambridge University Press, 1984).
da Vinci, Leonardo. *The Notebooks of Leonardo da Vinci* (Oxford: Oxford University Press, 1998).
Williams, Bernard. *Problems of the Self* (Cambridge: Cambridge University Press, 1973).

10b

Commentary on Reeve: *Blade Runner*: Becoming Human, Ready or Not

Mardy S. Ireland

The weave of Reeve's essay on the cult film *Blade Runner* is a rich one indeed. His close reading of the words of each significant character, and how he links their utterances to salient philosophical ideas, renders persuasive his interpretations of the movement and intent of this almost timeless movie. His composition reminds me as a psychoanalyst that some human knots can neither be completely untied nor finally understood by interpretation, but, rather, the threads of such human knots are worth exploring again and again over time. With this in mind, I offer a supplement to Reeve's essay by pulling upon three threads that he has articulately brought to our attention: what is human or not; freedom's limit; and time re-considered.

As a practicing psychoanalyst, I am drawn as much by what is unspoken as to what is. Deckard says to Bryant that he is "twice as quit" when he attempts to refuse his assignment, but we never actually hear why he quit in the first place. Is it in this "unsaid place" that an important question that Reeve raises really lives: Is Deckard truly human or another kind of Replicant designed to be a "one man slaughter-house"? Is he a Replicant evolving beyond the array of family photographs on his piano (perhaps they are not only the photographs of the Replicants he is hunting) and an implanted liminal image of a unicorn, or, is he truly just one of us?

Because I am not a philosopher, the issue of "soul" and who has it as a measure of humanness is "a little out of my jurisdiction," as Tyrell would say. (Perhaps if I were a Jungian analyst vs. a post-Freudian one I would have something to say!) Reeve believes, as do I, that the capacity for empathy and love are critical to answering the question of Deckard's humanness. I would add that the capacity to desire the desire of the other is also critical.[1] It is not enough that Deckard desires Rachael; he also needs her to desire him as well. This is so crucial because in the basement of the human psyche identity begins to organize itself around a kernel of real experience with the first caretaking "other." As a baby we begin to wonder and imagine what this earliest caretaker (usually a mother) wants/desires from us? This infantile unconscious fantasy will much later inform how we will desire another, and how, in turn, we want to be desired. And if there is no desire coming from the other for us (think here of an unwanted child)—bad things can often follow. We might even view Leon's shooting of Holden from this framework. Is it not after all cruel to be asked about a "mother" that Leon knows only too well he has neither had nor obviously been desired by. Thus, when Deckard asks Rachael to echo, "I want you," we see him at this basement level of human identity—either already human, or evolving to be so. Likewise, when Rachael moves from a "ventriloquist" response, that Reeve notes, to more of her own voice in saying, "Put your hands on me," we are reminded again that Freud said the first ego (first root of identity) is a body-ego that grows out of that first physically loving relationship.[2] Perhaps it is here in this beginning moment (from fear to tenderness) with Deckard that there lies the chance Reeve wonders about as to whether, and how, Rachael's love could become grounded despite not having received a mother's "real" love.

Another aspect of what makes us human is brought forward by how Reeve frames of the Voight-Kampff (V-K) test as a "psychoanalytic session." At one level the V-K appears as a mere test of socially appropriate emotional responses, as when Rachael fails because she does not show disgust with "boiled dog" as a dinner entrée. (Although there are cultures in which "boiled dog" would be an acceptable entrée.) And yet, when Rachael throws a question back to Deckard as to whether he is trying to determine if she is a "lesbian," she is highlighting an "other" level of this test, which is to look for evidence in the subject that she/he is aware and takes an interest in unconscious desires and processes. Admittedly in this instance Rachael is questioning the unconscious behind Deckard's curiosity rather than her own unconscious, but it does however take over a hundred questions to find her lacking, so to speak. If the lack of socially appropriate emotionality and empathy were the primary determinants of "passing" the V-K we might ask, as does she—how would Deckard do on the V-K test?

And even though we know the Replicant creator Tyrell is human, he certainly appears to be without empathy or emotional expressiveness. Would he pass the V-K test that clearly he did not design? From purely a clinical psychoanalytic perspective, Tyrell is only part human. In his conscious identification with, and striving for, omnipotence and perfection, he remains blind (unconscious) to the danger and vulnerability he is living within those final moments before Roy simply and easily crushes his skull. Not infrequently an important part of an analytic treatment is to assist a person, who may be wrapped up in godlike identifications like Tyrell, into the imperfect world of human feelings, values, and relationships so that she/he does not continue to endanger her or himself or others. What the analyst Wilfred Bion would say is that to be most fully human is to establish working "links" between feelings (as babies we feel first) and thoughts (which come later—first as image thoughts and then later in words) that will reliably connect us to ourselves, others, and move us into the world, for only then we can begin to construct a viable and ongoing life.[3]

A concomitant issue in Reeve's exploration of what it means to be human is the concept of "freedom." He wonders whether it really matters if there is "true freedom" if the choice would be the same either in the case of the Replicants as programmed beings or we un-programmed human beings. "Freedom" is a complicated issue between philosophical and psychoanalytic perspectives. Freedom in some sense is relative in psychoanalysis. On the one hand, is the "practical identity", as Reeve describes it, grounded entirely in the conscious ego, or, does "the freedom to choose" in fact always hover in the space that as human beings we are always living in—a "split identity" between the conscious ego and the unconscious?[4] At the same time there is a need for the "necessary fiction" of an ego that helps us feel "I am in control of my own mind." When, however, Pris (quoting Descartes) says, "I think therefore I am," as if to say I am human like you, she is absent to the lived twentieth-century knowledge that the psychoanalyst Lacan has underlined regarding the impact of the human unconscious upon "freedom of choice." To paraphrase Lacan, "Where I think, I am not, where I do not think, I am."[5] Both statements are true. I do wonder if the "implanted memories" Tyrell thought would "cushion" the emergent emotions of Replicants became instead seeds germinating an incipient unconscious in the Replicant-6 model. When Rachael has the "self-consciousness" to ask if it is her desire or that of Tyrell's niece, is this not similar to any human being's questioning of her/his own desire: "Is this what I really want or is it coming from somewhere else inside me?" As a Replicant, Rachael may not have as long to live, but the struggle with which she is engaged is as human as it gets!

Reeve also shows how time is an organizing element to the emotional landscape of *Blade Runner*. And as Einstein proved to us (and as Freud said)—time is always relative. What does a four-year life span really feel like? Clearly it is not enough time for the six who return to earth seeking to be "re-booted," even though they are risking immediate annihilation if caught. When Deckard leaves with Rachael we do not know how much time either of them or their relationship will have; we only know they are risking everything to experience this unknown amount of time. Reeve points to Roy's seeking of "more time" because past and current experiences will be lost forever and presumably meaning as well. This would put Roy on the side of philosophy and religion positing infinity as the only guarantee of meaning. And yet Roy's seeking of additional time may be as much an expression of his emerging humanness in his growing relationship with Pris—who he wants to save. We hear this in Roy's words, but we also see it in his physical emotional expressiveness toward Pris. From this vertex we see Roy more on the side of psychoanalysis where the role of human attachment, along with human beings' awareness of their own impending death, may combine such that individual choices can be given meaning. In saving the only life he can—Deckard's—Roy establishes an intense link through terror and gains an empathic witness to his short but evolving life. Perhaps this brief and searing link adds emotional weight to Deckard's decision in the end to flee with Rachael. So in the final analysis, is it about the quantity of time lived or the quality and with whom the time is lived?

All these prior comments are set in the context of conscious linear time. But non-linear or timeless time is equally compelling in *Blade Runner*. Unconscious time is not taken up by Reeve per se, so let me add a comment here. First, it has been more than thirty years since the film was made and one would think that everything about

Blade Runner would appear dated and stale. It doesn't. I believe this is true because *Blade Runner* touches on timeless conscious and unconscious conflicts belonging to both the individual and the group (society). Will we ever not want to be omnipotent? *Blade Runner* shows the unstoppable technological march we have been, and are still, on, of creating intelligent machines to do our work, all the time carrying the unacknowledged risk of what are "uniquely human values" slipping away. From one perspective *Blade Runner* appears to tilt toward nihilism as our inevitable *fate*; a place that Nietzsche suggested we must, following the death of God, finally arrive so humanity may be able create a new foundation.[6] From another perspective, however, we can ask if the escape of Deckard and Rachael is the mark of hope in a very dark landscape that a new *destiny* could be forged?

There is another kind of time illustrated in *Blade Runner* that the psychoanalyst Jacques Lacan called logical time.[7] It is obvious to us, the audience, that there is an immediate and compelling link made between Deckard and Rachael—neither could probably say what or why it is. They just see and feel it. In such an initial moment when any one of us encounters something familiar in a stranger that we just "have to" pursue it, we are experiencing "the instant of seeing" from an unconscious place. The remainder of what we watch unfold between Deckard and Rachael is in "the time of understanding" as they inescapably seek greater connection. When evolving self-knowledge (let's say through an analysis) leads to some understanding of the unconscious elements compelling such a connection, an individual reaches "a moment of conclusion" in time. We do not see this moment for either Deckard or Rachael in the film, thus it remains a mystery for us as viewers to imagine—are they doomed in their fate or are they going to be a part of forging a new destiny between human and machine?

Finally, to conclude on the hope vs. nihilism side of things, Reeve describes very nicely Gaff's role as marking for the audience the arc of Deckard's development. He offers us an engaging analysis of the small sculptures as symbolic evidence. A supplemental view here is that we are seeing a psychoanalyst (Gaff) conducting a brief analysis. If we hear the name Gaff as the word "gaffe," we might wonder if he, as an analyst, is consistently marking where there is a lack to be attended. If Gaff were an analyst of a certain British persuasion, he would be consciously and unconsciously "taking in" Deckard's experience, thinking about that experience, putting a shape to that experience (sculpted figures), and returning, or leaving them (sculptures) to be picked up and used—or not—by Deckard.[8] Gaff interprets Deckard's animal fear, confusion, and sense of helplessness to Bryant's command as a chicken made from a small piece of discarded paper. Deckard's coming to life with Rachael is expressed in the matchstick figure of a sexual desiring male. Deckard's emergent complicated feelings about his own survival while beginning to love and protect another are interpreted by Gaff in the final concrete metaphor of a unicorn made from more special shiny material. All of these small sculptures can be seen as complex mental emotional states belonging to Deckard that Gaff has been processing. It is significant here that the material of each sculpture is of a different quality and represents a higher order of psychic functioning—from a piece of trash paper, to matchsticks, to shiny aluminum. These different materials show how Gaff has metabolized Deckard's moving from chaotic intense emotions, to more organized modulated feelings, to finally being able to put feelings and thought together to act on his feelings of desire and attachment.

Often in any analysis, there may be a long period of time during which the analyst is primarily taking in the analysand's experience; there can be more time before a form can be given to it; and an even longer time before any form of understanding is offered to the analysand, be it in a spoken image or complete interpretive thought. In the film, Gaff's first two figures are made and placed, but not really in any way that they could be easily picked up by Deckard. We could say that this sequence illustrates an analyst's interior work during an analysis. It is usual for an image or reverie to emerge in the mind of the analyst in response to what she/he is hearing and experiencing in a session. It is sometimes only considerably later that words of an interpretation come into mind, and even then these words may not be spoken for a while. Sometimes holding these images and thoughts in mind is sufficient to move the clinical work along because the timing of actually speaking an interpretation is everything in terms of the analysand being able to use it. In fact Gaff only speaks around the time of the final sculpture of the unicorn. He first says, "You've done a man's job"—a job Reeve defines clearly in his essay. And then when returning Deckard's gun to him (because he needs, as we all do, an ongoing capacity to defend himself), Gaff says, "It's too bad she won't live. But then again, who does?" Now working as an analyst of a Lacanian persuasion, we could understand Gaff's words as simultaneously marking Deckard's desire having finally become embodied as well as the general importance of desire (not limited to sexual desire) as a prime mover in human life given the limited time any of us has. Deckard picks up the concrete metaphor of the unicorn sculpture, looks at it, recognizing it as part of himself (remember the dream image of the unicorn), crushes it—not to throw it away, I would say, but as if to digest it through his fingers—and then takes it with him as his talisman for beginning his new life with Rachael in whatever time remains. Perhaps now we have our answer as to why Deckard had quit his job—his work had rendered him numb, psychically dead, and without desire. Now we see him alive again. Perhaps then the conclusion of *Blade Runner* is not so different from an end of a successful analysis as seen from more than one analyst's theoretical perspective.[9]

Notes

1 J. Lacan (1964) *Seminar XI. The Four Fundamental Concepts of Psychoanalysis*, New York: W.W. Norton & Company, 1978.
2 S. Freud (1923) "The ego and the id," *Standard Edition* 19, London: Horgarth Press, 1986. See also D. Winncott (1972) "On the basis for self in the body," *International Journal of Psychoanalysis*, 1(1): 7–16.
3 W. Bion (1962) "A theory of thinking" in *Second Thoughts*, pp. 110–19, New York: Jason Aronson, 1967.
4 S. Freud (1915) "The unconscious," *Standard Edition* 14, London: Horgarth Press, 1986.
5 J. Lacan (1964) *Seminar XI. The Four Fundamental Concepts of Psychoanalysis*, New York: W.W. Norton & Company, 1978.
6 F. Nietzsche (1882) *Gay Science: With a Prelude in Rhymes and Appendix of Songs*, as translated with commentary by Walter Kauffman, New York: Vintage Books, 1974.

7 J. Lacan (1945) "Logical Time" in *Ecrits*, pp. 197–213, Paris: Seuil, 1966.

8 B. Joseph (1988) "Projective identification—some clinical aspects" in *Melanie Klein Today*, edited by Elizabeth Bott Spillius, pp. 138–50, New York: Routledge, 1988.

9 D. Winnicott (1962) "The aims of psychoanalytic treatment" in *The Maturational Processes and the Facilitating Environment*, pp. 166–70, New York: International Universities Press, 1962. See also J. Lacan (1964) "In you more than you" in *Seminar XI. The Four Fundamental Concepts of Psychoanalysis*, pp. 263–76, New York: W.W. Norton & Company, 1978.

Bibliography

Bion, W. (1962). "A theory of thinking" in *Second Thoughts*, pp.110–19. New York: Jason Aronson, 1967.

Freud, S. (1915). "The unconscious." *Standard Edition* 14. London: Horgarth Press, 1986.

——(1923). "The ego and the id." *Standard Edition* 19. London: Horgarth Press, 1986.

Joseph, B. (1988) "Projective identification—some clinical aspects" in *Melanie Klein Today*, edited by Elizabeth Bott Spillius, pp. 138–50. New York: Routledge, 1988.

Lacan, J. (1945). "Logical time" in *Ecrits*, pp. 197–213. Paris: Seuil, 1966.

——(1964a). "In you more than you" in *Seminar XI. The Four Fundamental Concepts of Psychoanalysis*, pp. 263–76. New York: W.W. Norton & Company, 1978.

——(1964b). *Seminar XI. The Four Fundamental Concepts of Psychoanalysis.* New York: W.W. Norton & Company, 1978.

Nietzsche, F. (1882). *Gay Science: With a Prelude in Rhymes and Appendix of Songs*, as translated with commentary by Walter Kauffman. New York: Vintage Books, 1974.

Winnicott, D. (1962). "The aims of psychoanalytic treatment" In *The Maturational Processes and the Facilitating Environment*, pp. 166–70. New York: International Universities Press, 1965.

Winncott, D. (1972) "On the basis for self in the body." *International Journal of Psychoanalysis* 1(1): 7–16.

Index

Please note that page numbers relating to notes will contain the letter 'n' followed by note number.

CPSIA information can be obtained
at www.ICGtesting.com
Printed in the USA
BVHW042133221119
564596BV00010B/93/P

9 780415 708166